Conceptual Nursing
in Practice

JOIN US ON THE INTERNET VIA WWW, GOPHER, FTP OR EMAIL:

WWW: http://www.thomson.com
GOPHER: gopher.thomson.com
FTP: ftp.thomson.com
EMAIL: findit@kiosk.thomson.com

A service of I(T)P

Conceptual Nursing in Practice

A research-based approach

Second edition

Mary Fraser

PHD, MSc, BSc (HONS), DIPN.ED, RGN, ONC, RNT§
Director, Research and Project Consultancy,
Stirling, Scotland, FK9 5NH

CHAPMAN & HALL
London · Weinheim · New York · Tokyo · Melbourne · Madras

Published by Chapman & Hall, 2–6 Boundary Row, London SE1 8HN, UK

Chapman & Hall, 2–6 Boundary Row, London SE1 8HN, UK

Blackie Academic & Professional, Wester Cleddens Road, Bishopbriggs, Glasgow G64 2NZ, UK

Chapman & Hall GmbH, Pappelallee 3, 69469 Weinheim, Germany

Chapman & Hall USA, 115 Fifth Avenue, New York NY 10003, USA

Chapman & Hall Japan, ITP-Japan, Kyowa Building, 3F, 2-2-1 Hirakawacho, Chiyoda-ku, Tokyo 102, Japan

Chapman & Hall Australia, 102 Dodds Street, South Melbourne, Victoria 3205, Australia

Chapman & Hall India, R. Seshadri, 32 Second Main Road, CIT East, Madras 600 035, India

Distributed in the USA and Canada by Singular Publishing Group Inc., 4284 41st Street, San Diego, California 92105

First edition 1990
Reprinted 1993
Second edition 1996

© 1990, 1996 Mary Fraser

Typeset in 10/12 pt Palatino by Mews Photosetting, Beckenham, Kent

Printed in Great Britain by St Edmundsbury Press Ltd, Bury St Edmunds, Suffolk

ISBN 0 412 60940 1   1 56593 418 0 (USA)

A catalogue record for this book is available from the British Library

Library of Congress Catalog Card Number: 96-068956

∞ Printed on permanent acid-free text paper, manufactured in accordance with ANSI/NISO Z39.48-1992 and ANSI/NISO Z39.48-1984 (Permanence of Paper).

Contents

Preface

Since 1990 there has been considerable development in research in nursing practice which uses a model of nursing. This is due to many reasons. However, the aims of this book remain the same as for the first edition – to present the reader with current reports of studies in nursing practice which use a model of nursing as their base. I will also criticize the research methods that the studies use, to give the reader an indication of the credibility of the findings, as well as commenting on the popularity of the model in different countries and cultures.

A development that is possible since the last edition is the ability to give some indication of why the model of nursing was used; in other words what was the author's intention in studying nursing practice in depth with the use of a model. This will give some indication of the implications of the authors' work; I will develop this point further in the Introduction to this edition. Therefore this edition is not simply an updating of further studies published since 1990.

Since the last edition there has also been some comment on the models that I included. I am grateful to Margaret Clarke (1991) and others who have pointed out that Neuman's model should be included, and there is therefore a chapter devoted to this in this edition.

The nursing models presented in this book are therefore:

- Roper, Logan and Tierney's model of activities of daily living
- Roy's adaptation model
- Orem's self-care model
- Johnson's model of behavioural systems balance
- Rogers' model of unitary human beings
- Neuman's health care systems model

REFERENCE

Clarke, M. (1991) Book review. *International Journal of Nursing Studies*, **28**(2), 204–5.

Preface to the first edition

As nursing models are currently being advocated for use in every practice setting, it was felt that the timing was right for a text which showed the potential in practice, through investigations of practice, of the best known of these models.

This book has therefore been compiled from a search of the literature where studies that are easily available to nurses in Britain are outlined. It is hoped that this compilation, with associated comment and analysis, will help nurses in practice to understand and to continue to develop their understanding of the conceptual basis of nursing practice.

There are many texts currently available that explain and outline nursing models for the beginner of nursing; this text is not one of these. It is aimed at the experienced practising nurse who realizes that her or his knowledge of the use of these models is insufficient. It is hoped that having achieved a certain level of understanding of the models, this text will then help the experienced practising nurse further to develop this understanding.

The nursing models presented in this book are chosen because they are the best known and therefore arguably the best understood in Britain. They are:

- Roper, Logan and Tierney's model of activities of living
- Roy's adaptation model
- Orem's self-care model
- Johnson's model of behavioural systems balance
- Roger's model of unitary human beings.

Introduction to the second edition

The aims of this second edition are the same as those of the first, but with some additions. In summary, the aims of the first edition were to help experienced practising nurses to make the link between an understanding of conceptual nursing models and the use of these models in patient care. Through a critical appraisal of the literature published up to that time, it was hoped that these nurses would be able to compare the results of their practice with the published results. However, there was no intention to compare the health outcomes from the use of one model against the outcomes from the use of another, as Clarke (1991) suggests. Indeed, I am not aware of any studies which attempt to do that. What the first edition and also this edition advocate is the use of multiple models, so that flexibility of nursing practice, according to the results of that practice, can be promoted. However, due to some of the results a healthy scepticism of the use of models in some aspects of nursing will delight some of their critics.

Since 1990 there have been many more studies of nursing practice using a model of nursing. These have been incorporated into the appropriate chapters. A new heading which clearly indicates the work since 1990 has been included where necessary. However, a simple updating of a book is never a very exciting proposition, nor would I have been very enthralled by doing such a thing. As the number of studies and the aims of the authors in conducting them and making them public have become clearer, it is now possible to give an assessment of the aims of research in nursing practice using a model – in other words, why have the authors of the articles used a model of nursing in their research of nursing practice? This is an addition to this text and will be given in a summary of each study and in a summary of the model at the end of each chapter. There were three papers that stimulated my interest in this area; the first two were by Fawcett and Tulman (1990) and Fawcett (1992), the third was by Draper (1993). These authors have very different views of the reasons to investigate nursing practice using a model of nursing.

Fawcett and Tulman (1990) and Fawcett (1992) have used Roy's model as the basis for their research programme. They state that this allows them to draw conclusions about the model's credibility; to this date they have found support for the concepts of primary, secondary and tertiary roles in the role function mode. They have also found support for the 'influence of environmental stimuli on adaptation' (Fawcett and Tulman, 1990, p. 724). Further evidence supports Roy's claims that the adaptive modes are related. In her 1992 paper Fawcett develops this further by claiming that a model specifies nursing practice, however systematic investigation of nursing practice using a model may lead to the discrediting of the model:

> The conceptual model is considered credible if patient outcomes are congruent with expectations raised by the model. If, however, patient outcomes are not congruent with expectations, the credibility of the conceptual model must be questioned.
>
> (p. 227)

Furthermore she states,

> Systematic and objective scrutiny of the outcomes of conceptual model-based practice is crucial, along with modifications in the model or even elimination of the model if the data warrant this.
>
> (p. 227)

It is clear from this that Fawcett is tending to use a positivistic stance in formulating the research question, to data gathering and analysis. In positivism, the testing of hypotheses is a key reason for research. Therefore, according to Fawcett, if a hypothesis is shown to be true, then it and the assumptions on which it is based are upheld; whereas if a hypothesis is shown to be false, this gives cause for concern that some parts, if not the whole of the theory on which it is based, should be viewed with caution, if not dismissed. Positivism is closely associated with the way that research is conducted in the natural sciences, such as biology, physics and chemistry, where there is considered to be one correct method of conducting research. However, positivism according to Popper (1978) is based on the rigorous testing of theories in order to try to disprove them; only in this way can they be seen as valid.

> All tests can be interpreted as attempts to weed out false theories – to find the weak points of a theory in order to reject it if it is falsified by the test. … But just because it is our aim to establish theories as well as we can, we must test them as severely as we can; that is, we must try to find fault with them. Only if we cannot falsify them in spite of our best efforts can we say that they have stood up to severe tests.
>
> (Popper, 1978, p. 18)

Positivism, therefore, has three main features; according to Von Wright (1978) these are:

- a single method – so the same method, which has been refined over a number of years, must be followed whatever the problem that is being investigated;
- that the phenomenon should be measured using mathematics – so descriptive studies have no validity here;
- that explanation of the phenomenon studied should be causal – in other words a cause and effect hypothesis must be generated and tested.

However, certain aspects of a positivistic approach to investigating social phenomena have tended to become discredited in the UK (Silverman, 1993). This rejection of positivism has, in some circles, been fierce and has led to an approach which is frequently seen as opposed to positivism – interpretive social science. Draper (1993) makes a clear distinction between positivism and the interpretive traditions. However, a clear distinction is not so easily found, as Silverman (1993) points out. Table 1 shows how Silverman (1993) sees the traditional difference between positivism and interpretive social science.

Table 1 Two 'schools' of social science

Approach	Concepts	Methods
Positivism	Social structure, social facts	Quantitative hypothesis testing
Interpretive social science	Social construction meaning	Qualitative hypothesis generation

Reproduced with permission from Silverman (1993, p. 21).

After an extensive study of the characteristics of positivism and the interpretive method, Silverman concludes that they should not be seen as direct opposites, as much current social research has elements of positivism. These elements, such as hypothesis testing and some use of numerical data, help to make social science rigorous, so that there should no longer be the criticism that 'anything goes'. Silverman prescribes four elements that should be evident in qualitative research: first, that it should be theoretically driven; second, that we should 'examine social phenomena as procedural affairs' (p. 29) by asking questions such as 'what do people have to do to be doing X?'; third, we must attend to and make problematic the commonsense reasoning that we use in the definition of variables; and fourth, the fundamental method is to examine people in their own territory, rather than to set up artificial settings, such as a laboratory, to examine them.

For the purposes of this book I will attempt to give some indication of the type of research method that each author or group of authors claim to use in the accounts of their research using a model of nursing. In making this kind of assessment of the authors' work, the criteria that I will use will attempt to combine the elements of positivism with interpretive social science in the way that Silverman suggests. These criteria are some of those that Silverman suggests should be the current way of conducting social research. They are shown in Table 2. Using these criteria I will be able to show whether testing the model is the authors' primary intention and if so how this is done; whether the research is a descriptive or an explanatory study; whether data gathering is within the field of nursing; and the extent of support for the model shown by the research.

Table 2 The criteria used in this book to make an assessment of the research methods used in the papers being analysed

- The method is theoretically driven. In other words it should be possible to see how the theory that underpins the research is being developed.

- There is an attempt to show the cause and effect of different aspects of the model. This should allow us to see, for example, that after identifying the patient's or client's needs, planning nursing care is an effective next step and leads to improvement in the patient's state; alternatively, that by planning nursing care, the intervention that is carried out by the nurse or significant others is effective in helping the patient's state.

- Is commonsense reasoning used to define the variables problematized? In other words, from the point of view of this book, has the model been taken directly from the theorists and used in an uncritical manner, or are we given a critical appraisal of the model through its use in the paper, which would help our understanding of the model in practice?

- Are the people examined in their natural environments? In other words, is the research conducted in the environment where nurses are practising nursing?

However, as I mentioned at the beginning of this introduction, my appraisal of each paper will also be the same as in the first edition. This is by assessing the effectiveness and rigour of the method used, which determines the credibility of the results, as well as commenting on the acceptability of the model in different cultures, depending on the country of origin of the published papers.

We are now ready to start this second edition. I hope you enjoy it and find it useful.

REFERENCES

Clarke, M. (1991) Book review. *International Journal of Nursing Studies,* **28**(2), 204–5.
Draper, P. (1993) A critique of Fawcett's conceptual models and nursing practice; the reciprocal relationship. *Journal of Advanced Nursing,* **18**, 558–64.
Fawcett, J. (1992) Conceptual models and nursing practice; the reciprocal

relationship. *Journal of Advanced Nursing*, **17**, 224–8.

Fawcett, J. and Tulman, L. (1990) Building a programme of research from the Roy Adaptation Model of Nursing. *Journal of Advanced Nursing*, **15**, 720–5.

Popper, K. (1978) The unit of method, in *Social Research: Principles and Practice* (eds J.M. Brynner and K.M. Stribley), Longman, New York.

Silverman, D. (1993) *Interpreting Qualitative Data: Methods for Analysing Talk, Text and Interaction*, Sage, London.

Von Wright, G.H. (1978) Two traditions, in *Social Research: Principles and Practice* (eds J.M. Brynner and K.M. Stribley), Longman, New York, pp. 11–16.

Introduction to *Conceptual Nursing in Practice: a research-based approach*   1

The aim of this book is to discover the knowledge that currently exists of the use of nursing models in the different areas of nursing practice. What is currently happening in Great Britain is that nursing models are being applied in practice settings, and although this is probably commendable, many of the practitioners have little idea of what can be expected from identifying patients' problems, planning their care, carrying out nursing care, or evaluating it using these models. It therefore appears to me that although practising nurses may have a conceptual understanding of some of the models of nursing, they cannot automatically make the link between their conceptual understanding and their work with their patients and clients.

It ought to be stated at the outset that the meaning of 'model' throughout this book is a set of concepts that have not yet been tested out in practice. Therefore the use of these models in practice remains speculative until it is shown by research. So it seems therefore that what is needed is a book to show practising nurses the knowledge gained through the use of some of the better known nursing models, the patient situations and the stage in the problem-solving process in which this knowledge has been gained.

It is expected that nurses reading this book will have some knowledge of the models presented, therefore it will not serve as an introductory text. However, to refresh the reader's memory of each model a few opening paragraphs are provided at the beginning of each chapter to outline the main ideas presented in the particular model, and the changes that have occurred in subsequent editions.

The approach to the use of nursing models in practice adopted in this text is that no single model will provide all the answers to the problems faced by nurses in clinical areas. Therefore a multiple-model approach to practice is considered the most appropriate. This approach was developed by Donald Schon (1983), although not specifically for nursing, when he analysed how practitioners solve practical problems in everyday work: experimenting using practical methods and assessing the results of these experiments. According to Schon this experimenting is carried out in a number of different ways; one way is to find out more about the situation through observation and/or questioning; another way is to take some kind of direct action and observe the results – now isn't that just what nurses do in their work with patients? However, practising nurses should be more aware of this process, in order to analyse their involvement with patients.

Schon considers that for practitioners to learn from their actions they must reflect on the effectiveness or the outcome of those actions. He suggests at least two ways in which this reflection might take place: first, through examining whether their framing (Schon's term for a conceptual model) of the situation was accurate; and second, whether the methods employed were appropriate to this framing. In nursing terms, if a nurse has noticed that a patient is very underweight, and has assessed through observation and questioning that this patient is able to feed herself without assistance, then using a self-care framing of the situation (Orem's model) the nurse would provide the patient with a balanced diet and with the cutlery and appropriate environment to eat this diet. However, if the patient did not eat the diet, the nurse might look for the reasons for this. Could it be that the patient was too emotionally distressed to eat, and had not sufficiently adapted to this stress in order to be interested in food (Roy's adaptation model), or are there other more subtle features of the situation that the nurse needs to find out about and take into account?

Schon's model is therefore useful in understanding how the practical nursing situation is used by nurses to find practical solutions to daily problems of patient care.

The idea of using multiple models in practice has also been discussed by Kristjanson, Tamblyn and Kuypers (1987). They say that while a single model may be useful in nursing education, in helping to plan a curriculum to 'organize' educational experiences 'so that students are provided with a systematic process that provides competence' (p. 525), this single-model approach to nursing practice is not appropriate. The reason for this is that nursing practice provides so many different situations, contexts and perceptions for both nurse and patient that a single model cannot cope with all of these. Nor should it have to, as a good model must have a consistent set of beliefs related to a particular aspect of the practice setting.

Therefore, to return to Schon's point, the experienced practitioner must learn to recognize and build up a repertoire of ways in which situations can be framed, and methods for dealing with situations. However, as stressed before, the practitioner who learns from practice will reflect on that practice and will constantly question and search for different and more effective methods of understanding situations and of achieving results.

Levels of understanding will not only help practitioners to be more reflective, through their broader and deeper understanding of different perspectives, but practitioners should also be able to use more discrimination between subtle differences in the practice setting. Therefore nurses who have taken a diploma or a degree course should be more able to choose between different models of nursing according to the situations, and be more able to select the appropriate activity to fit their framing of the situation at any particular time. Moreover, when things do not go as anticipated, they should be more able to examine critically what happened, and whether an alternative approach would have been preferable; therefore an analysis of alternative approaches to the problem can be made.

This book is to help nurses do just that. Through putting together much of the available knowledge from the use of some of the models, by organizing them into the various stages of problem solving, nurses in practice will be able to assess the researchers' framing of the situations, their actions and their outcomes against their own framing, actions and outcomes. Admittedly there is not a great deal of research available to date, but one of the more ambitious aims of this book is to stimulate practitioners to carry out and to write up their research into practice, to create further knowledge. Another area of great need in practice is for replication studies; as can be seen from many of the studies in this book the cultural setting in North America leads to many questions about whether the same patient or nursing problems arise in Great Britain. It would be refreshing therefore to think that some of the findings discussed in this book will be replicated in Great Britain.

I hope it is clear to the reader that including just a few selected studies from each model from those found in the literature would not have provided the richness and scope for nurses working in practice, and therefore would not have been as useful to them in dealing with their practical problems of patient care. This book can be used in a variety of ways: to learn more about models of nursing and how they can be used in practice, and the implications for their use; to assess the usefulness of these models in the nurse's own practice situation; to guide research into patient problems and nursing actions, where it is seen that a model of nursing can help to frame the situation; and to use the studies presented here to compare the findings with situations the nurse has dealt with, and perhaps is now considering or reflecting upon. To aid readers to locate studies particularly relevant to their area of practice, a table of studies outlining the topic and location of the study in the book is given in Appendix 1, on page 279. It may also be that some schools and colleges may want to use this book as a resource when planing their curriculum using a model of practice – although this is not seen as a primary aim of the book.

The idea for this book came from my own students who, during a four-year post-registration degree course in nursing, gain sufficient knowledge of the disciplines of biology, psychology and sociology to use in analysing nursing situations, with the knowledge of different nursing frameworks to aid this analysis. What we were unable to find in this level of work was a composite text which would help students to discriminate between the different ways nurses can frame a situation when dealing with pragmatic problems.

A further aim of this book is that the studies will help both to clarify and to deepen the knowledge of nurses in practice of the various aspects of each of the models presented. Therefore most studies have comments as to how central or peripheral the model is to the study. Each study is then outlined with the essential features of the problems, the method and the findings. Many of the studies are criticized in relation to the research design, in order to show how reliably the knowledge has been created, and therefore how much credence can be given to the results. Some of the studies have parallels in other research, but unless this other research has been designed specifically using a nursing model it has not been included here.

However, not all the studies in each of the chapters are empirical studies; some of the articles are literature searches that compile existing knowledge into a particular aspect of a model. An example or this is Davis-Sharts' (1978) article on the body's response to a raised temperature, which can be found in Chapter 3.

The ways in which nursing problems have been investigated in the studies in this book are wide and varied. This is seen as a strength in nursing that this variety of research methods can be sustained; the profession can feel proud of its versatility in this respect. This undoubtedly enhances the versatility of any practice-based profession. But as some of the terms, particularly in relation to research methods, may be unfamiliar to some readers, a glossary is included in Appendix 2.

The chapters of this book are organized as follows: a few biographical details of the appropriate author are given at the beginning of the chapters; this is followed by a brief outline of the model, then the studies using the model. The studies are organized so that those dealing predominantly with identification of problems are at the beginning of each chapter; a second section deals with planning of care; a third section with intervention; and a fourth with evaluation. As can be seen from the chapters, some of these sections have generated no research to date in some of the models, while others have generated much study in particular sections. Subsequent sections are needed in a few of the chapters where research in practice has been generated, but this is not directly related to the stages of problem solving, and these studies are included in a fifth section in the relevant chapters.

In order to help the reader who uses this text as a reference source, a diagram of the chapter contents is given on the first page of each chapter. This shows the stages of problem-solving as they are described by the model, and the studies that have been carried out in the different practice settings, with a note of the findings from each study.

Readers will find that the lengths of chapters vary considerably. This is not due to any bias on the part of the author, but is merely a result of the differing amounts of research that have been conducted using the various models chosen. However, this allows for some estimation of the popularity and the widespread use of these particular models.

Readers will also find that the language use by the models' authors has been adhered to in this book, so that readers can refer to the original sources.

The literature reviewed for each of the chapters was found through computerized searches, the Social Sciences Citation Index and the AJN International Nursing Index, as well as by following up references from chapters in books, from articles and from dissertations. A criterion for inclusion in this book is that the studies should be easily accessible in Great Britain through local or national libraries, or through inter-library loan systems. Those wishing to access primary sources can therefore do so without undue delays and frustrations.

A list of all the original references pertaining to the particular chapter is to be found at the end of each chapter, together with a list of further reading in the models concerned. This contains British and American publications which should be easily accessible, and covers publications devoted to explaining and analysing the model pertaining to the particular chapter.

It may interest readers to know that the original plan for the chapter titles was: Roper, Logan and Tierney's activities of living; Roy's adaptation model; Orem's self-care model; King's social systems model; Johnson's behavioural systems model; and Rogers' model of unitary human beings. However, a literature search revealed only one piece of research that met the criteria for this book using King's (1971, 1981) model, so this chapter had to be abandoned. For those interested in following up this particular study, see Luker (1979).

It may be worth mentioning at this point what this book is not. It is not intended as a book which analyses the models of nursing, as many such books are available – for example Chin and Jacobs (1983), Kim (1983), Fawcett (1984), George (1985) and Meleis (1985). Nor is it intended to be a statement about the state of the art of nursing models; its aims are as stated in the above paragraphs.

The work for this book has been immeasurably helped by the patience and continuing support of my husband, Sandy, without whom I would not have been able to even consider such an undertaking. Considerable help has also been given by Griselda Campbell of Harper and Row, who has given encouragement and support, and numerous cups of tea and coffee, as well as a considerable amount of constructive advice during the preparation of this book. My thanks also go to Professor Justus Akinsanya, for his considerable advice and comments on the text, and his many helpful suggestions, including those for a suitable title for the book. Reviewers' comments have also been of help and although I am not allowed to know who they are, I am most grateful for their considerable efforts and constructive advice. However, in the last analysis the errors and omissions are mine.

REFERENCES

Chin, P.L. and Jacobs, M.K. (1983) *Theory and Nursing: A Systematic Approach*, C.V. Mosby, St Louis.

Davis-Sharts, J. (1978) Mechanisms and manifestations of fever. *American Journal of Nursing*, November, 1874–1877.

Fawcett, J. (1984) *Analysis and Evaluation of Conceptual Models of Nursing*, F.A. Davis, Philadelphia.

George, J.B. (ed.) (1985) *Nursing Theories: The Basis for Professional Nursing Practice*, 2nd edn, Prentice Hall, Englewood Cliffs, NJ.

Kim, H.S. (1983) *The Nature of Theoretical Thinking in Nursing*, Appleton-Century-Crofts, Newark, CT.

King, I.M. (1971) *Towards a Theory for Nursing, General Concepts of Human Behaviour*, John Wiley, New York.

King, I.M. (1981) *A Theory for Nursing Systems, Concepts, Process*, John Wiley, New York.

Kristjanson, L.J., Tamblyn, R. and Kuypers, J.A. (1987) A model to guide development and application of multiple nursing theories. *Journal of Advanced Nursing*, **12**, 523–529.

Luker, K.A. (1979) Measuring life satisfaction in one elderly female population. *Journal of Advanced Nursing*, **4**, 503–511.

Meleis, A.I. (1985) *Theoretical Nursing: Development and Progress*, J.B. Lippincott, Philadelphia.

Schon, D. (1983) *The Reflective Practitioner*, Temple Smith, London.

Roper, Logan and Tierney's model of activities of living

2

Table of chapter contents

THE AUTHORS

Nancy Roper trained as a nurse at the General Infirmary, Leeds. She spent 15 years as Principal Tutor at the Cumberland Infirmary School of

Nursing. In 1964 she became self-employed as a writer. In 1975 she was awarded an MPhil based on her research from her fellowship of the Commonwealth Nurses' War Memorial fund. Between 1975 and 1978 she was Nursing Officer (Research) in the Scottish Home and Health Department. She has written widely on nursing.

Winifred Logan qualified as a nurse from the Royal Infirmary of Edinburgh. She graduated with a BA from the University of Edinburgh, where she was a lecturer and senior lecturer for 12 years. She worked in the Scottish Home and Health Department for 4 years, responsible for nurse education. From 1971 to 1972 she was Chief Nursing Officer at the Ministry of Health at Abu Dhabi, from 1978 to 1980 she was Executive Director of the International Council for Nurses and from 1981 to 1986 she was Head of Department of Health and Nursing at Glasgow College, Scotland.

Alison Tierney was one of the first graduates to the degree in nursing studies at the University of Edinburgh. From 1973 to 1980 she was a lecturer in the same department. She was awarded a PhD from the University of Edinburgh in the field of mental handicap nursing, for which she received a Scottish Home and Health Department nursing research training studentship. She was Director of the Nursing Research Unit at the University of Edinburgh from 1980.

THE MODEL

The first publication of this model was in 1980 when *The Elements of Nursing* made its first appearance (Roper, Logan and Tierney, 1980; second and third editions published in 1985 and 1990). This was followed by *Learning to Use the Process of Nursing* (Roper, Logan and Tierney, 1982) and *Using a Model for Nursing* (Roper, Logan and Tierney, 1983a).

This has become one of the best known and widest used models of nursing in Britain, mostly because it related well to the way British nurses understood nursing at that time. The authors attempted to explain their model to the profession at large after the publication of their third book in 1983, through a series of articles in the *Nursing Mirror* in May and June 1983.

The texts most frequently cited are *The Elements of Nursing* (Roper, Logan and Tierney, 1980, 1985, 1990) and *Using a Model for Nursing* (Roper, Logan and Tierney, 1983a). The model has had considerable analysis and application by various authors, including Aggleton and Chalmers (1986a,b), Kershaw and Salvage (1986) and the Open University (1984).

This chapter briefly describes the model, and then moves on to show its use through research in practice settings. However, the studies are few, which is sad. This is a considerable shortcoming, especially if nursing practice in many settings uses the model as a basis for nurse–patient interaction and for framing nursing needs.

Since the publication of the 1990 edition of this book, there is evidence from publications in the nursing press that this model is not as popular in practice as it was. Some authors (e.g. Parr, 1993) have made an evaluation of the model against other models. Parr (1993) came to the conclusion that a model generated in America suits his needs better.

SUMMARY OF THE ROPER, LOGAN AND TIERNEY MODEL OF THE ACTIVITIES OF LIVING

In *The Elements of Nursing* Roper, Logan and Tierney (1980) state that they are aiming this work at beginners in nursing. They base their work on the assumption that one of the concerns of living has to do with the activities people carry out regularly in their everyday lives. These 'activities of living' are therefore common to everybody, and are:

- maintaining a safe environment
- communicating
- breathing
- eating and drinking
- eliminating
- personal cleansing and dressing
- controlling body temperature
- mobilizing
- working and playing
- expressing sexuality
- sleeping
- dying.

The authors claim that conceptualizing living as a set of activities is a helpful start, but ' … the more one analyses these activities of living the more one realizes just how complex each one of them is' (p. 17). The inter-related nature of the activities adds to this complexity.

There are periods in life when some of the activities cannot be performed, therefore each individual could be said to be operating at certain levels of dependence or independence in each of the activities. Age is one factor that will affect a person's ability to carry out the activities of living; other factors are inborn disabilities and environmental conditions. Therefore developmental, biological and social factors are all extremely important.

As people grow and develop, they gain individual ways of carrying out their activities of living, their performance of each reflecting their individuality. The authors consider that the study of individual needs is a worthwhile undertaking, but these needs cannot be studied directly, only through the way the activities of living are carried out by the individual.

So important do the authors feel that developmental, biological and social factors are in influencing the activities of living that they devote a chapter to each of these.

'Biological aspects of living' takes the main tenets of theories from biology and discusses these in relation to health and illness. A systems approach is adopted, which builds understanding from the smallest to the largest structures in an hierarchical way. The biological tenets consist of the structure and activity of cells, including pathogens, inheritance and body tissues. Discussion of the latter also includes each of the human systems, pointing out a direct relationship to the activities of living, for example:

- the cardiovascular system is briefly explained – heat production is said to be distributed by the blood, and is therefore linked directly to controlling body temperature;
- the lymphatic system is described as indirectly linked to all the activities of living;
- the endocrine system is described as having overall influence on all the activities of living;
- the nervous system is said to coordinate all the activities of living;
- the musculoskeletal system structures are outlined and stated as facilitating the activity of mobilizing;
- the sensory system structures are outlined and are said to play an important part in communicating and maintaining a safe environment.

The other systems of the body are also described but have a more evident link to various activities of living, so therefore will not need further elaboration here.

Other biological tenets dealt with in this chapter are: bodily defence mechanisms including homeostasis; pain; and drugs and their actions. A table at the end of the chapter also outlines the broad side effects of drugs and how these influence the activities of living, and the resulting patients' problems. For example 'daytime sleepiness' affects maintaining a safe environment, working and playing, and mobilizing. These, in turn, produce problems of 'increased fire/accident risk, decreased concentration', and 'deprivation of driving/cycling' (p. 41), respectively.

The chapter dealing with development considers stages of fetal development, and development during infancy, taking into account physical growth and mentioning independence of the activities of living, particularly mobilizing, cognition, emotional and social development. Development in childhood (6–12 years) considers physical, intellectual, emotional and social factors. A section is devoted to adolescence (13–18 years), and again physical, emotional, intellectual and social factors are discussed. Maturity in early adulthood (19–30 years) is again concerned with physical, intellectual, emotional and social development. A brief section considers the settled nature of the middle years (30–45 years). In development of late adulthood (46–65 years) physical, intellectual and social changes are emphasized. Old age, considered as over 65 years, discusses physical and intellectual changes along with their implications for the health, social and emotional aspects of life at this age.

The chapter dealing with social aspects covers a variety of topics on society and socialization, culture and membership of a community. Housing is mentioned with the effects on the individual of poor amenities, high density housing and overcrowding. A section dealing with role discusses the concept of role set and the status attached to roles. Social relationships are discussed along with the interaction that takes place in social groups. The discussion of the organization of society centres around the interrelationship of the family, education, religion, economics, health and government. It outlines the basic features of each of these. Religion is given a more detailed outline informing the beginning student nurse of customs associated with a variety of religious beliefs as they affect health and illness. Social class is described and its relationship to health and illness outlined; social mobility in Western societies is compared with other cultures. The authors discuss the family as a unit and its effect on the socialization of children. Types of family are discussed, related to cultural variations: the extended family, the nuclear family and one parent families; also considered in this section is residential care and institutionalization with its effects on the residents.

The authors are now ready to state their model for nursing:

> Nursing is concerned with helping people at all stages of their lifespan to achieve their optimal level of health. It is also concerned with helping people to overcome, or adjust to and cope with problems in their activities of living caused by trauma, disease and so on.
>
> (p. 61)

They state that the activities of living create preventing, comforting and seeking activities in individuals, so nursing can be seen as concerned with preventing, comforting and dependent activities.

From ideas considered previously, each activity of living can be seen on a continuum of total dependence to total independence. Independence can be helped by the provision of suitable equipment; but sometimes patients need to be encouraged to withold their independence to promote health. Nursing should be concerned with assessing the individuals' level of independence in their activities of living, and then judging in which direction and by how much they should be helped to move towards dependence or independence.

Some circumstances can lead to a decrease in independence:

- the physical, psychological or social environment;
- congenital or acquired disturbed physiology which results in mental or physical dysfunction;
- pathological or degenerative tissue changes;
- accident;
- infection.

Nurses must think of these circumstances in relation to patient dependence/independence.

Nursing can help patients with particular problems by assisting them to carry out their usual activities of living as much as is possible. However, where these lead the patient to health problems, nursing should be directed towards changing the patient's habits or attitudes to develop a healthier lifestyle. Nursing is carried out in three ways:

- Prevention: hospitals have many potential sources of harm to patients, including stress and infection, but nurses can teach patients to alleviate these.
- Comfort: to promote the patient's maximum physical and mental comfort to aid coping. Such nursing activities would include ensuring the patient is able to eat meals comfortably, and to reach everything they need.
- Dependency: this assumes that when people are ill they seek medical help, therefore requiring nursing. An example of a dependent activity in nursing is giving drugs, carrying out wound dressings or assisting with physiotherapy – the 'technical' aspects of nursing.

The authors then move on to look at the stages of problem solving by the nurse when using the model, describing the stages as assessment, planning, implementation and evaluation. **Assessment** looks at each of the activities in turn and states that assessment is not a once-only activity, but should be continuous. The authors stress that the 'objective in collecting information about the activities of living is to discover' (p. 67):

- previous routines;
- what the patient can do for him/herself;
- problems;
- discomforts and previous coping mechanisms.

Planning is concerned with preventing potential problems or helping patients to cope with their existing problems. The resources that nurses use in planning are: consideration of where the patient should be nursed; the equipment that should be used; the staff available and their levels of expertise; the amount and type of support staff available; and the alternative nursing interventions. **Implementation** of the plan is briefly discussed, and **evaluation** centres on the benefits to the patient; however, this last section is very brief.

In *Learning to Use the Process of Nursing* (Roper, Logan and Tierney, 1982) the Roper, Logan and Tierney model is re-emphasized and its application made to a variety of patient problems in hospital and at home. These are arranged around a problem-solving approach.

In *Using a Model for Nursing*, Roper, Logan and Tierney (1983a) again re-emphasize their model without any change to its original form. The way the model can be used in many nursing settings is developed. The chapters are written by practising nurses.

In their paper 'Is there a danger of "processing" patients?', Roper, Logan and Tierney (1983c) show the shift of emphasis to increased participation by the patients: in identifying the patient's problems, where agreement about the problem is essentially a joint exercise between nurse and patient; planning that involves taking account of the patient's ideas; implementation that shows the patient as sometimes being entirely responsible for carrying out the plan; and evaluation that involves the patient's and significant others' opinions of the achieved outcome.

The second edition of *The Elements of Nursing* (1985) has a number of changes from the first edition. The emphasis is away from a disease-based model.

In part this move reflects that nurses ... have become increasingly aware that people's health and the illnesses from which they suffer are inextricably linked with their lifestyle and the activities of living.

(p. 63)

They restate their belief that their model is flexible enough to be used in any branch of nursing, or situation requiring nursing, and that it is deliberately uncomplicated, being written mainly for the beginning student of nursing.

The concept of nursing is changed from the definition given in 1980, the 1985 definition being: 'Nursing is viewed as helping patients to prevent, alleviate or cope with problems with the Activities of Living' (p. 65). The emphasis of nursing being on prevention remains, but the comforting and dependent activities of nursing are no longer seen.

One of the main factors contributing to dependence/independence of the activities of living is still age, or the individual's developmental stage. However, the factors influencing the activities of living have been expanded from three in 1980 – biological, developmental and social – to five in 1985 – physical, psychological, sociocultural, environmental and politico-economic. This change of emphasis and increase in the factors influencing the activities of living is probably due to the growing acceptance of psychology within nursing, and also to the focus of nursing being towards health rather than disease.

Analysis and criticism of the model has come from many sources. Aggleton and Chalmers (1986) comment that this model is primarily physiologically based, and will appeal to nurses who have a tendency to accept the medical model. Lister (1987) supports the model, and compares the activities of living with physiological systems, commenting that breathing, eating, eliminating and controlling body temperature strongly reflect the medical model; while other activities of living – namely communicating, mobilizing, expressing sexuality, sleeping and dying – have a strong physiological element.

Wilson-Barnett (1981), while commending the 1980 edition of *The Elements of Nursing* as a 'substantial contribution to the nursing literature' (p. 249), comments that the evaluation of care could have received more attention. Criticism of the weakness of evaluation in this model is also mentioned by Hunt (1983).

One of the best known criticisms of the model and the nursing process in particular, and one that is mentioned in the second edition of *The Elements of Nursing*, is that by Mitchell (1984). He comments that the model is too complex. He cites the 12 activities of living, each of which has a 40–50 item prompt list to help nurses to identify and record a patient's problems. Mitchell says that not only are these prompts unnecessarily lengthy, but some of them are incorrect. This will lead not only to confusion amongst nurses, but also to neglect of the patient in favour of the paperwork, which will demand a considerable amount of nursing time. Furthermore, the documentation does not reflect the differences in patient conditions and therefore patient needs.

Mitchell also argues for senior clinical nurses to work a similar system to medicine, which would mean working daytime hours rather than shifts; so facilitating continuity of patient care. He said this would ensure that the person who made the managerial decisions about patient care, where the 'checklists' were needed, was available when the decisions were being made. He argues that doctors care about nursing and would like to continue to contribute, particularly to nursing education, and to be involved in the nursing process, which to date they have not been asked to do. Mitchell feels that, using this system, there is a real threat of nurses spending a considerable amount of time away from the patient: 'The spectacle of rows of nurses beavering away at complex and irrelevant checklists fills me with gloom' (p. 219). Nurses may also become independent in their care of the patient and therefore possibly work in opposition to the medical diagnosis and plan. He calls for greater involvement by doctors and increased cooperation between doctors and nurses in the provision of patient care.

A reply to Mitchell's criticisms was published by Tierney in 1984. She feels his article to be 'deliberately contentious and unreasonably dismissive' (p. 835). She advocates some constructive dialogue between the two professions on the subject, despite this poor beginning. She defends the activities of living as being different from the medical diagnosis, by saying that the patient's medical condition will undoubtedly be responsible for the problems the patient has with the activities of living, but this diagnosis is not the only cause of the problems. Tierney says that nursing is concerned with more than care for patients in hospital and that the concept of disease is limiting. The activities of living is a more appropriate framework for nurses to use. To support this she cites the preventive role of midwives and health visitors, and the fact that nurses are also concerned with care of different age groups and people who are dying who have a legitimate need for nursing services. Tierney also says that nurses are concerned with caring for the handicapped, where the concept of disease is no longer appropriate, as nursing care incorporates those in the community who need help but are not currently receiving medical treatment. Three further groups for whom the medical diagnosis is limiting are patients who are in hospital where the medical diagnosis is unclear, but who still have problems in performing their activities of living; hospital patients who no longer have a need for medical attention but still need help to become independent before they go home; and finally, patients whose problems are caused by being admitted to hospital or being confined to bed – these problems are not derived directly from their medical condition.

Tierney refutes Mitchell's claim that nurses consider doctors not to be interested in the individual, as nurses' concern for the activities of living does not preclude interest in the disease, indeed in some areas of nursing the medical diagnosis and treatment are fundamental. She agrees that nursing documentation has become more complex, but argues that these documents now need to be fuller and more reliable than in the past, though this should not result in unnecessary complexity. She says that the two-page assessment form in *Using a Model for Nursing* could not be described as complex, and, as authors, they have painstakingly emphasized the need for simple documentation. She concludes that Professor Mitchell's comments on nursing documentation are 'inaccurate and exaggerated' (p. 837).

In 1990 the third edition of *The Elements of Nursing* was published. There are many alterations to this edition from the second edition. The title has now been extended to include the subtitle 'a model for nursing based on a model for living'. The authors say that this is to make it clear that this book incorporates their model for nursing. The emphasis continues to be on health rather than disease. Disease is seen as a problem of the activities of living caused by the illness. The chapters have been revised; the most noticeable difference is the omission of the chapters on biology, psychology and sociology, as these are felt to be more appropriately taught as foundation subjects to nursing. In this edition there is also acknowledgement of some of the internationally known models of nursing. However, in essence the model has not changed.

Having briefly described the model as presented by the authors, and some of the criticisms of their work, it is now time to examine some of the published work that uses this model as its basis. This part of the chapter will be organized, like subsequent chapters, into sections that concentrate mainly on identification of patient needs and problems using this model, followed by sections dealing mainly with planning, implementation and finally evaluation.

In this chapter, there is only one research-based study, by Allan (1987). The other papers are based on using the model in a practice setting. Also of significance is that no new papers were found since the publication of the first edition of this book in 1990. As I indicated at the beginning of this chapter, it is a shame that this model has not generated more research, particularly in the UK. In this respect the Roper, Logan and Tierney model falls behind its claimed counterparts in the USA.

IDENTIFICATION OF PROBLEMS USING THE ROPER, LOGAN AND TIERNEY MODEL

In this section four papers were found, each devoted to a different patient condition. Three papers used the Roper, Logan and Tierney model to assess patients (Bain, 1985; Webster, 1986; Heslop and Bagnall, 1988), a fourth developed an assessment tool for use with patients with multiple sclerosis (Allan, 1987).

IDENTIFICATION OF PROBLEMS WITH SLEEP

The paper discussed in this section (Webster, 1986) has only a small proportion devoted to the use of Roper, Logan and Tierney's model in relation to sleep. However, it shows a good knowledge base, and how this knowledge base can be integrated into the model.

In part of a lengthy paper, Webster (1986) considers Roper, Logan and Tierney's statement that individuals have certain routines before they go to sleep at night, therefore alteration of these may affect the patient's ability to sleep or to sleep well in hospital. She quotes Brezinova and Oswald (1972) who show that milky drinks can improve sleep, whereas Karacan et al. (1976) showed that coffee, and other drinks that contain caffeine, disturb sleep, although some of those who drink such beverages before going to sleep may not be aware of this.

The effects of alcohol on sleep have been studied by Williams, McLean and Cairns (1983). They showed that alcohol leads to more wakings during the night and also changes in the pattern of sleep. Palmer, Harrison and Horns (1980) found that the more alcohol that was consumed by habitual drinkers, the less they were able to sleep. Similar findings were also reported for smoking.

Other factors which affect sleep are exercise and general stimulation. Hobson (1968) found that excessive exercise before going to bed leads to increased levels of arousal and stress. Henderson and Nite (1978) support this and say that nurses should promote relaxation before patients go to sleep.

This is a useful compilation of knowledge, which if critically evaluated and used by nurses in assessing patients' sleep patterns, or claimed lack of sleep, may possibly lead to more predictable results of nursing actions when using this model.

ASSESSMENT OF PATIENTS WITH MULTIPLE SCLEROSIS

This paper (Allan, 1987) uses the Roper, Logan and Tierney model to show how assessment of patients with multiple sclerosis can be carried out. It uses the degrees of severity of the disease in order to demonstrate to the nurse a scaling system for dependence/independence which might be used.

Allan (1987) developed a tool to assess the quality of life of patients with multiple sclerosis. This was based on eight of the activities of living (maintaining a safe environment; communicating; eating and drinking; eliminating; mobilizing; personal cleansing and dressing; working and playing; and sleeping). He graded the patient's ability on a 7-point scale, from 1 = independent to 7 = very or totally dependent for each activity of living. Each of the grades specified the activity the patient would be able to carry out, for example;

	1	3	5	7
Maintaining a safe environment	Normal in all aspects in coping safely out of doors and alone at home.	Considerable difficulty alone outside. OK at home at own pace.	Wheelchair certainly outside. Ability to perform in home limited.	Totally unable to protect from or avoid any hazards. Essentially immobile/ quadriplegic.

(p.45)

The tool was used by a number of assessors, and the author claims good reliability between the assessors in its use, although no statistical measure of this is given. Allan also claims that the tool gave a 'sound basis for discussion for the person's adaptation to his disabilities' (p. 44) and that the activities of living were aspects of the patient's life which were important. However, one of the areas not included in this tool was 'expressing sexuality', which was found to be particularly important to the patients, and where nurses felt a trained counsellor had to be employed to deal with the issues which arose.

A problem for the patient which was displayed in many of the activities of living was fatigue. Talking with the nurse about the organization of their day to maximize their energy helped the patients to put their disabilities into perspective.

This tool was evidently based directly on the activities of living as identified by Roper, Logan and Tierney, and therefore makes a useful contribution to the use of this model in practice. The study is undoubtedly theoretically driven. However, it is unclear why only certain of the activities of living were chosen and not all of them. As Allan mentioned, expressing sexuality was an activity which was most pertinent to the patients. It might have been thought that breathing, controlling body temperature and dying would have been equally relevant; however the author gives no reason for not including these. Although the amount of testing this instrument received was not made clear from the article, the tool did appear to be of considerable use. It was also carefully designed for each of the activities of living used. It would be useful for such studies to be written up in a more rigorous manner, to demonstrate the ability of the model to be used with such groups of patients, particularly in relation to assessment of their needs. However, this was a descriptive study, and so did not test any of the aspects of the model in a cause and effect manner.

ASSESSMENT OF PATIENTS AT HOME WITH CHEST DISEASE

The authors in the following study were a team of doctors and nurses involved in a project setting up a support service for patients at home with chronic lung disease. The nurses worked as respiratory health workers (RHWs) during the time of the study. They carried out assessment of the patients using the Roper, Logan and Tierney model.

Bagnall and Heslop (1987), Cockcroft et al. (1987) and Heslop and Bagnall (1988) have written about their work as RHWs and how their role has developed. Heslop and Bagnall (1988) describe the assessments they made of patients using the Roper, Logan and Tierney model of nursing, and this aspect of their paper will be described here.

The RHWs identified between four and ten problems in the patients they visited. They found that these problems fell into four groups:

- physical health
- knowledge
- psychosocial
- sociodomestic.

Physical health

Most of the patients felt helpless and unable to have any effect on their state of health, having been progressively ill for a number of years. They had varying degrees of breathlessness for which some relied on oxygen cylinders, the most dependent of these being restricted by the length of the oxygen tubing. This inevitably had resulted in lessening exercise tolerance.

Knowledge

The level of knowledge of the patients about their illness was minimal; they also did not feel responsible for learning about their disease, nor how to recognize deterioration in their condition. This may have been partly due to learning being difficult for many of the patients who were elderly.

Psychosocial

Because many of these patients were elderly they had lost close relatives and friends, therefore combined with their incapacity many of them were very lonely and expressions of death occurred frequently. Their ability to cope with their illness depended on their personal resources and their ability to adapt, which had been developed over the number of years of this progressive illness.

Sociodomestic

Many of the patients had been rehoused, and many now lived in ground floor accommodation; however, some had not been rehoused. The existence of voluntary services was not always known to the patients, and even if known, the patients needed confidence in how to use them. Some patients needed help in knowing about benefits, and how to claim them. These problems were seen as common to many elderly patients, not merely this group with respiratory disease.

It is interesting that Heslop and Bagnall have divided the patients' problems into these four groups, as Roper, Logan and Tierney (1983a) have stated that biological, developmental and social factors are the influencing factors of the activities of living. They do not mention assessment of knowledge as a separate influencing factor. It may therefore be assumed that the Roper, Logan and Tierney (1983a) model, on which this study is based, will not be sufficient to meet the needs of nurses working with these patients, unless there is an addition to the assessment of each activity of living to allow the nurse to assess the patient's level of knowledge.

Heslop and Bagnall do not clearly state the method used to collect their data, therefore the method by which their four categories were arrived at remains unclear. The authors also do not comment on the usefulness, or otherwise, of the model in helping them to identify the patient's problems.

Therefore assessment using Roper, Logan and Tierney's model for this group of patients is not seen as totally inclusive. This study is also descriptive, and does not show any relationships between parts of the model. It therefore gives only very weak support to the usefulness of the model in this situation.

ASSESSMENT OF AN ELDERLY MAN FOLLOWING A STROKE

This study (Bain, 1985) looks in some detail at the problems for a patient suffering from a stroke and for a nurse caring for such a patient. The effects of the stroke produce difficulty for the patient in his level of under-standing and in his speech.

Bain (1985) conducted a nursing assessment on a 78-year-old man who had had a stroke which resulted in his initial inability to speak. Only some of the assessment of his activities of living appear in the article, but these give considerable detail.

The patient's abilities to communicate showed that he had two distinct problems. First, he was dysphasic, i.e. he had lost the ability to interpret and therefore to understand speech. He also could not form speech due to the loss of speech symbols. If this continued it could be a considerable frustration to the patient, the symptoms becoming worse when the patient was tired or emotionally upset. His second problem was dysarthria – he was unable to control his muscles used for speech, but with this patient the dysarthria only lasted for the first 2 days of his admission. A more detailed assessment showed that the patient was able to understand simple sentences and phrases which were related to the immediate situation, such as 'Do you want a cup of tea?'. However, generally his level of understanding of both speech and written communication was unreliable, with reading being worse than verbal understanding. His ability to speak showed he had marked difficulty with finding words, and was only able to speak a few non-fluent words. The patient's use of speech is summed up in a paragraph from the article:

> When asked to name an object he would stutter, 'Well it's … Well it's …' as if he knew what he wanted to say but could not find the word. When offered two words, 'Is it a towel or a flannel?' he would answer, rightly or wrongly, 'It's a flannel, flannel! It's a flannel!' On asking the name of another object, he would reply again, 'a flannel'.

(p.43)

The words he was able to say unprompted were combined into short sentences which contained no information such as 'Thank you very much!'

Further assessment, when the patient had been in hospital for a few days, showed that visual cues helped him to make a choice, and to under-stand what was being said to him. Therefore to offer him a choice of food or drink and to show him the different choices helped him to understand what was being offered. Nurses also found that facial expression helped his comprehension, therefore it was essential to face him when speaking to him. To promote his speech it was found necessary to emphasize an unhurried approach.

Due to the patient's communication difficulties the problems of potential social isolation and resulting depression were formulated. This was found to be a potential problem as during the first few days of his admission he took no interest in the other patients or in his surroundings. He chose to isolate himself by sitting by his bed for meals, rather than joining the other patients at the table.

The patient's mobility was assessed by the doctors and by the physio-therapists. This assessment found that the patient was able to feel touch on his limbs on his right side, but he did not know where on the limbs he was being touched. He also had a slight weakness in his right arm, and showed a preference for use of his left hand in spite of being right-handed. When he walked he was able to balance well and was independent, but he had a slight stoop to the right side, and guarded his right arm.

This study shows a detailed approach to assessment of communication abilities and mobility in a patient suffering from a stroke. The level of detail exceeds that given by Roper, Logan and Tierney, but in spite of this the assessment is seen to include the physical, developmental and social factors influencing these two activities of living. However, the same criticism can be made of this study as has been made of some of the others in this chapter, i.e. that the assessment is not written up in a way that would allow for replication. Therefore, although this is a good nursing care study, it does not necessarily support the use of the model. However, neither does it deny the model's usefulness in these circumstances.

This completes the studies which deal predominantly with assessment of patients/clients.

CONCLUSIONS

As I have shown, there is no study which gives an indication of whether assessment of patients using this model is valid, although there is some indication, from Allan, that assessment using some aspects of it are valid with patients suffering from multiple sclerosis. However, there is no indication of the relationship between the activities of living, nor between assessment and nursing activities.

PLANNING CARE USING THE ROPER, LOGAN AND TIERNEY MODEL

Two studies were found in the literature which developed this aspect of the model: one considers planning terminal care (Janes, 1986); the other plans the care of an immobile patient following traumatic spinal injuries (Harrison, 1986). Both these studies use the care study approach, and although demonstrating the wide use and therefore acceptability of this model in Britain, they do not test for its adequacy.

TERMINAL CARE PLANNING FOR AN ELDERLY MAN

This study, according to the author, is 'loosely based on Roper's activities of daily living nursing model' (p. 27). It describes the care given to an elderly terminally ill man in hospital until he died.

Janes (1986) describes the assessment of a 79-year-old man admitted to hospital from home. His wife had died of cancer the previous year, and he had looked after her at home until she died, with the help of a close friend. The latter found the patient to be unkempt with increasingly incoherent speech. His general practitioner admitted the patient to hospital immediately.

The nursing assessment carried out on admission found the patient to have good functioning in all his activities of living, apart from speech where it was noted that he had 'expressive dysphasia on admission' (p. 25) whereas his previous speech pattern had not shown this. He also complained of an occasional headache. As his problems were not severe at this time the plan was for the patient to maintain his independence as much as possible.

Within a few days the patient's condition deteriorated, beginning with vomiting. Nursing goals were to relieve vomiting and prevent dehydration by ensuring he had the necessary equipment within reach, that his intake and output were monitored, that he was given antiemetics and dexamethasone, and that fluids and diet were given in the quality and quantity which could be tolerated. Soon after admission a medical diagnosis of carcinoma of the bronchus with widespread cerebral secondaries was made. This altered the nature of the nursing care given, and preparation for continuing deterioration was planned.

When the patient's level of communication deteriorated so that he had difficulty articulating his needs, a picture board was used and the patient was able to indicate his needs using this. Communication skills by nurses were emphasized by frequently initiating conversations with the patient, and by encouraging him to participate as much as possible.

The patient developed problems of mobility on the tenth day after admission; this was shown by a marked hemiparesis which gradually increased in severity. Planning to help the patient to cope with this involved the physiotherapist in teaching arm and leg exercises, and the nurses helping the patient when he was walking, placing his locker and possessions on his non-affected side and within reach, and giving mouthwashes after meals to cleanse the affected side of his mouth.

Problems developed for the patient with swallowing food and a potential problem of choking on food was identified. Apart from ensuring that the patient received antibiotics following aspiration of food into his lungs, the nursing plan was to ensure he received a 1500 calorie intake daily, orally, as he enjoyed food. This was achieved through planned monitoring of his food consumption and by giving food in small enough pieces for him to eat; he needed to be fed when he became too weak to do so for himself.

Personal cleansing and dressing gradually became an increasing problem: the goal of meeting the patient's usual standard of hygiene was achieved through assisting him with the washing routine he observed at home, and helping him to change his clothes while teaching him to cope with his paralysed limbs. When the patient became bed-bound this care was continued in a more dependent manner.

When the patient's condition continued to deteriorate the nurses discussed the question of dying, although when the patient indicated no readiness to do so the nurses felt some sense of failure. When his friend took on this role nursing goals became to prevent further psychological deterioration by encouraging visits from friends and family, to organize weekend leave, and to encourage mixing with other patients in the ward.

Pain as a problem was identified as separate from the other activities of living. The goal was to relieve the pain, and to this end two types of medication were given to aid relief before an effective analgesic was found. Nurses aimed to give this as prescribed and to note its effect, to ensure a comfortable position for the patient, and to reassure him that his pain could be relieved.

With continued deterioration in his condition the patient developed pressure sores and retention of urine. The former was overcome by use of a Ripple mattress and changing position every 3 hours combined with the application of lotions. Urinary retention necessitated catheterization with observation of the patency of the catheter and colour and consistency of the urine. Recording of fluid intake and output and catheter toilet to prevent urinary tract infection were undertaken.

The last problem identified was when the patient attempted to resist nursing care when he was close to death. The goal was to keep him comfortable and free from distress by giving his care needed for the next 3 hours at one time, so that he could rest in between these periods of care, and to explain the necessary care.

This study shows an approach that resembles Roper, Logan and Tierney in that many of their activities of living are used, although Janes found it necessary to use a separate heading for pain. The biological, developmental and social factors are loosely used for assessment and problem identification. The nursing action is not based on knowledge from research, nor are the nursing actions based directly on preventing, comforting and dependence, although some evidence of this is seen. Although the study is based on the first edition of *The Elements of Nursing*, a further factor influencing the activities of living is seen – psychological. No substantial rationale is given for these changes, but with the growing acceptance by nurses of the influence of psychology it is impossible to ignore this.

Again, with this study there is no evidence of systematic collection of data which would allow for testing of this model, through either a deductive or inductive approach. The fact that this model was used for this patient shows its general acceptability in this situation.

THE MAN WITH COMPRESSION FRACTURES OF THE THORACIC VERTEBRAE

This study, based on Roper, Logan and Tierney's model, considers problems with activities of living that are caused by, or develop as a result of, being hospitalized by a traumatic compression fracture of the thoracic vertebrae.

Harrison (1986) describes the care of a 46-year-old man who fell 3 m (10 feet) from a ladder and subsequently found he was unable to lift his head and shoulders from the ground.

On admission to an orthopaedic ward the patient was assessed according to his activities of living, in some of which he had problems. He had no difficulty with breathing and so needed no nursing intervention with this activity.

The patient was unable to fully maintain his own safe environment due to loss of mobility and being in a strange environment. The nurses planned to overcome this by introducing him to other patients and placing his call bell and other necessary items near to hand.

The patient was articulate, although at first he seemed withdrawn; the nurses attributed this to his pain and anxiety due to his accident. The plan was to involve the patient and his wife in all decisions about his care which resulted in the maintenance of good communication between the three parties.

Eating and drinking observations established that the patient was suffering from a paralytic ileus 6 hours after admission. This was diagnosed due to vomiting, nausea, a distended and tense abdomen and the absence of bowel sounds. In planning to prevent inevitable dehydration and the risk of inhalation of stomach contents, a nasogastric tube was passed with continuous drainage of stomach contents, and an intravenous infusion was commenced, while the patient was to take nothing by mouth until his bowel sounds returned. To monitor the situation the nurses instituted a fluid balance chart, ensuring care of the patient's mouth, while no fluids were being taken orally, and being aware of the potential risk of infection from the invasive procedures. Nursing care was gradually withdrawn as bowel sounds returned and the patient began an oral intake of food and fluids. However, a further problem emerged of eating while lying flat. This was planned to be overcome by rolling the patient on his side, where if his food was cut up and he was given a fork, he could eat it when it was placed alongside him on the bed.

Disturbance of elimination was an inevitable consequence of both the accident and of lying flat in bed. The patient found it very difficult to micturate in bed; to help him to achieve this his bed was moved into the bathroom, to ensure privacy, where the taps were turned on and he was rolled onto his side. These measures produced the desired effect. Planning care also ensured the patient's urine was tested for blood, as a positive result could have been the effect of trauma.

Planning to overcome the patient's constipation involved the use of laxatives, and equipment which made minimal movement of the spine possible.

Care of the patient's personal cleansing and dressing showed the patient to be completely dependent on others for this activity. Planning to help the patient the nurse assisted him to wash and clean his teeth and comb his hair. The physiotherapist was involved in advising the patient on ways of dressing while he was immobile.

The patient's lack of mobility meant potential problems of pressure sores, respiratory and circulatory damage, loss of independence, boredom, frustration and apathy. Planning to overcome pressure sores was managed through turning the patient every 2 hours and providing adequate pain control for this procedure. Respiratory and circulatory damage was minimized by active leg exercising combined with information on the importance of this activity. Gradual mobilization was planned and commenced, each stage of movement being explained and developed. It is interesting to note that although boredom and frustration were potential problems, the article did not mention ways of overcoming this.

The patient was able to return to work, and planning was developed to ensure he could drive in safety and comfort as this was essential to his job.

Night sedation was prescribed for the patient as he had difficulty sleeping at night; it had the desired effect.

This study was evidently based on the activities of living, and apart from controlling body temperature, expressing sexuality and dying, each seemed to have been useful for this patient. There is also evidence that developmental and social as well as biological factors were taken into account in considering the patient's situation. However, as with many of the other studies in this chapter, data collection was not sufficiently rigorous to lead to conclusions about testing the model; also the planning of care was not based on research findings, therefore the effectiveness and efficiency of the nursing actions cannot be estimated in the care carried out. Finally, the article did not mention overtly the role of the nurse as preventing, comforting and dependent, although it appeared that much of the care planned could be considered to be either preventive or comforting.

CONCLUSIONS

Janes considered planning terminal care for an elderly hospitalized patient, and Harrison planned care for a man suffering from acute spinal injuries. Although these are good nursing care studies, and were evidently written as such, neither of these authors problematized the model or the care they gave to these patients using the model, therefore the adequacy of the model is not evident from the articles.

The authors also did not collect data in a systematic or rigorous way so that conclusions cannot be made about the adequacy of the parts of the model for these patients. However, that the model was used in these settings shows a good level of its acceptability at the time that the papers were written.

IMPLEMENTING CARE USING THE ROPER, LOGAN AND TIERNEY MODEL IN PRACTICE

In this last section three studies were found. Each of them deals with a very different area of nursing, and some cover topics not seen before in this chapter: movement of a mentally handicapped man into the community (Ford, 1987); infection control (Webster and Bowell, 1986); and care of a patient with respiratory failure due to chronic bronchitis (Ledger, 1986).

PREPARATION OF A MENTALLY HANDICAPPED MAN TO BE DISCHARGED FROM HOSPITAL INTO THE COMMUNITY

The patient discussed in this study had spent many years in a hospital for the mentally subnormal, and, using a token economy scheme, nursing intervention was aimed at helping him to return to the community, despite the patient's resistance and fear of this move.

Ford (1987) assessed a 51-year-old patient who had lived in an institution for the mentally handicapped for 26 years. An assessment of his abilities in relation to the skills necessary for the outside world used the Roper, Logan and Tierney format. This showed he was unsafe in the environment outside the hospital as he had no road sense, but he could use electrical appliances with safety. He could communicate adequately enough to live independently, he could use the telephone, read and write.

He had no respiratory problems. He was able to eat in a socially acceptable manner, to buy and to cook simple foods. He had no evident problems with elimination.

The patient's level of ability to wash and dress himself showed meticulous cleanliness which was unprompted and he had an immaculate appearance; he was also able to adjust his clothing according to the ambient temperature. In mobility, he had no physical difficulties and was able to travel independently into the town using public transport. At work he was found to be able to carry out tasks in the industrial therapy department, but was frequently late arriving and wandered off during his time there. He had problems with recognizing large amounts of money. In playing activities he was able to visit the local pub independently, but had difficulty forming relationships and had little confidence in himself. His sexuality was expressed by his good dress sense, but he showed little evidence of interest in the opposite sex, saying he preferred to be alone.

In order to gain the skills necessary to live in the community the following intervention was set up for the patient.

- He should attend the adult education department for 1½ days a week to develop his social skills, to enable him to make relationships, and to improve his reading and writing ability to a level which would enable him to live independently in the community.
- He should visit the local town with the adult education department to practise buying goods and recognizing prices in the shop windows, especially larger prices.
- A token economy scheme was to be started to increase his motivation to work, and particularly to get to work when in the community. Nursing staff would act as counsellors in this area.
- His fear and lack of confidence at leaving the hospital would be overcome by increased visits outside the hospital, for a longer time, to his community placement, and ensuring adequate support for him from the community team.

However, the paper gives no evaluation of the effectiveness of these interventions. This is consistent with the model's weakness in evaluation.

The study showed a knowledge of the literature, as Elliott and Mackay's (1971) work structured some of the intervention strategies. The model helped with assessment of this patient; problems were found with most of his activities of living, and included biological, developmental and social factors. However, it does not appear that token economy methods are consistent with this model, particularly as psychology and behaviourism do not form part of the 1980 model on which this study is based, nor its application to a psychogeriatric unit as shown in *Using a Model for Nursing*. It is also difficult to see how the model's definition of nursing as being preventing, comforting and dependent in relation to the patient's problems are met using token economy.

PREVENTION OF HOSPITAL CROSS-INFECTION

The model is used to discuss problems of infection in hospitals and measures to prevent cross-infection between patients and from staff. The authors particularly consider the preventive aspect of the nurses' role outlined by the model as being crucial to this area of nursing.

Webster and Bowell (1986) consider patient needs and nursing intervention in prevention of infection. They feel that the use of the Roper, Logan and Tierney model will help to identify those patients most at risk of infection.

The three main sources of infection (the authors state) are exogenous, endogenous and latent (Lowbury et al., 1975). The preventive role of the nurse is seen in a number of nursing activities that can minimize the risk of exogenous infection, including the position of the patient in the ward, where it should be considered that infected patients will also be a source of infection and therefore a risk to other patients. The nurse should make sure that communal equipment is scrupulously clean and dry to prevent coliform organisms being transmitted between patients (Collins, 1981). Handwashing has been well documented by Lowbury et al. (1975) as the most important procedure in preventing cross-infection. Webster and Bowell (1986) suggest that this should be reinforced at each staff handover.

A further procedure to minimize infection through decontamination of the hands is suggested by Hoffman (1982), where an alcohol solution is rubbed on the hands until it evaporates. This may be useful between procedures. Protective clothing such as plastic aprons should be renewed whenever they are used with the patient at risk; the aprons should not be reused.

Patients can act to prevent or minimize their own infection levels by hand-washing, especially where invasive procedures have been used, for example bladder catheters or intravenous infusions. Equipment for this should be made available for immobile patients. Showering, to rinse off dead skin and bacteria, is preferable to bathing. Daily showering increases hygiene and reduces the risk from transient organisms.

Reducing the risk of infection from faecal organisms and skin, with associated bacteria, is also helped by careful and daily change of bed linen.

This well-researched article also specifies the mode of operation of the nurse as that of 'preventing'. The article takes the model and develops it in relation to one area of nurse/patient interaction, thereby showing how knowledge can be used in the context of the Roper, Logan and Tierney model, with both nurse and patient in the preventive role.

THE PATIENT IN RESPIRATORY FAILURE DUE TO CHRONIC BRONCHITIS

This study (Ledger, 1986) takes the basis of a good level of knowledge of respiration, its function and effects, on the maintenance of the other activities of living. The study is impressive for its level of knowledge, and the application of this to the study of the patient in respiratory failure who is being nursed in an intensive care unit (ICU) using an intermittent positive pressure ventilator (IPPV).

Ledger takes each of the activities of living and shows their use in caring for a patient in respiratory failure being nursed in an ICU. Maintenance of a safe environment for the patient involved complete dependence on the nursing staff. The patient was intubated and ventilated, therefore his safety would be helped by being cared for by nurses with a high level of knowledge and ability; by their continuous observation of him and his equipment; by their quick action when his stability altered; by their careful use of problem-solving skills; by minimizing the risk of infection using aseptic techniques and changing equipment regularly; and by early detection of the signs of infection and obtaining specimens for culture and sensitivities.

Communicating with the patient is essential to prevent sensory and perceptual deprivation, which Ashworth (1979) said contributed to hallucinations and perceptual disturbances. Worrell (1977) outlined seven factors to prevent sensory deprivation in patients who are intubated:

- organizing the work so that the patient has periods of rest;
- encouraging the patient to understand what is happening to him/her;
- involving the patient in his/her own care where possible;
- orientating the patient in time and place;
- explaining unfamiliar sounds to the patient;
- orientating the patient to their environment;
- minimizing sensory deprivation or overload.

The nurse can provide for the patient's needs in these areas. Worrell suggested using the five methods of communication outlined by Borsig and Steinacker (1982); speech, writing, symbols, skin contact and mime. The nurse must learn which method is most appropriate for the patient being nursed according to his/her abilities and preferences.

In this study Ledger considered a number of aspects of breathing as the patient was maintained on IPPV. For the nurse to understand intervention in breathing using such equipment, she must understand the effects of IPPV, which, according to Bushnell (1973), are threefold:

- a reduction in pulmonary blood flow is produced as the pulmonary capillaries are compressed;

- the negative intrathoracic pump is prevented – the action of the negative intrathoracic pump is normally to help venous return, therefore on IPPV the venous return is reduced;
- positive intrathoracic pressure acts like a cardiac tamponade, leading to increased atrial pressure, again reducing venous return to the heart.

This reduction in venous return during inspiration lowers the stroke volume of the heart which leads to a fall in blood pressure. As a result of this, according to Green (1977), sympathetic activity increases to produce vasoconstriction, in an attempt to raise the blood pressure; this produces a fall in peripheral temperature and urine output.

The nurse would frequently need to take and record the patient's blood pressure, apex rate and rhythm, central venous pressure and respiratory rate, and also temperature and urine measurements.

While being ventilated a patient will need muscle relaxants. This produces potential hazards for the patient if he/she is disconnected from the ventilator. Observation of the paralysed ventilated patient will need to take account of rate and pattern of respiration and the patient's colour, and also ensure that any respiratory effort by the patient is synchronized with the ventilator. Observations of the ventilator will need to include (Green, 1977, p. 39):

- the preset respiratory rate (and the patient's rate if different);
- inspired and expired minute volume;
- forced intake of oxygen (FIO_2);
- airways inflation pressure;
- use of the sign mechanisms;
- frequency of endotracheal tube suction.

Observation of the 'airways inflation pressure' is in case of serious complications. These could be where the inflation pressure is high or low. Where the pressure is high possible reasons are that the patient is breathing against the ventilator; that the tube is partially blocked by kinking or being bitten by the patient; that the tube is in the right main bronchus; that the cuff is over the end of the tube; that the lung has lost some of its functioning due to pulmonary oedema or pneumonia; or that there is increased resistance from the patient to the airflow due to bronchospasm, obstruction or a tension pneumothorax. Where the inflation pressure is low this could be due to an air leak in the ventilator or around the endotracheal tube; this would produce a serious risk for the patient of underventilation, inhalation of saliva or regurgitated gastric contents.

Where there is no synchrony between the ventilator and the patient's breathing, it may be supposed that the patient is either in pain or anxious, has hypoxia or hypercapnia, metabolic acidosis, or a pneumothorax.

Where the patient starts to breathe against the machine, the action by the nurse should be to talk to the patient, to detect why this has happened, to recommence the regular breathing pattern by hand ventilation for a short period; suction of the patient's endotracheal tube; to give intravenous sedation, and muscle relaxants if necessary; to check the patient's blood gases, and if necessary to ask the anaesthetist to reassess ventilation; and to look for signs of pneumothorax, and if these are positive obtain urgent medical help.

The function of the upper respiratory passages as an air filter, warmer and moistener are diminished during intubation. Therefore the nurse will need to institute a mechanical means of filtering and humidifying the air. The temperature the air is warmed to is important, as temperatures below 40°C may cause colonization of the water by *Pseudomonas aeruginosa*. However, the temperature of the water should not rise above 60°C as this may damage the patient's lung tissue. Further efforts to reduce infection involve changing the ventilator tubing every 24 hours.

Endotracheal suction is associated with a variety of hazards for the patient. First, damage to the respiratory mucous membrane and ciliated epithelium results from high negative suction which causes ulceration (Young, 1984a, b). These effects cause a reduction in the clearance of mucus, and the retained secretions act as a further potential source of infection. When suctioning a hypoxic patient the nurse should remove as little air from the lungs as possible with suction, using small catheters, and the maximum length of time suctioning should occur is 30 seconds. The patient being nursed in the study had thick secretions, so 2 ml sterile normal saline was introduced into the endotracheal tube before each suctioning. The patient and his relatives were also instructed about the procedure, and warned each time when it was about to be performed.

The patient could not be fed orally, therefore a fine-bore nasogastric tube was used; this is more comfortable for the patient than a larger bore tube, and is less likely to produce aspiration of gastric contents. The amount of feed and liquid was 2500 calories in 2000 ml fluid in 24 hours. Bowel sounds were checked every 4 hours to ensure functioning.

Urine measurements were taken hourly; renal functioning was good as the patient's urine output was over 30 ml/hour. Catheter care was given every 6 hours, reducing the risk of ascending urinary tract infection. Bowel functioning was not mentioned in the article.

Control of body temperature was dependent on the environment and the amount of clothing worn. Fanning was needed initially to reduce the patient's pyrexia.

Mobility was dependent on nursing care. Risk of pressure damage was high. Torrance (1981) outlined eight predisposing factors to pressure sores: pyrexia, moist skin, anaemia, poor nutrition, reduced mobility, vascular problems, neurological problems and friction. The Norton scale

(Norton, McLaren and Exton-Smith, 1975) was used to assess the patient's risk of developing pressure damage; this necessitated that he was turned every 2 hours and that care consistent with overcoming Torrance's factors was given. Equipment to relieve pressure was also used.

Working and playing were encouraged through watching television and listening to the radio. The study stated that he enjoyed this activity. No indication was given of the effect on his occupation of his current hospitalization.

Expressing sexuality is taken in the study to be direct sexual activity: 'The patient had limited opportunity for this whilst on ICU; he sometimes held Mrs Carter's hand' (p. 41).

The work in the ICU was arranged so the patient had maximum periods of rest day and night. Night sedation was given only whilst he was being ventilated in order to prevent the risk of depressing the respiratory centre. Repetitive noise was kept to a minimum, as EEG changes within 30 min have been shown when a patient is subjected to these noises every second (Liberson, 1960).

Dying was not indicated by the patient until after extubation, when he said he realized how ill he had been. He asked to see a priest which was arranged. No reference is made in the article that this was something discussed with his wife, or that support for her was provided in this area.

This study not only shows a good knowledge base, but also demonstrates the role of the nurse in an ICU using Roper, Logan and Tierney's model to show nursing intervention; however, the comforting aspect of nursing does not seem to be very much in evidence. Perhaps it is more the relatives who are in need of this while the person they love is in the ICU, but the model does not allow for comforting to be included at any stage in problem solving.

The use and acceptability of the model in such a situation is well demonstrated by Ledger's study, but as with nearly every other study in this chapter it has not demonstrated testing of the model.

CONCLUSIONS

Three studies were found which dealt predominantly with the implementation of nursing care using the Roper, Logan and Tierney model. Although each included a good literature search of the area, none of them demonstrated testing of implementation using the model. The model was also not problematized in any of the studies, so comment on its usefulness in helping to implement nursing care was not given. However, that these studies were from a variety of settings shows the acceptability of the model in the UK at the time that the studies were published. It also shows the acceptability of the model to a UK audience at that time.

It is interesting to note that no studies were found which developed the evaluation stage of the nursing process, nor which considered the link between implementation of nursing care and its evaluation. Therefore the effectiveness of nursing care using the Roper, Logan and Tierney model is still speculative. That studies of evaluation or of implementation to evaluation have not been found may reflect the weakness of the evaluation section in the main texts by Roper, Logan and Tierney. This has also been pointed out by Wilson-Barnett (1981) and Hunt (1983).

OVERALL CONCLUSIONS

Although the Roper, Logan and Tierney model of nursing has been used in many settings in Great Britain, as shown in the literature, there has been only one study that has systematically studied an aspect of the model in practice (Allan, 1987). This study shows how patients with multiple sclerosis can be assessed for independence/dependence using a 7-point scale. It also shows the development of an assessment tool for this purpose. The other studies in this chapter show a good level of literature review and the use of this literature within the model. However, these studies are more like nursing care studies, which do not problematize the model, therefore giving the reader little indication of the effectiveness of the model with the patients that were cared for.

A further aspect of the studies in this chapter is that they did not link any of the aspects of the nursing process in order to test for cause and effect. So, for example, the link between assessment and planning has not been tested using this model, nor has the link between planning and implementation of nursing care. Therefore, we do not have any idea if the model is appropriate for nursing care, or what problems it causes.

Furthermore, there is some evidence from the literature (for example Parr, 1993) that Roper, Logan and Tierney's model is being seen as rather too simplistic for trained nurses. Parr shows how he is trying out alternative, American-generated, models and comparing them with Roper, Logan and Tierney, to the detriment of the latter model. Coupled with this is the indication from the literature that no new studies have been published since 1990 using the Roper, Logan and Tierney model in practice. These two factors could show the decline of this model's popularity. There is also little evidence from the literature that Roper, Logan and Tierney's model has been used in settings outside the UK.

REFERENCES

Aggleton, P. and Chalmers, H. (1986a) *Nursing Models and the Nursing Process*, Macmillan Education, Basingstoke, pp. 27–36.

Aggleton, P. and Chalmers, H. (1986b) Nursing research, nursing theory and the nursing process. *Journal of Advanced Nursing*, **11**, 197–202.

Allan, S. (1987) Arms extended. *Nursing Times*, **83**(43), 44–5.

Ashworth, P. (1979) Sensory deprivation – the acutely ill. *Nursing Times*, **75**(6), 290–4.

Bagnall, P. and Heslop, A. (1987) Chronic respiratory disease: educating patients at home. *The Professional Nurse*, June, 293–6.

Bain, J. (1985) Communication breakdown. *Nursing Mirror*, **161**(17), 42–6.

Borsig, A. and Steinacker, I. (1982) Communication with the patient in the Intensive Care Unit. *Nursing Times, Supplement*, **78**(12), 1–11.

Brezinova, V. and Oswald, I. (1972) Sleep after a bedtime beverage. *British Medical Journal*, **2**, 431–3.

Bushnell, S.S. (1973) *Respiratory Intensive Care Nursing*, Little Brown, Boston, pp. 112–13.

Cockcroft, A., Bagnall, P., Heslop, A. *et al.* (1987) Controlled trial of respiratory health workers visiting patients with chronic respiratory disability. *British Medical Journal*, **294**, 225–8.

Collins, B.J. (1981) Infection and the hospital environment. *Nursing* **1** (Suppl.) (9), 1–3.

Elliott, R. and Mackay, D.N. (1971) Social competence of subnormal and normal children living under different types of residential care. *British Journal of Mental Subnormality*, **17**, 48–53.

Ford, S. (1987) Into the outside. *Nursing Times*, **83**(20), 40–2.

Green, J.H. (1977) *An Introduction to Human Physiology*, 4th edn, Oxford Medical Publications, Oxford.

Harrison, A. (1986) Compression fractures of the thoracic vertebrae. *Nursing Times*, June 25, 40–2.

Henderson, V. and Nite, G. (1978) *Principles and Practice of Nursing*, Macmillan, New York.

Heslop, A.P. and Bagnall, P. (1988) A study to evaluate the intervention of a nurse visiting patients with disabling chest disease in the community. *Journal of Advanced Nursing*, **13**, 71–7.

Hobson, J.A (1968) Sleep after exercise. *Science*, **162**, 1503–5.

Hoffman, P.N. (1982) *Transient Contamination on Hands*, in *ICNA Thirteenth Annual Symposium Papers* (ed. D.J. Cheesbrough), ICNA Publications, pp. 29–30.

Hunt, J. (1983) Book reviews. *Journal of Advanced Nursing*, **8**, 550–1.

Janes, G. (1986) Planning for terminal care. *Nursing Times*, April 23, 24–7.

Karacan, I., Thornby, J.I., Anch, M. *et al.* (1976) Dose-related sleep disturbances induced by coffee and caffeine. *Clinical Pharmacology and Therapeutics*, **20**, 682–9.

Kershaw, B. and Salvage, J. (1986) *Models for Nursing*, John Wiley, Chichester.

Ledger, S.D. (1986) Management of a patient in respiratory failure due to chronic bronchitis. *Intensive Care Nursing*, **2**, 30–43.

Liberson, W.T. (1960) Electroencephalography. *American Journal of Psychiatry*, 116–584.

Lister, P. (1987) The misunderstood model. *Nursing Times*, **83**(41), 40–2.

Lowbury, E.J. *et al.* (1975) *Control of Hospital Infection – A Practical Handbook*, Chapman and Hall, London.

Mitchell, J.R.A. (1984) Is nursing any business of doctors? A simple guide to the "nursing process". *British Medical Journal*, **288**, 216–19.

Norton, D., McLaren, R. and Exton-Smith, A. (1975) *An Investigation of Geriatric Nursing Problems in Hospital*, Churchill Livingstone, Edinburgh.

Open University (1984) *A Systematic Approach to Nursing Care.* Module 1.

Palmer, C.D., Harrison, G.A. and Horns, R.W. (1980) Association between smoking and drinking and sleep duration. *Annals of Human Biology*, **7**, 103–7.

Parr, M.S. (1993) The Neuman Health Care Systems Model: an evaluation. *British Journal of Theatre Nursing*, **3**(8), 20–7.

Roper, N., Logan, W.W. and Tierney, A.J. (1980) *The Elements of Nursing*, Churchill Livingstone, Edinburgh.

Roper, N., Logan, W.W. and Tierney, A.J. (1982) *Learning to Use the Process of Nursing*, Churchill Livingstone, Edinburgh.

Roper, N., Logan, W.W. and Tierney, A.J. (1983a) *Using a Model for Nursing*, Churchill Livingstone, Edinburgh.

Roper, N., Logan, W.W. and Tierney, A.J. (1983b) A Nursing Model. *Nursing Mirror*, 25th May, 17–19.

Roper, N., Logan, W.W. and Tierney, A.J. (1983c) Is there a danger of 'processing' patients? *Nursing Mirror*, 1st June, 32–3.

Roper, N., Logan, W.W. and Tierney, A.J. (1983d) Problems or needs? *Nursing Mirror*, 8th June, 43–4.

Roper, N., Logan, W.W. and Tierney, A.J. (1983e) Identifying goals. *Nursing Mirror*, 15th June, 22–3.

Roper, N., Logan, W.W. and Tierney, A.J. (1983f) Endless paperwork? *Nursing Mirror*, 22nd June, 34–5.

Roper, N., Logan, W.W. and Tierney, A.J. (1983g) - with diversity. *Nursing Mirror*, 29th June, 35.

Roper, N., Logan, W.W. and Tierney, A.J. (1985) *The Elements of Nursing*, 2nd edn, Churchill Livingstone, Edinburgh.

Roper, N., Logan, W.W. and Tierney, A.J. (1990) *The Elements of Nursing*, 3rd edn, Churchill Livingstone, Edinburgh.

Tierney, A. (1984) A response to Professor Mitchell's "Simple guide to the nursing process." *British Medical Journal*, **288**, 835–8.

Torrance, C. (1981) Pressure sore predisposing factors: the 'at risk' patient. *Nursing Times*, **77**(8), 5–8.

Webster, O. and Bowell, B. (1986) Thinking infection. *Nursing Times*, June 4, 68, 70, 74.

Webster, R.A. (1986) Sleep in hospital. *Journal of Advanced Nursing*, **11**, 447–57.

Williams, D.L., McLean, A.W. and Cairns, J. (1983) Dose response effects of ethanol on the sleep of young women. *Journal of Studies on Alcohol*, **44**, 515–23.

Wilson-Barnett, J. (1981) Book review. *Journal of Advanced Nursing*, **6**, 249.

Worrell, J.N. (1977) Nursing implications in the care of the patient experiencing sensory deprivation, in *Advanced Concepts in Clinical Nursing* (ed. K.C. Kintzel), J.B. Lippincott, Philadelphia, 618–38.

Young, C. (1984a) A review of the adverse effects of airway suction. *Physiotherapy*, **70**(3), 104–6.

Young, C. (1984b) Recommended guidelines for suction. *Physiotherapy*, **70**(3), 106–8.

FURTHER READING

Aggleton, P. and Chalmers, H. (1986) *Nursing Models and the Nursing Process*, Macmillan, London.
Chapman, C.M. (1985) *Theory of Nursing: Practical Application*, Harper and Row, London.
Kershaw, B. and Salvage, J. (1986) *Models for Nursing*, John Wiley, Chichester.

Roy's model of adaptation

3

Topic researched	Model components	Results
3. Outcomes for the baby	Focal and contextual stimuli	Improvement for baby when birth is vertical
Care of long-term diabetic patients	Evaluation of nursing intervention	Outcome for patients shown
Comparing women's functional abilities after Caesarean or vaginal delivery	Assessment of physical energy	Physical energy regained quicker in vaginally delivered women
Comparing physical energy following childbirth	Longitudinal assessment at 3 weeks to 6 months	Increased physical energy from 3 weeks to 3 months
Mothers' views of breastfeeding in a neonatal intensive care unit	Assessment of mothers' views in all 4 modes	Many problems for mother and father described in all 4 modes
The functional status of fathers	Primary, secondary and tertiary role activities	Development and testing of assessment tool
Giving information to Caesarean birth mothers	Four adaptation modes	Contradictory findings between the control and the experimental group

THE AUTHOR

Callista Roy is a member of the Sisters of St Joseph of Carondelet. She was born in 1939 in Los Angeles, California. She obtained a BA in Nursing in 1963 from Mount St Mary's College, Los Angeles and a Master of Science in Nursing from the University of California in 1966. Her PhD was in Sociology from the University of California in 1977.

She began to develop her concepts of nursing while studying for her Master's degree.

From 1968 to 1982 she was Associate Professor in the Department of Nursing, Mount St Mary's College, Los Angeles. Between 1983 and 1985 she was the Robert Wood Post-Doctoral Fellow at the University of California, San Francisco.

She appears in the *World Who's Who of Women, Personalities of Americas*.

THE MODEL

The Roy adaptation model was conceived by Sister Callista Roy in 1964, and has been developed, mainly as a basis for a curriculum for students of nursing, since 1968. Roy has published two volumes of her model (Roy,

1976, 1984) in which she describes the components of nursing using her framework. These have been further developed in a joint publication with Andrews (Andrews and Roy, 1986). Another joint publication with Roberts (Roy and Roberts, 1981) explores the construction of the model and its use.

Less well-developed texts have shown the model in its initial stages of development (Roy, 1970, 1971), and a jointly edited book with Joan Riehl briefly describes and analyses a wide variety of models of nursing by American authors (Riehl and Roy, 1977, 1980). A text by Randall, Tedrow and VanLandingham (1982) shows the application of the Roy model in a number of practice settings.

The Roy adaptation model is now described, followed by the practice-based research which has resulted from this model.

SUMMARY OF THE ROY ADAPTATION MODEL

Roy (1976) sees her model as having three elements: the recipient of nursing care, the goal of nursing, and nursing activities. The recipient of nursing care she describes as 'a biosocial being in constant interaction with a changing environment' (p. 11). In this constantly changing environment people cope through innate and acquired biological, psychological and social mechanisms. An example she gives of innate biological mechanisms is blood clotting following injury; an example of an acquired mechanism is learning.

This positive response to the changing environment Roy calls adaptation. She uses Helson's (1964) work to describe this process. He calls the ability of the person to adapt in the face of change the individual's 'adaptation level'. The adaptation level results from three stimuli: the focal stimulus, that immediately confronting the individual; the contextual stimuli, all the other stimuli present and relevant to the individual at the time; and the residual stimuli, the factors the individual brings to the situation such as attitudes, beliefs, experiences, traits, etc.

An individual's adaptive response has the function of maintaining the person's integrity, while a maladaptive response disrupts integrity.

Roy identifies two major adaptive mechanisms: the regulator, which works through the autonomic nervous system; and the cognator, which is the level of recognition and understanding of the situation.

Roy sees humans as adapting in four ways:

- **physiological**: exercise and rest; nutrition; elimination; fluid and electrolytes; oxygen; circulation; temperature regulation; the senses and the endocrine system;
- **self-concept**, divided into two aspects – the personal self, consisting of the moral–ethical self, self-consistency, self-ideal and self-esteem, and the physical self;

- **role function;**
- **interdependence.**

The role function and interdependence modes are related to the need for social integrity. All the modes are seen as interrelated, therefore change will create the need for adaptation in more than one mode.

Internal or external environmental changes create a need that results in the individual making an internal and/or external response; this is seen in behaviour and is activated in order to reduce the need.

The goal of nursing is to promote or sustain adaptation in each of the modes; this is where needs have resulted from situations which create deficits or excesses in the individual.

The way the nurse works is through the nursing process. This approach, using Roy's model, has six stages. The first stage is first level assessment in the four modes and involves the nurse observing the patient's behaviours and questioning the patient in order to measure the internal and external responses of the patient to change. This stage ends when a judgement is made of whether the individual's behaviour is adaptive or maladaptive and will depend on whether the behaviour promotes integrity. The second stage involves assessment of focal, contextual and residual stimuli where the behaviour is maladaptive or needing reinforcement. The four further stages of the nursing process involve the diagnosis of adaptation problems, which involve criteria for setting priorities; establishing goals for removal of the focal stimulus, or changing the contextual or residual stimuli; intervention, where the nurse manipulates the stimuli by removing, increasing or decreasing them; and evaluation of the effectiveness of the intervention by enabling the patient to adapt.

Roy recognizes that much of the knowledge needed to use this model effectively is not known as yet, and that whereas normal states are known in some areas of the biological mode, in the self-concept, role function and interdependence modes knowledge is sketchy or absent at present.

In Riehl and Roy (1980) the model remains essentially unchanged. The adaptive modes are enlarged. The physiological mode remains the same as in Roy (1976), but the self-concept mode now includes the physical self, the personal self and the interpersonal self. The role mastery mode now has two categories: role function and role conflict; and the interdependence mode contains a similar list of examples as seen in Roy (1976).

In the second edition of her model (Roy, 1984) there is again essentially no change, but there is fuller development than in the first edition. One development is the adaptive mechanisms of the regulator and the cognator. The regulator is defined as (p. 31): '...[receiving] input from the external environment and from changes in the person's internal state. It then processes the changes through neural–chemical–endocrine channels to produce responses.' These changes and responses are then more clearly outlined. The cognator is also developed and enlarged (p. 33):

> The internal and external stimuli trigger off four kinds of processes: perceptual/information processing, learning, judgement, and emotion. Under perceptual/information processing, we may consider the person's internal activity of selective attention, coding, and memory. Learning involves such processes as imitation, reinforcement, and insight. The judgement process includes problem-solving and decision-making. Through the emotional pathways, the person uses defenses to seek relief and effective appraisal and attachment.

Other amendments to the 1984 edition of her model are in the adaptive modes. The physiological mode has been reduced to five categories which are oxygenation, nutrition, elimination, activity and rest, and skin integrity. The self-concept mode is reduced to two modes, physical self and personal self; the role function and interdependence modes remain essentially unchanged.

Despite the considerable amount of written work and development of the model, the research in practice settings using this framework has been slow, particularly when one considers that the model has been in existence for well over a decade. I also found that unpublished higher degree work was sparse. However, at least one study was found in each of the areas of identification of patients' problems of adaptation, planning, nursing intervention and evaluation; but unfortunately none have been conducted outside North America. The main text referred to by the researchers is Roy (1976).

The sequence of this chapter is the same as for all chapters in this book – the sections follow the format of identification, planning, intervention and evaluation.

IDENTIFICATION OF PATIENTS' PROBLEMS OF ADAPTATION

There are five studies in this section: adaptation problems in the elderly; the needs of patients with arterial occlusion before vascular surgery; problems of patients with right hemispheric lesions; the mechanics and manifestations of a raised temperature; and the needs of Caesarean birth parents. It is interesting to note that four out of the five studies investigate long-term problems of either adaptation to chronic disease or of old age.

Although these studies investigate very different problems associated with illness or ageing, the method of investigating them is predominantly through the use of questionnaires. In some cases these have been designed by the researcher, in others a rather more *ad hoc* approach is taken.

ADAPTATION PROBLEMS IN ELDERLY PEOPLE

A single paper analyses the perceived problems of the elderly and their significant others, describing the factors that influence the elderly, or those close to them, in deciding to apply for permanent residence for the elderly person to live in a nursing home.

Farkas (1981) studied a group of 22 elderly people of both sexes, over the age of 75, who were living at home, and had applied for admission to a nursing home. She compared these with a control group of 22 elderly people who were matched for sex and as closely as possible for address. The control group were of a similar age and ethnic background but had not made an application to a nursing home. The main differences between the experimental and the control groups were that 41% of the experimental group were living on their own, compared with 55% of the control group, and 73% of the experimental group had children living nearby, compared with 55% of the control group.

Farkas' research question was three-fold:

- How can an adaptation framework help us to understand the problems faced by this group of people?
- What adaptation problems are there which make the difference between the two groups of elderly people?
- What are the problems encountered by either the elderly person or the significant other which make for the application to a nursing home?

These research questions assessed particular factors in the situation of the elderly person or the significant other which led to an application to a nursing home. These factors were:

- overall adaptation problems – this could be related to all four modes in Roy's model;
- a sense of powerlessness – Roy's 'self-concept' mode;
- role reversal by either the elderly person or the significant other or both – Roy's 'role function' mode;
- a sense of guilt by either party – Roy's 'self-concept' mode;
- the level of knowledge and use of services provided in the home of the elderly person – Roy's 'interdependence' mode.

Two structured questionnaires were used to interview all members of the two groups and their significant others. A chi-squared test was used for analysis of the data. However, no mention was made of testing the questionnaires for validity with this group.

The results relate to the factors in the situation of the elderly person or their significant others.

1. Overall adaptation problems. Farkas found that the number of physiological problems encountered by the elderly was not

significantly different between the two groups, but the perception of these problems was greater in those making an application to a nursing home. This showed that their physiological problems caused them to have greater loss of self-esteem and a greater dependence on others than those not seeking residence in a nursing home. Only one of the physiological items was statistically different between the two groups; this was checking things over and over again. In relation to Roy's model, this finding shows validity for her assumption that the modes are interrelated, so that a problem in one mode will have an effect on the need to adapt in the other modes.

When the difference between the total number in the study (440) and those in the experimental group was analysed, statistical differences were found in a number of areas: sight, hearing, getting up at night, incontinence of urine, difficulty in using stairs and forgetfulness; also in the experimental group bereavement was more often of a spouse or relative, whereas in the control group bereavement was more often of a friend. A further significant difference between the total sample and the experimental group was that the latter worried more about their health, had more ritualistic behaviours, and preferred things to be done for them. However, assessment of physiological difficulties from an interview questionnaire would seem a somewhat dubious method of obtaining this type of information.

Analysing the responses from the significant others showed that they perceived the same level of difficulty that was felt by the elderly person. This would help to verify the extent of physiological problems, provided there was good communication between both parties about the exact nature of the problems. Significant differences in the perception by the significant others of the waiting list elderly compared to the control group showed that incontinence of urine, frequency of falling, difficulty in managing stairs and the elderly person doing more or less than expected were the main areas of difficulty. These results show the difference between their perceptions of the elderly person's problems and those of the elderly people themselves.

2. A sense of powerlessness. This was tested by asking the elderly people in both groups how much say they felt they had in the decision to apply for residence in a nursing home. The difference between the answers each group gave was not statistically different. Therefore a sense of powerlessness was not felt significantly more by those applying for residence in a nursing home.

3. Role reversal by either party. Farkas measured this in three ways: first, whether the significant other felt more like a parent than a child or a friend; second, whether the elderly person was dependent on the significant other; and third, whether the significant other felt it necessary to know where the elderly person was. One statistically signifi-

cant difference was found: when the significant other felt more like a parent than a child. A difference in this factor led more often to the significant other making an application for the elderly person to live in a nursing home. The other two indicators were not significant but results were in the predicted direction.

4. A sense of guilt. Initiation of application for residence in a nursing home had most frequently come from a doctor, with the significant other agreeing. This meant that guilt was not felt by the significant other.

5. Knowledge and use of services. Farkas expected that those with less knowledge of services would not only use them less, but would be more likely to make an application for residence in a nursing home. She tested for knowledge of 10 specific services. The reverse was found to be the case – the experimental group had more knowledge of services and were also making more use of them than the control group.

The most significant factors from the elderly person's perspective in an application to a nursing home was their perception of their level of disability and reliance on others. Farkas reports that they had a sense of being unable to control their own level of ability, but felt able to control what happened to them. However, from the perspective of the significant others the extent of the role reversal (daughters feeling more like mothers to the parent, and finding it necessary to adopt a nurturing role) was the most significant factor associated with the significant other making a nursing home application.

If these findings hold true for Britain, nurses will be paying great attention to the interaction between the elderly person and their significant other, where a significant other exists and visits frequently.

This study set out to test the validity of Roy's model in such a setting. The findings are shown to support the model in being able to identify changes that have occurred in the lives of the elderly living at home. These changes are seen to have created maladaptive states that their own resources and those of their significant others are unable to meet. First and second level assessments found maladaptation in all four modes of adaptation which shows the validity of these modes in assessment of the elderly living at home. As mentioned above, it also shows that the claim by Roy that her model as a systems model is valid, as changes for these elderly people in one mode have also created problems of adaptation in other modes.

So, in testing Roy's model, the study used a cause and effect design by showing the factors that caused maladaptation in the elderly and their significant others which was sufficient to lead them to make an application to live in a nursing home. However, the article is not specific in the nature of the questions asked, nor whether all aspects of each of the modes were covered. Therefore assumptions about the adequacy of every aspect of the model for these people in this situation will need to be tempered with caution.

THE PRE-OPERATIVE NEEDS OF PATIENTS WITH ARTERIAL OCCLUSION

The chronic nature of this disability means that adaptation problems of patients are going to be long term and sometimes radical. There will be a strong emphasis on inability of the condition and its consequences to be reversed, and admission to hospital for surgery may precipitate the patients' continued and worst fears for their well-being. The process and outcome of previous surgery will also be an important factor in the patients' optimism.

Leech (1982) studied a sample of 60 patients (40 men and 20 women) with arterial occlusive disease from four hospitals in Canada. She addressed the question of what needs these patients had during the pre-operative period, and specified four questions.

- What physiological, psychological and sociocultural needs do patients with the disease experience pre-operatively?
- Are there differences in the level of satisfaction between male and female patients' body image?
- Are there differences between (a) male and female, and (b) older and younger patients?
- How are the patient's needs, or the needs as identified by the researcher, associated with the patient's (a) body image, (b) perceived severity of illness, (c) physiological severity of disease, (d) adaptation, (e) previous vascular surgery and (f) type of surgical procedure?

The data were obtained from three sources.

- A 48-item structured interview schedule of mainly closed questions, based on a review of relevant literature, the conceptual framework of adaptation to chronic illness, and the clinical experience of the researcher. It explored any potential imbalance between physiological, psychological and sociocultural domains, and the patient's level of adaptation and perception of the severity of the disease. Leech states that the data were collected when her instrument was at the first stages of design, therefore no tests of validity or reliability were conducted. She pretested with 10 subjects and found that no revisions were necessary, so face validity did not appear to be a problem.
- Secord and Jourard's (1953) body cathexis questionnaire, where answers are ranked by the subject on a 5-point scale of satisfaction/ dissatisfaction with parts and functions of their body.
- The patients' personal details were collected: age; other diseases; length of time of vascular disease; previous vascular surgery; severity

of the disease according to an aortogram; and the type of surgery to be undergone on the current admission.

The paper gives a detailed summary of the method, without being unduly lengthy.

As the sample studied was a convenience sample collected over a 4-month period, the patients' personal details were analysed. The patients had a mean age of 61.5 years and were from the lower socio-economic classes. Their disease patterns showed that they also suffered from an average of 2.2 other diseases, and were not working at the time of the study due to arterial disease; they had all experienced symptoms for more than a year, such as difficulty with bending and climbing stairs, and they could only walk a few metres; and their level of disease was moderately severe according to aortogram results. Approximately half of the sample had previously undergone some kind of vascular surgery.

The results from the questionnaire in the physiological mode showed that all patients had a history of smoking; 85% considered that cutting down or stopping smoking was important, but this was due to their fear of lung cancer rather than vascular disease; 26% had stopped smoking. More than 80% of the sample did not see the benefits of altering their diets or of regular foot care in relation to vascular disease, and had not adopted any of the suggested practices. Twenty per cent were taking large amounts of analgesics at home without realising the side effects. Patients also stated that they had been inadequately prepared for the discomfort of an aortogram.

In the physiological and social modes 83% of patients showed difficulty in coming to terms with the changes that resulted from the disease; they spoke at length of feelings of frustration, uselessness and depression with their situation and their perceived inability to cope with it. All the patients saw a need to have a sense of control over their future; this may have been linked to their anxiety over the effects of surgery on the progress of their disease. Patients were not anxious about their hospital admission *per se*, and 70% indicated that pre-operative information would be helpful; 83% indicated that a positive and friendly atmosphere would help them; and 28% expressed loneliness due to separation from their families.

Analysis of the questionnaire revealed the needs identified by the patients. The need for active emotional support by the nurses was identified; a higher proportion of men felt the need for this type of support than women, which Leech found surprising. There was also the need for fostering a sense of control; helping to reduce the patients' level of anxiety; and enhancing family support. The patients also expressed the need for support with perceived changes in their self-concept and their role relationships, support with the effects of surgery on their prognosis, and general pre-operative information.

The unexpected finding that more of the male patients wanted emotional support than the female patients, Leech says, shows the need for a detailed nursing assessment. She believes this will test the nurses' abilities to pick up cues and know how to ask appropriate and non-threatening questions, as this need may not be openly expressed.

Analysis of the body image questionnaire showed a significant difference between men and women, women having a significantly greater level of dissatisfaction with their body structure and function. They felt the disease not only affected themselves but their life in general. However, men were three times more likely than women to have financial worries because of loss of income; men also tended to express concerns relating to work and the ability to drive. Leech also found differences between older (over 65 years) and younger patients (under 65 years). Older patients saw less need to follow a special diet, showed less awareness of the relationship between smoking and circulatory disease, saw general nursing support as more helpful, and wanted less pre-operative information with less detail.

When correlating all factors together it was found that patients with the most severe disease did have the perception of their disease as severe, had low levels of adaptation, and had negative perceptions about changes to their self-concept and role relationships. It can be assumed from this that patients' ability to adapt becomes increasingly poor as the disease progresses. Possibly those who have made greatest and more satisfactory adaptations in the early stages of the disease will be more easily able to continue to adapt as the disease progresses.

Leech also found that with increasing perceptions of the severity of the illness came increased perception for the need for a special diet, and also the greatest likelihood of financial insecurity. It may be that for these patients the reality of finance to buy a special diet on a small income will mean increasing frustration and powerlessness.

Leech says that these findings show clearly that giving patients instruction in relation to preventive health practices is of little use, as patients indicate their wish to have control over their lives. However, she says the lack of understanding by patients of the relationship between their lifestyle and their disease process should be the subject of nursing intervention. If nurses were able to inform patients of this relationship in a manner acceptable to the patients, it would give them a basis on which to make informed decisions, which must then be respected by the health professionals. She also states that the patients in her study did not have a realistic expectation of their prognosis, or the effects of surgery on it, and that they felt a need to be able to examine this realistically in the presence of active emotional support.

This study showed clearly the changes that occurred to patients with progressive arterial occlusion. These changes can be seen as both internal, related to both their physiological and their self-concept mode, and also external as related to their role function and interdependence modes. The external changes are seen as those in their relationships with their families, their abilities to provide for their families, and their increased reliance on others to provide for them. Therefore the first level nursing assessment has shown that adaptations these patients face are considerable and are linked with each other.

In this paper the patients' needs were noted in relation to their forthcoming surgery and their prognosis. Using this level of knowledge about these patients' expressed needs provides some evidence of validity for Roy's model.

Roy's second level of assessment does not appear to be so comprehensive in this paper, as little mention is made of the adaptations these patients have already made. However, one is left with the impression that many of their resources to aid adaptation have already been used up during the progress of the disease.

The research method in this study is well described, so the findings can be assessed in the light of the method. Despite the fact that the questionnaires used closed questions, Leech evidently spent much time with the patients during the study, talking with them about worries relating to their disease. It is to her credit that she included these findings in the study, and noted them in the analysis. As well as being a very humane approach this adds to the validity of the questionnaire. However, Leech admits that the validity and reliability of the questionnaire are not yet fully tested. This study does not set out to test for cause and effect; it is a descriptive study. Despite this, Leech is able to give some advice to nurses on the types of care these patients need in order to meet their problems of adaptation.

PROBLEMS OF THE PATIENT WITH A LESION OF THE RIGHT HEMISPHERE

The paper discussed in this section claims that little research to that date has been conducted to show the kinds of behavioural changes occurring in patients following a right hemispheric lesion. As there was a movement at the time in America towards the development of nursing diagnoses, this paper can be seen as a contribution to this movement, as well as to the development of Roy's model.

Norman (1979) reviewed the literature and conducted a small clinical study (four patients) to assess the types of behavioural changes found in patients with a right hemispheric lesion. Although the sample size was small, it is to the credit of the researcher that she did not merely conduct a literature review, but also tested the findings with a group of patients.

She found that the behavioural changes described in the literature were grouped under four headings:

1. visual–spatial misperception;
2. body scheme disturbances;
3. impaired cognitive processes;
4. alterations in the levels of emotions.

Norman then made a patient assessment of the signs and symptoms related to each of these headings, using an interview questionnaire on four patients each of whom had a lesion of the right hemisphere confirmed by computerized tomography, and who had been discharged from acute care at least 6 months previously. She also interviewed the patients' families.

It is unclear at this point whether the researcher intended to elicit the perceptions of the patients to their behavioural changes, or whether she was aiming at a more behavioural assessment, or combining the two. It can only be assumed that by obtaining information by interview from the patients and their relatives, she aimed to compare the perceptions of these groups.

The findings from the literature under the four headings mentioned above are then expanded.

The visual-spatial group contained the following consequences of right hemispheric lesion:

*   loss of vision in the left visual field of each eye (left homonymous hemianopsia);
*   inability to recognize an object or 'mind blindness' (visual agnosia);
*   ability to recognize only part of a complex visual stimulus, not the whole of it (simultaenagnosia);
*   inability to recognize people's faces, or in extreme cases one's own in a mirror (prosopagnosia);
*   inability to perceive or carry out activities requiring a three-dimensional relationship (constructional apraxia);
*   visual distortion of objects where judgement of distance, speed of movement and relationship between objects are concerned; spatial perception is also a problem, for example being unable to distinguish up from down, inside from outside, left from right (metamorphopsia) – difficulties associated with metamorphopsia, Norman says, will cause particular problems for the patient and their carer(s) with dressing, reading and writing, and mobility.

When patients with a right hemispheric lesion were interviewed by Norman, they had a varying level of acceptance of their disability. One patient appeared unaware of her level of difficulty; another described the problems clearly and her coping strategy when she was put in a situation where she was likely to incur harm.

The literature also identified body scheme disturbances, i.e. patients had difficulty in distinguishing self from non-self (agnosia). The body image may be distorted so that a patient becomes unaware of particular parts of his or her body, and may neglect these parts, or feel they do not exist. This results in the position of the ignored part not being considered by the patient, who rarely compensates for the deficit and tends to deny any problem.

Norman says this tendency to denial may be explicit or implicit. Where explicit denial occurs, this may be complete denial of any form of physical difficulty, or denial of the most significant feature of the disability. With this lack of adaptation the patient tends to concentrate on some minor aspect of the illness, but denies any major difficulty; or patients attribute their difficulties to some other cause, for example saying that they can move their arm but they do not want to at that moment. Other strategies involving explicit denial are projection by patients of their disability, for example saying that their limb does not belong to them; or displacement of the disability in time, for example saying that they did have a disability, but are now recovered.

It is unclear whether Norman found any of these signs of body schema disturbances in the four patients she interviewed; she certainly makes no mention of these types of statements made by the patients in her sample, nor by their relatives.

The literature further identifies impaired cognitive processes as a problem. Patients with right hemispheric lesions were found to have the following types of behaviours:

- trial and error does not produce learning;
- patients are impulsive and attempt tasks beyond their capabilities;
- patients have a short attention span and are easily distracted from the task in hand;
- there is poor insight, noticeable in situations of danger; patients have difficulty with abstract thought and integration of facts which may be associated with visual impairment;
- patients have decreased reasoning in a creative or intuitive sense.

Norman again does not appear to have gained information about impaired cognitive processes from the interviews she conducted with patients or their relatives to support the literature.

Another aspect identified from the literature was alteration in the levels of emotions. This was found to be the least well defined in the literature. Norman says this important aspect of the patient's life is shown by lack of concern for the usual social norms, which poses one of the most difficult problems for nurses and a distressing problem for families when the patient is discharged from the acute care setting. An indication of the patient's personality and the coping behaviours before the lesion occurred may not mean that the patient will necessarily use these in recovery from illness, because adaptive processes may become disorganized as a result of the lesion.

Norman uses the information from her interviews with patients' relatives to show the distressing impact on the family of these changes in levels of emotions:

> one patient's husband stated 'she takes her teeth out at the most inappropriate times and when I ask her to put her teeth back in her mouth, she says that she didn't take them out'.

(p. 2130)

This paper shows the changes that occur in the acquired mechanisms, such as learning, in patients suffering from a right hemispheric lesion. It is also clear that external changes are created for patients with this condition. What is unclear is the internal changes, apart from the evident physiological change of the lesion itself. It is therefore left to the nurse to judge the appropriateness of the patient's adaptive mechanisms, using the cognator, by observation of their behaviour, and therefore to diagnose adaptation or maladaptation mainly on this basis. Assessment of the adaptive mechanism using the regulator would seem to be easier, as Norman shows the literature to refer to frequent emotional changes with this group of patients.

A further difficulty for the nurse is to make an assessment of the focal and contextual stimuli for these patients, as Norman has shown that there is frequent denial. Also Norman says that their coping behaviours may become disorganized following this condition, so assessing the residual stimuli will not be reliable if based on the patient's previous coping behaviours.

This article shows that some of Roy's adaptive modes are valid for these patients. Surprisingly, however, no note is made of physiological changes occurring in these patients, although this must be one of the main effects of the condition. Also, assessment of the self-concept and interdependence modes is not shown as a strong feature of the literature review conducted for this article. The sample chosen by Norman appeared to be aimed more towards confirming the findings from the literature than towards testing Roy's model, therefore the appropriateness of Roy's modes of self-concept and interdependence for patients suffering from a right hemispheric lesion has not been shown by this article. The design of the study was exploratory, maybe leading to a larger study later, but was at the level of description, as no attempt was made to show cause and effect using the model as a guide.

For these reasons the efficacy of Roy's model for this group of patients is questioned, particularly as one of the two ways in which the patient adapts – through acquired mechanisms – has been destroyed to some extent in these patients. The way the nurse uses this model in these circumstances has also not been convincingly shown by Norman's article.

THE MECHANISMS AND MANIFESTATIONS OF A RAISED TEMPERATURE

The fourth paper in this section (Davis-Sharts, 1978) deals with a further aspect of the identification of problems using Roy's framework. This paper draws on the knowledge of biology and bacteriology in order to explain the mechanisms and reasons for a raised temperature. Empirical data collection is not part of the study, but it does demonstrate how a good knowledge base in an area relevant to nursing can be used effectively to understand the assessment of a patient.

Davis-Sharts (1978) defines fever as 'a rise in deep body temperature in response to an inflammation, an infection, or both' (p. 1874). She sees it as a particular type of hyperthermia that results in the body thermostat being raised; it still regulates the body heat but at a higher temperature than normal, due to circulating toxins from an inflammatory process.

The site for thermoregulation is in the preoptic area of the hypothalamus, where most of the neurons are sensitive to changes in blood temperature. This area functions as a thermostat by stimulating the anterior and posterior hypothalamus to produce appropriate behaviours to either gain or lose heat, in order to maintain the body temperature constant at 37°C. When a fever develops, the thermostat changes to a higher setting. This allows body heat to be produced and conserved until the higher temperature setting is reached, and subsequently maintained through the normal regulating mechanisms.

Substances that cause fever are pyrogens, and these can be endogenous or exogenous. Endogenous pyrogens develop from within the body from damaged tissue, cell necrosis, malignancy and tissue rejection. Atkins and Bodel (1972) believe that the substance most responsible for fever in humans is an endogenous pyrogen found in various body tissues, for example blood leucocytes and monocytes, peritoneal and alveolar macrophages, and liver Kupffer cells. It is probably stimulated by an exogenous pyrogen or by endogenous stimuli such as inflamed or necrotic tissues. All endogenous pyrogens contain essential peptide bonds as well as small amounts of carbohydrates and lipids, and they become less active at an alkaline pH, or at a temperature of 56°C.

Exogenous pyrogens are substances which, when introduced into the body from outside, produce a fever; these could be Gram-negative or Gram-positive bacteria, viruses, yeasts, fungi or protozoa. Davis-Sharts describes endotoxin, an exogenous or bacterial pyrogen which has been extensively studied (Milton, 1976). She describes it as a lipopolysaccharide which forms part of the cell wall of Gram-negative bacteria. Of its three regions, it is region 'lipid A' which is responsible for the pyrogenic activity. Endotoxin causes prolonged fever of rapid onset, the area of the body most sensitive to its influence being the preoptic area of the hypothalamus.

Rosendorff (1976) has shown that factors which prevent or lower the action of calcium in the hypothalamus result in a rise in the thermo-regulatory setting, which in turn produces fever.

Davis-Sharts describes three distinct stages of fever. The first stage is when the body temperature is rising due to the resetting of the hypothalamic thermostat. The patient feels cold, and finds it necessary to conserve heat as much as possible. This stage lasts from 10 to 40 minutes, with a rise in temperature of 1–4°C.

The mechanisms for raising the temperature are by raising the metabolic rate and through vasoconstriction. The metabolic rate is increased by stimulation of the sympathetic nervous system, which releases adrenaline into the circulation and has a direct effect on the rate of cell metabolism; impulses from the preoptic area of the hypothalamus stimulate the thyroid gland to secrete increased amounts of thyroxine. The vaso-constriction resulting from stimulation of the whole body by adrenaline produces massive decreases in blood flow to the skin to prevent heat loss; this is accompanied by stimulation of the shivering centre in the posterior hypothalamus which causes increased muscle cell metabolism and there-fore increased heat production. Gooseflesh may also occur and sweating ceases, both being a further attempt to conserve heat.

The second stage begins when the body temperature has reached the new level set by the hypothalamic regulating mechanism, when many of the mechanisms used by the body in the first stage are reversed; for example the skin becomes flushed, as vasoconstriction ceases, and feels warm. The patient also complains frequently of feeling hot. Sweating returns, and with the increased fluid loss the patient complains of thirst. Where there is a raised temperature over a period of time, fluid and electrolyte imbalance become evident resulting in mild to moderate dehy-dration: dry skin with a loss of skin turgor, dry and coated mucous membranes, cracked lips, sunken eyes and increased urine concentration. As the basal metabolic rate remains high to maintain the raised tempera-ture, there is tachycardia and tachypnoea.

A further feature associated with a prolonged rise in temperature is a changed neurological response. Davis-Sharts says that this is probably due to increased nerve cell irritability as a direct result of the increased body temperature. This may cause restlessness, delirium or, at its most severe, convulsions, which usually occur when the temperature is over 40°C, but will depend on the age of the patient. Photophobia or headache may also be present. It is important for the nurse to be able to distinguish the cause, as all these signs may be due to factors other than a raised tem-perature. For example, herpes simplex may be activated by a sustained high temperature, usually developing after 48 hours.

The longer the second stage of fever lasts, the more likely it is that more profound changes will occur; these involve tissue destruction, where body proteins are catabolized and the parenchymal tissue of the cells is destroyed. The patient becomes increasingly lethargic, and exhibits general malaise with muscle aching and weakness, accompanied by albuminuria. Anorexia is a common feature, and there may be increased breakdown of body fat, which, if rapid, causes ketosis and acidosis.

The third stage of fever begins when the hypothalamic thermostat is reset to normal – when the underlying cause of the fever is removed. The reduction of heat occurs through the body heat loss mechanisms: peripheral vasodilatation, due to inhibition of the sympathetic nervous system and reduction in impulses from the hypothalamic centre; and increased sweating, triggered by stimulation from the hypothalamus through the sympathetic neurons which in turn causes stimulation of the sweat glands. This can further aggravate dehydration. There is also inhibition of shivering through direct hypothalamic inhibition, so muscle tone throughout the body will be decreased, and body metabolism and heat production decreased.

Davis-Sharts briefly describes nursing activity to help the patient adapt to these stages of a raised temperature. She says the usefulness of a raised temperature is not well understood and therefore its role in disease is unexplained. The nurse needs to be able to assess the patient's response to a fever accurately, in order to plan effective care.

The fever can be reduced by the use of antipyretics such as aspirin, which inhibits the synthesis of prostaglandins (Brobeck, 1973); cooling the surface of the body by sponging with cold water or alcohol to increase heat loss, although some patients may be unable to tolerate alcohol fumes; also rubbing the skin stimulates heat loss. More profound cooling may be through the use of a hypothermia mattress, but the nurse will need to be aware of and prevent any skin damage due to extreme cold; alternatively the patient may be placed in an iced water bath. Replacement of fluids, electrolytes and proteins and treatment of the cause of the raised temperature is essential.

This paper makes no claims, as did Norman's paper, to assess the acquired mechanisms of adaptation, nor does it attempt to collect empirical data from patients or nurses working with patients with a raised temperature. But it shows very effectively how a knowledge base of physiology can be used in assessing the innate mechanisms of a patient with a raised temperature. It shows the focal stimuli of possible reasons for a raised temperature and the effects seen and felt by the patient. Contextual stimuli are less easily detected in this paper, although some can be inferred; residual stimuli would possibly be of little note in such situations, although preferred behaviours and health beliefs in infection may be considered as relevant residual stimuli.

The adaptive mechanisms of the regulator are shown well by Davis-Sharts. The mode of assessment of adaptation using Roy's physiological mode is seen as totally appropriate, with the effects of a raised temperature on each of the categories of the physiological mode, and their interaction with each other.

Using the knowledge from this paper the nurse can make a first level assessment to measure both internal and external responses to infection, and therefore to judge whether the patient's behaviour is adaptive or maladaptive in the circumstances. Although this paper was written some time ago, so some of the physiological knowledge may have been superseded, it does give an excellent example of the use of one aspect of the model. However, confusion arises in the change from measuring temperature in degrees centigrade at the beginning of the paper to measurement in degrees Fahrenheit towards the end.

This paper does not make any claims to be testing Roy's model, although, as I have indicated, it does so in some areas very effectively. The way it tests the model is by incorporating a sound knowledge base into some of Roy's concepts. It therefore shows that patient assessment of adaptation and maladaptation can be carried out in patients with a raised temperature using a combination of Roy's model and this level of knowledge. However, there is little attempt to move beyond the assessment stage, as this is not the purpose of the paper, although some indication is given of actions that the nurse might take to relieve some of the patient's symptoms.

THE NEEDS OF CAESAREAN BIRTH PARENTS

Fawcett (1981) is the only paper that I found which uses empirical data collection to assess the problems of short-term adaptation. It surveys the needs of both parents before, during and after a Caesarean birth.

Fawcett (1981) states that the problems of both parents towards a Caesarean birth have not been identified. She claims that in the past the needs of the mother have usually been inferred from her reaction to the birth, but the needs of the father have only been identified through interviews with his wife. Fawcett undertook a survey to elicit the needs of both parents.

The method adopted in this retrospective survey was to determine the reactions of both parents to Caesarean birth, their expressed needs during the experience, and their suggestions about changes that could be made. Fawcett implies that the experience is not a totally positive one.

Her survey comprised a convenience sample of 24 married couples, three of whom were her professional colleagues. The ages of the women ranged from 22 to 39 years (mean 29 years); the ages of the men ranged from 23 to 42 years (mean 30.8 years).

The spread of primiparous and multiparous couples is shown in Table 3.1. The births occurred between 1973 and 1980. This time lapse between the births of the first and last children means a far greater opportunity for a shift in opinion about the birth to have occurred with some couples than with others; this problem is not considered in the article.

Seventeen of the couples attended classes preparing them for childbirth, 14 of whom indicated that the classes included some information on Caesarean births; one of the couples had attended Caesarean birth classes.

Table 3.1 Distribution of Caesarean births in Fawcett's (1981) study

	Method of delivery		Total sample
	Emergency Caesarean	Planned Caesarean	
Primiparous couples	13	4	17
Multiparous couples	5	3	8

Each parent was given a questionnaire with open-ended questions, which asked them to identify both physical and emotional reactions to events surrounding the birth, and to identify their greatest needs during this time. They were also asked to identify what they felt could have been done, and by whom, to improve their experience. This question implies bias.

Content analysis of the responses identified needs relating to Roy's concepts of deficits and excesses in the four adaptive modes.

Analysis showed the mother to have several physiological need deficits. Mothers who had experienced labour felt extreme fatigue; some mothers were very frightened when told they had to have a Caesarean section; pain was experienced, but mothers reported this was relieved when they found they had a healthy baby. During the post-partum period most mothers said they needed rest. The fathers who stayed with their wives for the duration of labour and the Caesarean section needed sleep and food, and a few felt extreme physical and emotional exhaustion both before and during the delivery.

Analysis of the self-concept mode found many of the mothers to be profoundly disappointed that they had been unable to deliver in a more conventional manner; some felt anger towards the obstetrician. Mothers also frequently expressed the feeling of loss of control over themselves and events, particularly in the case of an emergency Caesarean. The fathers felt no direct threat to their self-concept, but supported their wives' views and feelings that their capabilities were undermined. Both parents expressed anger that neither obstetrician nor nurses were sensitive to their needs during the Caesarean.

In the role function mode the failure felt by the mothers was frequently expressed. Mothers were very aware of the delay in mothering due to the effects of the general anaesthetic, and the discomfort some felt, which interfered with their mothering role. Fathers also felt a sense of failure in being unable to perform the coaching role they had been prepared for during classes. The extent of preparation for the Caesarean seemed to be important in whether role failure was strongly felt; this was minimized if parents were able to be together during the delivery. Most parents said they needed more information about what to expect, to help them cope with the process and the outcome.

The interdependence mode showed that all parents wanted to be together and with their baby. They frequently expressed resentment at being forced into a dependent role during the birth, and made comments relating to lack of information from the obstetrician and the nurses.

This study shows Roy's model being used to assess both innate and acquired mechanisms of adaptation. The changes to the parents caused by the Caesarean birth are clearly identified, and the adaptive mechanisms, mainly of the cognator, are shown. These responses confirm previous findings of studies of bonding and attachment behaviours, which could be interpreted as attempts to maintain the integrity of the individuals and the family unit.

The four modes of adaptation are seen to be valid for such situations, as both internal and external needs were reported. In each of the modes the focal, contextual and residual stimuli are seen; it can therefore be inferred that the nurse can make a judgement of adaptation or maladaptation on the basis of these data.

Despite showing good and valid use of the Roy model, the study had at least two methodological problems which will affect the validity of the results. First, the length of time that elapsed between the birth and the data collection for some of the couples was considerable. There is therefore bound to be some alteration in their perceptions of events, particularly those which occurred nearly 7 years previously; it is therefore difficult to use all responses to make statements about the group as a whole. The second problem is the sample. Fawcett says that some of the parents were known to her personally; this would tend to bias the quantity and quality of data received from these couples when compared to data received from couples who were not known to the author. No indication is given by Fawcett that she allowed for these problems.

The study was clearly theory led. It was also an explanatory study, as it looked at the perceptions of the parents to their adaptation to a Caesarean birth, while attempting to show what helped or hindered the parents to adapt. However the results are somewhat suspect, due to the research design.

CONCLUSIONS

Five studies were found (Davis-Sharts, 1978; Norman, 1979; Fawcett, 1981; Farkas, 1981; Leech, 1982) that investigated adaptation or maladaptation to changes. Farkas showed Roy's model to be useful in helping to identify adaptation and maladaptation in the elderly, leading to those who had more maladaptive behaviours applying for residence in a nursing home. This shows support for Roy's model in the situation studied. Leech found considerable maladaptation by patients with arterial occlusion. Greater adaptation problems were found in patients with the more progressive disease. Roy's model was also supported by this study. Norman shows that some parts of some of the adaptive modes are useful when assessing patients with right hemispheric lesions, although emphasis seemed to be on confirming the search of the literature. This study, at best, shows weak support for Roy's model in assessing adaptation and maladaptation with these patients. Davis-Sharts showed how a good literature search and analysis could enable Roy's model to be used effectively to identify adaptation and maladaptation in patients with a raised temperature. This gave some support to identifying patients' adaptation and maladaptation using Roy's model in this area. Fawcett showed the adaptation and maladaptation problems of both parents following a Caesarean birth. However, the methodology used leads to some questions about the findings, so few conclusions can be made to support Roy's model in this area.

All the studies were conducted in North America.

PLANNING NURSING CARE

In this section of the Roy model the nurse must plan to help the patient to adapt to the current situation or maladaptive state. The model, if used strictly as Roy intended, is by manipulation of the focal stimuli in the first instance, where this is possible, otherwise by manipulation of the contextual or residual stimuli.

A single paper was found which addressed the issue of planning nursing care in order to achieve the maximum adaptive responses to health or illness; it dealt with adaptation to chronic illness (Pollock, 1986).

PHYSIOLOGICAL AND PSYCHOSOCIAL ADAPTATION TO CHRONIC ILLNESS

Pollock (1986) examines three chronic illnesses or patient conditions – diabetes, hypertension and rheumatoid arthritis – and views them from the potential of the patient to adapt. The adaptation is seen within physiological and psychosocial perspectives.

Pollock hypothesized that there was a difference in personality of patients with chronic illnesses between those who had adapted to their illness and those who exhibited maladaptive behaviours. She called this difference in personality 'hardiness', and suggested that this characteristic may have an effect on the individual's coping ability and use of social support. It is evidently important for the nurse to be able to plan to help patients with chronic illness to adapt to their conditions.

In studying patient adaptation to chronic illness, Pollock took the focal stimulus as the threat to the individual of each of the three chronic illnesses. The contextual stimuli she used were variables of: age; sex; race; social class as measured by Hollingshead (1978); level of education about their condition which included involvement in a patient education programme; and self-initiated behaviours related to their condition, for example exercise, stress management or psychotherapy. The residual stimuli she assumed were the genetic patterns which accounted for the hardiness characteristic. She therefore felt that adaptation to chronic illness would be the result of its chronic nature, the stress associated with this, the adaptive behaviour of the individual, and the hardiness characteristic.

Her sample was 60 individuals with at least a 1-year history of the illness: 20 of these had been diagnosed as suffering from insulin-dependent diabetes, 20 suffered from hypertension and 20 had rheumatoid arthritis (Table 3.2).

Table 3.2 Demographic details of patients with chronic illnesses in Pollock's (1986) study

	Arthritis (n = 20) (%)	Diabetes (n = 20) (%)	Hypertension (n = 20) (%)
Sex			
Male	15	40	55
Female	85	60	45
Ethnic group			
White	85	85	100
Black	–	10	–
Other	15	5	–
Marital status			
Married	75	65	70
Unmarried	25	35	30
Time since diagnosis			
1–2 years	5	–	15
2–5 years	35	–	25
5–10 years	30	45	25
Up to 20 years	25	55	35
Employed	80	85	100

The measurement of physiological adaptation was according to the diagnosis. The scales used were the Physiological Adaptation to Diabetes Mellitus scale (PAD), the Physiological Adaptation to Rheumatoid Arthritis scale (PAR) and the Physiological Adaptation to Hypertension scale (PAH). These measures were developed by a team of six experts including nurses and physicians who specialized in the areas. The measures were felt by Pollock to be the most reliable way of assessing physiological control by the patient. In a pilot study of five subjects, experts rated patients' physiological adjustment to illness; Pearson's correlations of the experts' ratings against the ratings from the scales devised by Pollock were $r = 0.95$ for the PAD scale, $r = 0.90$ for the PAH scale and $r = 0.92$ for the PAR scale; all were significant beyond the 0.01 level. Each scale had seven criteria measures, each criterion being given a score of its importance from 0 to 10 by the experts.

The hardiness characteristic was also measured using a scale devised by Pollock. Development of the scale used Rotter's (1975) internal–external locus of control as a guide. Pollock's scale contained 48 items, all of which were measured on a 6-point Likert scale; 15 items were designed to measure commitment, 15 items to measure challenge, and 18 items to measure control. Inter-rater agreement by a panel of judges of the measures was 0.85. Comparison was made with Kobasa's (1979) hardiness scale using a pilot study of 50 subjects, to whom both scales were administered. Alpha coefficients for both the entire scales and also subscales indicated better reliability and internal consistency for Pollock's scale. In addition, a panel of experts from faculty and doctoral students with expertise in adult health evaluated the appropriateness of Pollock's scale against that of Kobasa. Agreement was 100% that Pollock's scale was more appropriate.

The third scale used to measure adaptation to chronic illness was the Psychosocial Adjustment to Illness Survey (Derogatis, 1983). The scale has 31 items divided between five scales; each item is rated on a 4-point Likert scale. A previous study using this scale (Morrow, Chiarello and Derogatis, 1978) found inter-rater reliability to be 0.83 for the whole scale, and alpha coefficients for the subscales ranged from 0.62 to 0.83, adding support to construct validity. Criterion validity had previously been established by Kaplan DeNour (1982) who correlated patients' self-report of distress with the scores obtained from the Psychological Adjustment to Illness Survey. The scale had also been shown to have good reliability when administered to renal dialysis patients (alpha coefficient 0.8), lung cancer patients (alpha coefficient 0.83) and cardiac patients (alpha coefficient 0.78) (Derogatis, 1983).

The results were analysed using the Statistical Package for the Social Sciences (SPSS). Internal consistency was checked for the PAD, PAR and PAH scales and was found to be good for these patients, as was correlation between ratings by experts of the adjustment by the patients as compared to the adjustment shown by the three scales.

Correlations between measures showed a significant relationship between hardiness and psychosocial adaptation (Pearson's correlation $r = 0.42$, $p = 0.01$). However, the relationship between physiological and psychosocial adjustment was not significant; neither was the relationship between hardiness and physiological adjustment.

Results by diagnostic group showed that the hardiness characteristic for rheumatoid arthritic patients was not significantly correlated with either physiological or psychosocial adaptation. In patients with diabetes the hardiness characteristic was significantly related to physiological adaptation ($r = 0.43$, $p < 0.05$) and psychosocial adaptation ($r = 0.62$, $p < 0.01$). Physiological and psychosocial adaptation were also significantly correlated for diabetic patients ($r = 0.35$, $p < 0.05$). Patients with hypertension were found to have the hardiness characteristic significantly related to physiological but not to psychosocial adaptation; there was also no correlation between physiological and psychosocial adaptation for the hypertensive group.

Analysis of demographic factors in relation to adaptation showed that sex and social status were significantly related to both psychosocial and physiological adaptation, and to the hardiness characteristic. Unfortunately Pollock did not state which sex was found to have significantly better adaptation, nor from which social group they came. Other significant variables were marital status and days lost from work. Also, having attended a patient education programme specific to their illness related significantly to the amount of physiological adaptation by the patient. This last finding may say something about the nature and content of the education programme.

This study, and the method of constructing the scales, was obviously thorough and rigorous at every stage. However, it failed to show a significant correlation between the level of adaptation of patients with rheumatoid arthritis or with hypertension and the hardiness factor, which Pollock hypothesized was a personality characteristic in those who adapted to chronic illness. Her comment on the lack of support for her hypothesis in these two diseases was that a small sample size could have been a contributing factor, as could the nature of the diseases which have different symptoms. This last factor may have been a serious omission in the research design, as measuring the hardiness characteristic with a single scale for diseases with such different effects on patients may have been a reductionist approach. Pollock comments that patients with different diseases had different personalities, and one might assume that some of their overt behaviour was as a result of the effects of prolonged pain (as with the rheumatoid arthritis patients) or as a result of constantly being aware of what they ate in relation to exercise (as with the diabetic group). Future studies of this nature need to take this into account, and to investigate what predominant characteristics patients need and what coping mechanisms they adopt in order to cope with the symptoms of their particular disease.

It is naive, with our current state of knowledge, to think that identifying the hardiness factors in patients with long-term illnesses can be easily resolved; there will have to be a great deal more observation of behaviour of these patient groups before this can be attempted. The cynics amongst us might even say that there is no such thing as enduring personality characteristics anyway, and that any kind of adaptation must be the result of the situation in which the patients find themselves and their response to that situation.

Also of interest in this study is the lack of correlation between the physiological and psychological adaptation in patients with both rheumatoid arthritis and hypertension. This does not show support for Roy's statement that her model is a systems model, as it could be expected that measures on one indicator would be likely to show effects on another indicator if this statement were true. This lack of correlation could imply that patients either cannot or do not know how to control their physical symptoms, but accept their disease process and its limitations; this would be unlikely, as chronic debilitating diseases usually cause a further loss of self-concept at each crisis. Alternatively, the patients are able to control their physical symptoms, for which they may have received good instruction, but are unable to come to terms with the impact of their disease on themselves and their lives. This latter hypothesis is far more likely to be the case, as knowledge of most health care systems shows they are geared more towards symptom control than to helping the patient to come to terms with the psychological and social problems associated with their disease.

This study was not primarily based on Roy's model. However, the theoretical base used concepts that are indistinguishable from some of Roy's concepts, for example adaptation. Therefore results from the study can be seen in the light of support or denial of Roy's model.

The study was certainly a cause and effect study, as the disease from which the patient suffered was what caused their maladaptive state; the extent of their adaptation to the illness was the result of the hardiness characteristic.

This study by Pollock is the only one that considers care planning for patients using the Roy model. Its lack of success with two of the three diseases investigated shows the very complex nature of adaptation to chronic illness. Increased efforts in research are needed to establish the nature of adaptation to acute and chronic illness if Roy's model is to be accepted as a valid method of conceptualizing nursing practice. It may be that, as Pollock implies, for the time being these factors are too complicated to unravel.

PROVISION OF NURSING CARE

This section of the Roy model deals with how the nurse provides care in order to help the patient to adapt to stimuli. According to Roy, when stimuli are outside the individual's zone of adaptation they are unable to adapt to them and therefore nursing care is indicated.

In this section of the model are three studies conducted by the same investigators. Each one uses Roy's model to analyse the effects on the mother and her baby at the birth using the birth chair. The papers investigate three different problems in the process of birth in relation to the outcome of the birth using the birth chair. The studies follow from provision to evaluation of care, and so also form a useful tool for evaluation of the effects of the model in the situations described.

THE EFFECTS OF THE BIRTH CHAIR DURING THE SECOND STAGE OF LABOUR

The birth chair was obviously being widely used in North America before the first of these studies was published (Shannahan and Cottrell, 1985); however, its effects had not been well documented. The three studies in this section were conducted by the same researchers, who published their findings within a 2-year period. They considered the focal stimulus to be the birth, which was uncomplicated in their sample, so they did not want to manipulate this stimulus. The position of the mother was considered to be one of the contextual stimuli, and this they sought to manipulate.

Shannahan and Cottrell (1985) retrospectively examined the records of 60 primiparous women who gave birth in a medical centre in Florida, USA, between 37 and 41 weeks' gestation; 30 of the births were on the traditional delivery table, and 30 used the birth chair. Each of the women had a normal pregnancy and spontaneous onset of labour. Data were collected from the patients' records.

As labour was seen as the focal stimulus, the researchers felt that the position of the mother was one of the contextual stimuli, and sought to manipulate this in order to improve the outcome for both mother and baby. Their specific hypotheses were that women who deliver in the birth chair, compared with those who deliver by more traditional methods, will have:

- a shorter second stage of labour;
- a better fetal outcome;
- more maternal blood loss.

Differences between the mothers who delivered on the delivery table and those who delivered in the birth chair were not found in demographic data from the mother, which included marital status, ethnic origin and length of pregnancy. Neither were differences found between the groups in mean birth weights of the infants.

Difference in the length of the second stage of labour was found between the groups. For women using the birth chair the mean pushing time was 28 minutes in the labour room and 43 minutes in the birth chair. For women using the delivery table the mean pushing time was 20 minutes in the delivery room and 34 minutes on the delivery table. This was not found to be a statistically different length of time between the two groups, but the trend was clearly in the opposite direction from the hypothesis.

Fetal outcome was assessed through Apgar scores at 1 and 5 minutes. Differences between the two groups were not seen: the mean 1 minute score for the birth chair group was 8.7 and the 5 minute score was 9.4; for babies born on the delivery table mean score at 1 minute was 8.8 and at 5 minutes 9.4. From this evidence, although a crude measure, there is no difference to the baby between the two methods of delivery.

Maternal blood loss was assessed from the records through haemo-globin levels on the first and second days following delivery. On admission the group being delivered in the birth chair had higher mean haemoglobin (13.3 g) and haematocrit (39.5%) levels than their counter-parts who were delivered on the delivery table (haemoglobin 12.8 g, haematocrit 37.9%). Following the birth the mean levels were found to be significantly lower in the birth chair group (haemoglobin 11.3 g, haemato-crit 33.7%), than the mothers delivered on the delivery table (haemo-globin 12.1g, haematocrit 36%). This shows that the level of blood loss from the women using the birth chair was significantly higher ($p < 0.025$) than the women being delivered on the delivery table, therefore this hypothesis was supported.

The birth chair was introduced because it was thought to have the advantages of giving birth in the upright position. This would make uterine contractions more effective and enlarge the pelvic outlet; the force of gravity would also be used to expel the fetus. Roberts (1980) also showed that psychological advantages of the birth chair include increased comfort in the second stage of labour and a better response by the mother to the infant.

It is unclear from this study alone how the contextual stimulus of the birth chair was manipulated by the nurse; however, this will become clearer as the series of studies progresses. The study only considered Roy's physiological mode.

This study showed that the birth chair was a safe method of delivery, but no benefits to either the mother or infant could be detected; indeed a problem for the mother through increased blood loss was evident. However, using records only prevents psychological benefits from being detected. The method of allocating women to the birth chair or the deliv-ery table was not clear to the researchers from the records they studied; as they indicate, the obstetrician may have suggested the birth chair to women who were experiencing a more prolonged second stage of labour.

As a first stage in a series, these findings pose more questions than they answer. The research method appeared sound but more information is needed about factors that contribute to blood loss in the mother and the nursing interventions that might reduce this; also more sophisticated measures of infant status are needed to ensure their well-being using the birth chair.

The second study in this series (Cottrell and Shannahan, 1986) considered more fully the question of maternal blood loss and associated factors when delivering in the upright position.

This prospective study was conducted with 55 primiparous women, 33 delivered in the birth chair and 22 on the delivery table. Demographic details were: age range 14–35 years; 44 were white and 11 black; labour was spontaneous and between 37 and 41 weeks' gestation. These details were not significantly different between the two groups. The differences hypothesized between the groups were:

- that the women who delivered in the birth chair would have a shorter second stage of labour than those delivered on the delivery table;
- that women delivered in the birth chair would have a higher incidence of perineal swelling, episiotomies and lacerations, from which there would be a greater blood loss, and a greater incidence of haemorrhoids than the women who were delivered on the delivery table;
- that bleeding would be greater from the women using the birth chair than those being delivered on the delivery table.

A quasi-experimental design was used to compare the outcome.

Observation of the births was by staff nurses who recorded duration of pushing in the labour room and in the delivery suite, and frequency of episiotomy, laceration, perineal swelling and haemorrhoids. The position of the fetal head and the baby's weight were also noted. Maternal blood loss was again from comparison of admission and post-delivery haemoglobin and haematocrit levels. The researchers collected data from the charts recorded by the staff nurses. No indication was given in the article that these staff nurses were informed that their recordings were to be used in this way, nor whether they were given any instruction on how to record, therefore an assessment of recording bias is not possible. Also unclear is what was recorded in relation to pushing, i.e. its duration and whether the women were coached by the midwives to do this. This is crucial to the statements made by the researchers.

No significant differences were found between the groups in relation to marital status, length of pregnancy, position of the fetal head, the need for instrument-assisted delivery, the weight of the baby, or the mean time when the membranes ruptured.

Also, no significant difference was found between the groups in the length of the second stage of labour. Women delivering in the birth chair had a mean of 60 minutes pushing time of which 33 minutes was in the delivery room. The women who were delivered on the delivery table had a mean pushing time of 53 minutes, of which 30 minutes was in the delivery room. However, black women were found to have a significantly shorter pushing time ($p = 0.009$) and duration of second stage of labour, regardless of their delivery method. The first hypothesis – that women delivering in the birth chair would experience a decrease in the length of the second stage of labour – was not supported. As with their previous study, sample selection by the obstetrician may have influenced this result.

The incidence of episiotomies, lacerations and haemorrhoids was found to be increased in women using the birth chair, but this incidence was not significantly different between the groups. However, a significant difference in perineal swelling ($p = 0.05$) was found between the women delivered in the birth chair (incidence of 26) and those delivered on the delivery table (incidence of 10). The researchers consider this difference may be due to the upright position of the women in the birth chair when compared with women on the delivery table; they also note that women pull on the handgrips of the birth chair which may have caused trauma to the perineal area by pushing the buttocks into the rim of the seat. Three factors which the researchers also felt contributed to increased perineal swelling in the birth chair group were: an early transfer to the delivery room; pushing encouraged regardless of fetal descent in the delivery room; and prolonged breath-holding while pushing, i.e. exceeding 6 seconds. However, from records alone this is likely to be pure conjecture, as there is no information in the article of the extent of encouragement to push in the delivery room.

Differences in blood loss between the two groups were compared using levels of admission and post-delivery haemoglobin and haematocrit, but these were not significant. This finding is different from their previous study, where the angle of the birth chair was not tilted to a more horizontal position after delivery. During the present study the position of the birth chair had been tilted towards the horizontal after delivery in 88% of cases. The angle of the birth chair is considered further in the third paper in this series.

This second paper demonstrates how manipulation of the contextual stimuli (use of the birth chair) will affect the outcome of giving birth for the mother, as in the incidence of perineal swelling, episiotomies, lacerations and haemorrhoids. This shows good support for Roy's model in this situation, as manipulation of the contextual stimuli (the level that the chair was tilted) by the midwives is evidently beneficial to the mothers delivering in the birth chair. However, increased confidence in the results would have followed if bias in documentation could have been ruled out.

The third study in this series (Cottrell and Shannahan, 1987) considers the condition of the baby following birth in the birth chair. An upright position has been associated with a reduction in supine hypotension and aortic compression (Carr, 1980). The position in the birth chair should therefore promote both maternal and fetal adaptation.

The hypothesis was that fetal outcome would be improved by birth chair delivery. Improvement would be measured by time of first cry, 1 and 5 minute Apgar scores, and umbilical artery and vein pH and pO_2. The findings from the birth chair babies would be compared with those born on the delivery table.

The method was a prospective study of 55 women with normal pregnancies, a spontaneous labour and uncomplicated vaginal delivery. All were primiparae with an age range of 14–35 years, delivered between 37 and 41 weeks' gestation, 33 in the birth chair and 22 on the delivery table. No significant difference was found between the demographic factors of the two groups.

Data were obtained from the nurses' recordings, which were as follows.

- Categories of the angle of the birth chair: specific categories were defined by the researchers for this purpose and a drawing of the angle was included with the categories; also a protractor was placed in each delivery room. However, inter-rater reliability was not established; we are told that nurses had been prepared by the researchers to use the forms, but we are not told how this preparation was conducted or its extent.
- Categories of pushing were defined by the researchers as breath-holding for less than 5 seconds or for more than 6 seconds. The primary position for pushing was also documented, from four possible positions.
- Nurses counted the number of seconds which elapsed before the baby's first cry; researchers were present to verify these recordings.
- Researchers collected samples of venous and arterial blood from a clamped section of the cord; quality-controlled standard equipment was used to analyse the blood samples.

The results showed that there was no significant difference in the 1 minute Apgar score between the babies in the two groups. However, whether the baby was born in the birth chair or on the delivery table, the 1 minute Apgar score was significantly improved ($p = 0.038$) when the angle of the chair or table was more than 30° upright. This supports the hypothesis that an upright birth position is more beneficial to the fetus, and that positions lower than 30° put direct pressure on the mother's abdominal aorta which reduces the blood supply to the fetus. This is consistent with the findings of Carr (1980).

A further significant difference was found to be arterial pCO_2, which was significantly lower ($p = 0.023$) for the babies born in the birth chair. This supports the findings of Carr (1980) and the hypothesis that less transient cord compression occurs in a more upright position. With the birth chair angle being more than 45° a significant increase in pO_2 was found ($p = 0.007$), compared with when the angle of the birth chair was less than 45°. This supports the hypothesis that with the mother in a more upright position there is a greater oxygen supply to the fetus. No significant differences were found between the other measures.

This study has shown how manipulation of the one of the contextual stimuli, the angle of the birth chair, has affected the status of the baby. This provides good support for Roy's statement by showing that manipulation of stimuli by the midwife will lead to adaptation.

This study showed good experimental design, although reliability between the nurses' methods of documenting would have increased the confidence with which results are interpreted. The study showed that the fetus does tend to be compromised when a more horizontal position is adopted by the mother. The researchers admit to having the samples chosen for them by the physicians; however, the effects of this selection on the outcome to the mother have not been fully explained.

Therefore, taken as a whole these three studies show good support for Roy's model with these mothers and their babies. They show that the link between identification of potential maladaptation and the manipulation of stimuli by the midwife is effective in producing a better outcome for the mother and her baby in certain circumstances. Therefore the cause and effect design used by the researchers has given strong support to Roy's model in linking identification with nursing actions in this area of work.

In these studies Roy's model was very central to the design of the research. This also means that giving birth in the birth chair was problematized for the women and their babies and also that the model was similarly problematized by the investigations. That the women were studied in their natural environment, rather than being given questionnaires to complete after the event, is also a strength of the studies.

CONCLUSION

In a series of studies Shannahan and Cottrell showed how the contextual stimulus of giving birth – the position of the mother during the birth process – could be manipulated. This demonstrated resulting levels of adaptation in the mother and baby. These studies gave good support to Roy's model.

EVALUATION OF THE LEVEL OF ADAPTATION

In this phase of Roy's model the nurse should be concerned with how much adaptation has occurred in the patient or client. As adaptation can be viewed in the physiological mode as achieving and maintaining homeostasis, it is interesting to note that no studies dealing with physiological outcomes were found in the literature, apart from the three above which investigated the use of the birth chair in relation to mother and baby outcomes.

However, a single study was found in the literature which attempted to outline the evaluation of care in diabetic patients.

DIABETIC PATIENTS

The study in this section is not strictly based on research. However, as a case study it does have some benefits in outlining the changes that can be achieved in patients with long-standing chronic illness. The means by which the results were obtained are impossible to isolate from the article, and I cannot make an attempt to do so; also description is not sufficiently detailed to use any form of qualitative analysis on the text. In spite of this, nurses could develop the particular techniques outlined in the paper to produce some good research questions and results.

Miller and Hellenbrand (1981) showed what can be achieved by nurse practitioners in North America. They worked with two diabetic patients over a period of time. One was a 50-year-old black man from a low socio-economic group who had been a diabetic for 15 years; 3 years previously he had developed resistance to beef insulin that resulted in very high blood sugar levels; changing to pork insulin improved the situation although complications persisted. The other patient was a 63-year-old black woman, also from a low socio-economic group, who had been a diabetic for 26 years; she had experienced poor diabetic control since her diagnosis was made; she frequently said she did not understand diabetes or its control and had a fatalistic attitude to the condition.

The strategies used by Miller and Hellenbrand for the first patient are outlined as teaching him the pathophysiology of diabetes and its long-term effect on his state of health. They reviewed his diabetic control and his knowledge of diet, and assisted him with problem solving and recognizing the effects of his actions. They taught him how to prevent problems through foot care, and the effects of his levels of activity on his diabetic control as well as where he could seek help.They also taught him how to monitor his own body signs.

A second strategy was persuasion, which was used to encourage the first patient to have a more positive response and to take a more active role in his care. The third strategy was entitled 'facilitation and support', and entailed weekly follow-up visits aimed at fostering his self-concept and giving continuity to his care plan; encouraging his participation in his care, particularly during visits to the doctor; and supporting his behaviour by pointing out its direct effects on his health state.

The effects of these nursing strategies were divided into 'clinical outcomes' and 'behavioural outcomes'. For this patient the former were:

- a decrease in the number of hypoglycaemic episodes over a 4-month period;
- a decrease in foot pain due to the discovery that eating beef caused increased pain (the patient also reported increased sensory perception in both feet accompanied by an increased ability to walk).

The behavioural outcomes were:

- increased self-esteem and positive self-concept which was shown by a willingness to share his concerns and to make decisions about himself;
- an increased interest in his physical condition, demonstrated by asking relevant questions and seeking advice to help him to make decisions;
- reduced level of disability, and a much healthier interdependence with others;
- a better understanding of the values of foods;
- he demonstrated the skills of being able to prevent further problems.

Although these strategies and their evaluation are very broad, and one cannot demonstrate any detailed link between process and outcome, it is clear that this patient did adapt to diabetes, probably due to nursing intervention. However, the Roy model had not been used in its strictest sense here. There was no defining of stimuli and no expression of manipulation of the stimuli, and on occasions one has the impression that the goal of self-care and teaching the patient to self-care was more the conceptual framework that the authors had in mind.

With the second patient a similar set of strategies was used: a teaching plan, which also had the aim of building the patient's self-esteem to increase her receptiveness to the teaching; assistance with her adaptive resources to cope with her lack of understanding of the disease; encouragement of her work role as improving her self-care and knowing how and when to seek professional help.

As with the first patient, persuasion was used. This included moderating her health beliefs from her existing ones which accepted obesity as a sign of good health and weight loss as a sign of illness; and helping her to become less defensive about diabetes so that she could develop the ability to learn from others with the same problems. The third strategy used by the nurses was facilitation and support; this used three methods: understanding her family situation with its many life stresses; promoting her family support by involving her husband and daughter in her care, and supporting her interest in God; encouraging her to improve her self-esteem so that she would be motivated to improving her self-care.

Various outcomes were seen as a result of these nursing strategies, similar to the first patient. These were again divided into 'clinical outcomes' and 'behavioural outcomes'. The former were:

- less frequent hyperglycaemic episodes;
- an unchanged level of both retinopathy and foot numbness.

Behavioural outcomes included:

- verbalizing and demonstrating more control, particularly in relation to food;
- finding a part-time job which improved her self-esteem;
- beginning to take a more active role in managing her illness;
- her compliance with drug and diet regime improved, as shown by urine and blood sugar readings;
- attendance at out-patient appointments regularly;
- she demonstrated continuing development of her self-management abilities.

Although each of the claims made in the article is in very broad terms, and no specific indication of the extent of achievement with these diabetic patients is given, it allows practitioners researching their own practice to broadly compare their results with those outlined in this article. The nature of the problems for poorly controlled diabetic patients is clearly evident here. However, to what extent differences in culture and health care systems between North America and Great Britain would contribute to different types of problems for diabetic patients such as these can only be the subject of conjecture.

Roy's model is used in its broadest sense in this article. The acquired mechanisms of learning are easier to isolate than the innate mechanisms, and some of the stimuli influencing maladaptive behaviour can be seen in both patients. Also shown, to some extent, are the adaptive mechanisms of the cognator, as they relate to cultural factors. However, adaptation in the adaptive modes is not clearly isolated, although maladaptive behaviour is stated. Manipulation of the stimuli by the nurse practitioners results in the patients showing increased adaptation to their condition.

The number of patients in this study causes problems for generalizing any results, as do the problems of the exact length of time over which any of the results were achieved. Also, the detailed nature of any intervention given is not expressed specifically, or of any barriers the nurse had to overcome to achieve the results. Furthermore the model was not problematized, so any indication of its effectiveness with these types of patients is difficult to assess.

CONCLUSIONS ON THE USE OF THE MODEL TO 1990

Several studies have been found that demonstrate the use of Roy's adaptation model in a wide range of practice settings.

Roy's model has been used and developed in the areas of identification of adaptation and maladaptation in the four modes, using both first and second levels of assessment, and identifying the influencing stimuli (Davis-Sharts, 1978; Farkas, 1981; Fawcett, 1981; Leech, 1982; Norman, 1989). A single paper has also been published that shows planning to remove or change the stimuli (Pollock, 1986). A series of three papers published by Shannahan and Cottrell between 1985 and 1987 showed how manipulation of the stimuli is a successful method of providing intervention; and a single paper (Miller and Hellenbrand, 1981) claimed a good level of adaptation achieved following nursing intervention.

All the studies give some level of support to the use of Roy's model. None of the studies showed the model to be inappropriate or to be unable to deal with the problems posed by the types of patients, people or situations being investigated. However, all the papers originated in North America, so the use and attractiveness of this model in other cultures is, up to 1990, untested.

DEVELOPMENTS SINCE 1990

A further edition of the Roy model has been published since 1990. Roy and Andrews (1991) have now produced a definitive statement on the model. This has confirmed many of the statements in Roy's (1984) second edition of her model. The Roy model, therefore, remains substantially unchanged.

An interesting feature of the use of the model in research and practice is that it is now being claimed to be the focus of a research programme. Fawcett (1990) shows how an area of nursing practice can be systematically studied through the use of Roy's model to provide new knowledge. I have also commented on Fawcett's approach to testing models of nursing in the introduction to this edition (pp. 1–3).

Fawcett is also regularly publishing papers of her joint research work with other researchers using Roy's second edition (1984) as their basis (e.g. Fawcett and Tulman, 1990).

BUILDING A PROGRAMME OF RESEARCH FROM THE ROY MODEL

Roy's model has been used in a number of studies to investigate childbirth and the post-partum. The model has helped in the development of instruments and in the conduct of the research programme. Fawcett has concluded that in her studies to date the credibility of the model has been supported.

Fawcett and Tulman (1990) say that far from lacking influence, conceptual models can have a real impact on the design and methods of research into nursing. They say that these research designs and the methods used are usually specified in the model itself. Their research has been: 'to enhance our understanding of how people adapt to environmental stimuli, how adaptive processes affect health, and how nursing can enhance adaptive life processes and functioning' (p. 721). They see clinical research as studying the effects of nursing on the person's ability to adapt. Their particular area of interest is in how women adapt in the role function mode during the post-partum. They have developed the core variable which they call the functional ability, defined as 'the ability to perform role activities' (p. 721). However, they later redefined this as 'the current status of role performance' (p. 721) or functional status. So functional status became 'the degree to which new role responsibilities and usual role activities are performed' (p. 721). This, they claim, captures the essence of Roy's adaptation in role function.

Their programme of clinical research began with the development of an instrument to measure the adaptation to the roles that society defines. According to Andrews and Roy (1986) most people have three roles: a primary role, which fundamentally affects behaviour according to age and gender; a secondary role which is taken on at a particular stage in life to complete the tasks that are needed, for example someone's job; and the third role which is freely chosen as a result of the second role, for example joining special interest groups. Fawcett and Tulman's research was based on measuring these roles as performed by women following childbirth.

Substantive studies by Fawcett and Tulman to date have included the following.

- A comparison of women's full functional abilities following either Caesarean or vaginal delivery (Tulman and Fawcett, 1988). In this study physical energy was considered to be an indication of functional status. The focal stimulus was the childbirth, while the contextual stimuli were the mother's demographic and health levels. The study was conducted by survey which relied on the mothers' memories of the post-partum up to 5 years previously. However, according to Oppenheim (1992) this is testing the memory of subjects beyond what could be reasonably expected. The findings were that 72% of the vaginally delivered women said they regained their usual level of physical energy by the end of the sixth post-partum week, while only 34% of the Caesarean delivered women had done so. They also found a similar level of abilities and differences between the two types of delivery in taking on the care of their infant, resuming household tasks and socializing. They concluded that the usual 6-week recovery period after childbirth should be reconsidered.

- A longitudinal study to investigate the changes in functional status during the 6 months following childbirth (Tulman *et al.*, 1990). In this study, physical energy was considered to be a health variable. A number of factors associated with the adaptive modes were tested as well as the influence of a large number of contextual stimuli on adaptation. The study examined the changes in the functional status at 3 weeks, 6 weeks, 3 months and 6 months post-partum in 97 women with healthy full-term infants. Results showed a steady increase in functional status from 3 weeks to 3 months, but no statistically significant increases thereafter. However, even at 6 months post-partum they found that many women had not resumed some of the maternal and female roles, such as infant care and household activities.

As I have indicated above, the design for the first study could be criticized as expecting too much from the memory of those surveyed.

Fawcett and Tulman claim that their findings support Roy's model, particularly in the influence of environmental stimuli on adaptation as well as that the adaptive modes are related to each other.

This paper, as well as setting out the research programme and the studies completed to date, also indicates that Roy's model is being applied to the clinical area. In this sense the clinical areas simply provide the data to either support or overturn the model, but the clinical area gains to a certain extent in that the results of the research feed back into practice to show the practitioners what could be the outcomes of their actions. However this approach can assume a hierarchy, where research can be more important than practice.

This last point is not lost on Draper (1993), who says that Fawcett is working with the 'belief that models can be applied to practice ...' (p. 560). He also notes that this view 'can be seen in her [Fawcett's] view of nursing models in directing nursing practice' (pp. 560–1). A further criticism by Draper of Fawcett's approach to research is that she is looking for confirmation of the model. He links Fawcett's approach to positivism.

However, according to Silverman (1993), and the approach this book has also taken, we should not be making such direct opposites as positivism and interactionist forms of theory and research. According to Silverman, it is now high time that we started to test some of the hypotheses that have been produced through inductive research; we cannot go on for ever merely generating hypotheses, but never testing them. I would suggest that this is precisely what Fawcett, in her programme of research, is doing. It is therefore very useful, not only to the practitioner, who may want to use a model of nursing, to know that some aspects of it are valid, but it is also very good for the model to show that it is being systematically tested and being shown to be useful and valid.

There have been two other papers published since 1990 which develop Roy's model in the area of assessment. One of these is by Tulman *et al.* (1990). These two papers will be outlined and commented upon below. I also found one further paper that developed the evaluation stage of Roy's model; this was by Fawcett *et al.* and is outlined in a later section of this chapter (pp. 85–87).

ASSESSMENT USING ROY'S MODEL

The first paper published since 1990 is an assessment of mothers' views of feeding their babies in a neonatal intensive care unit (NICU). However, this paper goes far beyond simply asking the mothers their views; it also develops the notion of models in a practice setting and what they can hope to achieve.

MOTHERS' OPINIONS ON THE NICU

This paper, by Nyqvist and Sjoden (1993), as well as developing Roy's model in the substantive area of mothers' views on breastfeeding in a NICU, also shows the use of Roy's model in a Swedish setting. The aims of the study were to classify the mothers' views according to Roy's model, while testing for reliability between those who were classifying the interview data.

Nyqvist and Sjoden obtained the names of mothers from their medical records. The infants whose mothers were selected had to be a single infant delivered at full-term who was admitted to the NICU on the first day of life and was discharged within 6 days. The infants were not chosen if they had a congenital malformation or a severe disease or were treated by ventilation or total parenteral nutrition.

A total of 178 mothers and infants met the criteria. Of these, 92 were boys and 86 were girls. One hundred and two mothers were primiparous, 51 had had their second child and 25 of the mothers already had two or more children.

The data were collected by telephone interviews with the mothers who had agreed to participate after receiving a letter asking for an interview and detailing the contents of the interview. However, we are not told how many mothers were asked to give an interview in order to arrive at the final total of 178. The interviews were conducted when the babies were 3 months old, so this research design relies heavily on the mothers' memories over a substantial period of time when a lot could have been happening to them. This could make one question the validity of their replies in relation to the events in the NICU.

The interviews aimed to answer two questions:

1. what advice can you give me as a nurse on how we can facilitate the initiation of breastfeeding in the NICU, and
2. what advice would you like to give another mother in the same situation as you were, trying to start breastfeeding in the NICU?

(p. 56)

The answers that the mothers gave were written down verbatim or as notes during the interviews. Mothers were asked to check the accuracy of the recording by the interviewer repeating their response and then asking them whether it had been correctly recorded.

Responses were then classified according to Roy's model. This was done independently by Nyqvist and by two research assistants who were also registered nurses working in the NICU but who did not know Roy's model. Agreement on the categories between the raters was between 74.3% and 92.5%. Where agreement was reached between two or more raters this was used in the findings. The analysis also showed that only 31% of the themes were assigned to only one of Roy's modes; therefore 69% of the themes overlapped between the modes.

The data obtained from the mothers showed maladaptation in a number of areas and in all the modes. In the physiological mode the mothers' needs were the following.

- Diet and fluids – mothers had difficulty in keeping to mealtimes and often needed drinks in the NICU.
- Protection – pain meant the mothers needed help to care for their baby in carrying and positioning it as well as comfortable chairs and somewhere to lie down in the NICU. Prevention of breast soreness was also needed.
- Exercise and rest – the distance between the mothers' ward and the NICU and the lack of privacy in the NICU made rest difficult.
- The senses – the environment of the NICU negatively affected the mothers' senses.
- Endocrine functions – the pain, lack of rest and stress due to the infant being in the NICU negatively affected milk production and the let-down reflex.

In the role function mode the mothers' needs were the following.

- Maternal role – there were obstacles to the mothers' role, such as feelings of unreality about the birth, separation of the infant from the mother which delayed the first contact, embarrassment in front of others, the behaviours of the nurses and the hospital routines.
- Mothers as patients in the maternity ward – as they spent much time in the NICU, mothers missed information in the maternity ward and felt they did not fit in with the other mothers. They also may not have

asked for help or asked questions and therefore felt denied the role of a patient, unlike other mothers.

- Role of parent of a patient – mothers needed to know the NICU routines, their role and visiting arrangements. Mothers also needed to be prepared for discharge of their baby.

In Roy's self-concept mode the researchers found that the mothers needed the following.

- Physical self – they needed the opportunity to talk about a difficult or unplanned delivery, to regain their self-confidence. Incorrect bodily concepts may be preserved by lack of breastfeeding or the opportunity to do so.
- Personal self/self-consistency – mothers not only needed to feel wanted and respected in the NICU but they also needed to feel they could carry out a normal mothering role in private. They needed to be given relevant information and feel able to ask questions.
- Self-ideal – mothers needed to feel capable of meeting their infant's needs; obstacles such as pain, tiredness, distance from the NICU incurring transport problems, and also the nurses taking over their role, needed to be overcome.
- Moral/ethical self – mothers felt guilty in a number of ways: about delayed contact with their infant and about being missing from the maternity ward for information and routines.

In the interdependence mode the mothers relied on the nurses for their own and their infant's physiological needs; also for permission from them to care for their infant and to have the confidence to do this on discharge.

The paper also gives the needs of the infant and the father, classified according to Roy's model. For the infant the needs were assessed as:

- the physiological needs of fluid and electrolyte balance and nutrition;
- protection;
- exercise and rest;
- the senses;
- endocrine functions;
- the infants' role and self-concept;
- the infants' interdependence.

The fathers' needs were classified according to Roy's model as:

- physiological needs for information to reduce their anxiety;
- role function, by being present and helping the mother by giving her information and taking an active part in infant care;
- interdependence – the fathers needed specific instruction on visiting and the care and condition of their infant which would inspire confidence that the infant was in good hands.

Lastly, Nyqvist and Sjoden classify the role of the nurse according to the interview data and to Roy's model. They found that the mothers saw the nurses as needing to be assigned to particular patients in the NICU and the maternity ward. They should also be flexible in their approach to the mothers and infants to allow for the needs of both. Nurses should have a clear sense of roles between themselves and the mothers while encouraging mothering and parental responsibilities.

The reasons for conducting this study, according to Nyqvist and Sjoden, were not only to improve service delivery, but also to assess the usefulness of Roy's model in this situation. Therefore the study was driven by the model, and the authors clearly state that they wished to test the model by their study. The authors state that the model was useful in an NICU setting but needed to include the attitudes, behaviour and role functions of nurses and the ways in which these were perceived by patients and their families.

The nurses who classified the interview data had a high level of agreement between themselves and with the researcher. As the nurses were not familiar with Roy's model this level of agreement is very encouraging for the use of the model and the recognition of its components by practising nurses. However, the authors state that because of the amount of overlap between the modes and their lack of clarity, this could cause difficulties in the classification of the data. For this reason there could be considerable confusion for nurses working with the model on a daily basis. They suggest that the model should therefore be confined to the design of assessment tools that nurses could use in their work with patients.

This study is evidently descriptive, as the researchers describe the views of the mothers by assessing them using the model. There is no attempt in the paper to plan for nursing care as a result of assessing the mothers' levels of adaptation and maladaptation. Therefore the link between assessment and planning is not tested by this study.

The design of the study encourages the expression of commonsense views and experiences by the mothers. One of the strengths of the study is that these views are problematized through the use of Roy's model. However, the study did not examine these mothers in their natural environment, while they were in the hospital. Instead it chose to ask for their views some 3 months after the baby was born. Therefore, it could be that some of their memories have changed during this time.

THE FUNCTIONAL STATUS OF FATHERS

The second paper on assessment since 1990 is again based on Tulman and Fawcett's work. Tulman, Fawcett and Weiss (1993) look at how the father's functional status increases or continues during their partner's pregnancy and after the baby is born. They developed a tool to measure the man's activities in the home and outside it, as well as with the baby.

In a strict sense the title of this section is incorrect, as fathers are in no sense 'patients'. However, the following paper addresses identification of adaptation and maladaptation by fathers to their partner's Caesarean section.

Tulman, Fawcett and Weiss (1993) developed the Inventory of Functional Status – Fathers (IFS-F) which they state was developed from the role function mode of Roy's model. Role function they represent as functional status, as in previous work, by primary, secondary and tertiary roles. The inventory was designed to measure the functional status of the father during his partner's pregnancy and post-partum. The role function of the father is measured in such activities as their personal care activities, household activities, child care, occupation and educational activities as well as social and community activities.

The IFS-F contains 51 items and is self-administered; many of the items ask for a response on a 4-point scale. A helpful aspect of this paper is that some of the items are given as an appendix. Content validity was judged using Popham's (1978) criteria and expectant and new fathers acted as judges for content validity by comparing the items on each subscale with the definition of that subscale. For the ante-partum section an 82% congruency was achieved; for the post-partum section this rose to 86%.

Internal consistency was tested to check reliability by involving 125 expectant fathers and 57 new fathers. The final IFS-F scale contained 51 items. Correlation was assessed using Fisher's z. The correlations between each subscale ranged from 0.54 for household activities to 0.75 for social and community activities. Correlation was also carried out for each subscale with the total IFS-F score. Correlations ranged from 0.31 for the subscale Social and Community Activities, to 0.61 for the subscale Child Care Activities. This shows that although the social and community subscale was internally consistent, it had only a low consistency with the scale as a whole. The researchers felt these levels to be satisfactory.

Construct validity of the scale was also undertaken by using Pearson's correlations between the subscales. It was expected that the correlations would be low, as each of the subscales was theoretically independent. As expected most of the correlations were low, ranging from –0.02 to 0.3; however, two subscales correlated highly – household activities and child care activities – and it was therefore assumed that these two scales were, to a certain extent, dependent on each other. The researchers were again satisfied with this level of validity, as they noted from Weiss (1991) that child care and household activities loaded onto a single factor when factor analysed.

Due to the rigorous nature of testing, the authors were confident that the scale tested the domains of primary, secondary and tertiary role activities of the functional status of the men sampled at this stage in their lives. However, the researchers do recognize the potential difference between what people say they do, in response to a questionnaire, and what they actually do in a situation. Tulman, Fawcett and Weiss therefore recommend that observation might be conducted and compared with the results from the questionnaires. This enhances the quality of any research where views of respondents are sought.

As with their other papers, this study is driven by the model and therefore the findings support the model in this setting. This is a descriptive study, so there is no attempt to link the assessment of the fathers' role function with planning or with implementation or evaluation of the effectiveness of the role.

The commonsense reasoning of the fathers is evidently problematized by the use of the model. The Inventory can be used anywhere, however an instrument based on a questionnaire format implies that it is usually administered in a wide variety of situations and, if it is a self-administered questionnaire, there is no advantage to be gained from this being completed in the environment on which the questions are based.

EVALUATION OF THE LEVEL OF ADAPTATION

There has been a single paper published in this section since 1990. It compares the effects of giving information about Caesarean births to two groups of mothers. The difference between the groups was the depth and extent of information given to them.

THE EFFECTS OF GIVING INFORMATION ON ADAPTATION TO CAESAREAN BIRTHS

Fawcett et al. (1993) compared giving information at antenatal birth preparation classes in two different ways. One group (the experimental group) had comprehensive Caesarean birth information, while the second group (the control group) comprised women who attended the traditional childbirth preparation classes, and received limited information about a Caesarean birth. A number of outcomes for the mothers were investigated. The four modes of adaptation to Caesarean birth were used: the physiological mode included pain and physical distress; the self-concept mode included self-esteem; the role function mode included functional status; and the interdependence mode included feelings about the baby and changes in the marital relationship. Adaptation was assessed through perception of the birth experience. The contextual stimulus was nursing intervention through the experimental and control groups. The focal stimulus was the Caesarean birth.

A total of 122 women agreed to take part in the study; 74 were allocated to the experimental group and 48 to the control group. Teaching of each group took place in separate hospitals so that contamination would be less likely. The experimental group parents received a guide to Caesarean births which contained detailed information on the procedure, the sensations and how to cope with them from labour through to the post-partum. This group were also involved in discussion about Caesarean births during classes. The control group received the standard childbirth preparation which included factual information on what a Caesarean is and the reasons for it as well as how it is carried out.

Following the birth all the Caesarean birth mothers were given seven different scales to complete at different times. Within the first 2 days of delivery, while the mothers were still in hospital, they were given the Perception of Birth Scale, the Pain Intensity Scale and the Distress Scale. At the sixth week post-partum all mothers received, through the post, the Pain Intensity Scale, the Distress Scale, the Self-Esteem Scale, the Inventory of Functional Status After Childbirth, the Feelings about the Baby Scale, the Relationship Change Scale and a background data sheet. Of the total number of women in the study, 106 (87%) completed the scales during the first 2 days post-partum. However, after 6 weeks the number of respondents had dropped to 88 (72%) despite personal contacts, follow-up telephone calls and reminders sent through the post. Attrition rates were higher for the control group women than for the experimental group women.

From the analysis of the scales there was found to be no support for a difference in the perception of the birth between the experimental and the control group ($p = 0.055$). There was also no statistical difference between the two groups on pain intensity or on physical distress. However, pain intensity was different for women in the experimental group who reported no change over the 6 weeks, whereas the control group mothers reported a decline in pain. Other findings show that the groups of women did not differ in their self-esteem, their functional status, their feelings about the baby or in changes in the quality of their marital relationships.

However, although the response rate was good, the number of scales sent to the mothers was very large. One wonders if they were filled in as diligently as they might have been, particularly as they were sent to the mothers' homes.

This paper is quite a challenge to Roy's model. According to Fawcett *et al.*, Roy's model says that manipulation of the contextual stimuli leads to adaptation. Therefore it could be assumed that giving more teaching to one group of women than to another, as a deliberate ploy to manipulate the contextual stimuli, would lead to differences between the groups. However, the findings do not support this, as there were no significant differences between the groups at 6 weeks post-partum. As Fawcett *et al.*

say, this raises the question of the credibility of the model, as manipulation of the stimuli with these two groups of women did not lead to a different outcome. An alternative interpretation could be that the level of teaching to both groups was not sufficiently different, which is suggested by Fawcett. However, this study does not allow us to tease out which is causing the problem – the research design or the model.

CONCLUSIONS ON THE USE OF THE MODEL FROM ITS DEVELOPMENT TO 1995

Between 1990 and 1994 continued work on the development of Roy's model has taken place, with the publication of practice-based research using the model. Another development is that published research from countries outside North America has started to appear, for example the study by Nyqvist and Sjoden (1993) from Sweden. Therefore there is evidence that this model is starting to be used in other cultural settings.

The use of the model to guide research in the practice of nursing has been enhanced by Fawcett and Tulman's claims to be basing their research programme on Roy's model. In most of their research the model has credibility, as they are able to show that their findings are in line with the model's assumptions. But when it comes to evaluating the effectiveness of teaching as a nursing intervention, results suggest that there is no difference between in-depth teaching and more superficial teaching of mothers about Caesarean birth and the effects that this has on the mothers.

Therefore to date the use of Roy's model has been in all the four areas of identification, planning, intervention and evaluation. I will now summarize the knowledge that has been created so far in each of these areas and how this relates to the model. I will then assess how the model stands up to this level of testing in practice and the implications of this.

Investigations that identify adaptive and maladaptive behaviours have shown the following.

- The perceived abilities of the elderly to adapt. Those who lived alone were compared with those who had made application for residence in a nursing home. Both the elderly and their significant others were assessed for the elderly person's abilities to adapt. Maladaptation was found to be greater in those applying for nursing home residence and their significant others, than in the elderly not applying for such residence.
- Maladaptation was found in all four modes in identifying the behaviours of patients with arterial occlusion before surgery. In this type of progressive disease it is possible that many of the patients' abilities to adapt have already been used up.

- The behaviour changes that occur in patients with a right hemispheric lesion are identified from the literature. A small group of patients verified this. However, the use of Roy's model in helping to identify adaptation and maladaptation is less clear for these patients. It is also unclear how identification of the focal, contextual and residual stimuli can take place, due to patient denial and disorganized coping as a result of the condition. Therefore this model is less efficient than some others when used with these patients.
- Adaptation to infection through a raised temperature. Adaptation is identified mainly in the physiological mode.
- Identifying the adaptations by parents to Caesarean births. Adaptation or maladaptation were identified in all the four adaptive modes where the focal, contextual and residual stimuli are clearly seen.
- Identifying the maladaptations of mothers, babies, fathers and nurses to breastfeeding in an NICU in Sweden.
- The development of an instrument to measure the functional status of fathers following their partner's Caesarean section.

Therefore Roy's model has the potential to be able to identify adaptive and maladaptive behaviours in many situations with both ill and well people. However, where the patient is less than rational or has a recent behaviour change, such as in a right hemispheric lesion, the model is less well able to be used by nurses to make an assessment.

The Roy model's ability to plan in helping patients to adapt by manipulating the stimuli has been used in one study. Adaptation to three chronic conditions was studied, i.e. diabetes, hypertension and rheumatoid arthritis. The levels of adaptation were measured using scales designed for the study. Results failed to show a correlation between hardiness, the residual stimulus, and the patients' abilities to adapt in rheumatoid arthritis and hypertension. Therefore in this study manipulation of the stimuli was felt to be a difficulty in helping patients to adapt to their conditions.

Therefore, from the one study conducted in planning to help people with chronic conditions to adapt, the Roy model has been found to be ineffective at present.

In the area of providing care there has been a series of three papers all produced by the same authors. Provision of care according to Roy's model helps the person to adapt to the stimuli. This has been investigated in the effects of the birth chair in the second stage of delivery of a baby. In these studies the position of the mother was the contextual stimulus which, it was felt by the researchers,was appropriate to manipulate. Manipulation of the angle of the birth chair was found to make a significant difference to the baby. However, the mother was found to have increased perineal swelling when compared with those mothers delivered on the delivery table.

From these three studies we can see that manipulation of the contextual stimuli can have a considerable effect in a number of different directions. These studies not only add credibility to the model but also give useful advice to those carrying out care as to how to be most effective.

Evaluation of nursing care using Roy's model has only been studied systematically in one published work. This showed the effects of manipulating the stimuli through teaching; mothers who received greater and more focused teaching to prepare them for a Caesarean birth showed either no differences or differences in the opposite direction in pain intensity following the birth when compared with mothers who had received routine teaching.

This study throws doubt on the link between nursing intervention and evaluation using teaching as a way of reducing maladaptation in these women. Therefore this stage of the Roy model is in doubt.

We can conclude from the published practice-based research studies that identification of adaptation in the four modes is appropriate and possible in many patient and client situations. Also appropriate and possible is identification of maladaptation along with identification of the influencing stimuli. However, from here through planning, provision and evaluation of nursing there are many difficulties to be overcome. Some of these difficulties were overcome by persistence in the case of the three studies investigating the angle of the birth chair, but other studies, such as investigating the adaptation of people with chronic conditions, have been less successful in showing the usefulness of the model. Therefore, at present the model provides more questions than answers in its ability to interact with nursing in an effective way.

Despite these various difficulties for the model, it is becoming more widely known as a guide to research in practice in an international context.

REFERENCES

Andrews, H.A. and Roy, C. (1986) *Essentials of the Roy Adaptation Model*, Appleton-Century-Crofts, New York.

Atkins, E. and Bodel, P. (1972) Fever. *New England Journal of Medicine*, 286, 27–34.

Brobeck, J.R. (ed.) (1973) *Best and Taylor's Physiological Basis of Medical Practice*, 7th edn, Williams and Wilkins, Baltimore.

Carr, K.C. (1980) Obstetric practices which protect against neonatal morbidity: Focus on maternal position in labour and birth. *Birth and Family Journal*, 7, 249–54.

Cottrell, B.H. and Shannahan, M.D. (1986) Effect of the birth chair on duration of second stage labor and maternal outcome. *Nursing Research*, 35(6), 364–7.

Cottrell, B.H. and Shannahan, M.K. (1987) A comparison of fetal outcome in birth chair and delivery table births. *Research in Nursing and Health*, 10, 239–43.

Davis-Sharts, J. (1978) Mechanisms and manifestations of fever. *American Journal of Nursing*, November, 1874–7.

Derogatis, R. (1983) *Psychological Adjustment to Illness Survey. Administration, Scoring and Procedures Manual*, Clinical Psychometric Research, Baltimore.

Draper, P. (1993) A critique of Fawcett's conceptual models and nursing practice: the reciprocal relationship. *Journal of Advanced Nursing*, **18**, 558–64.

Farkas, L. (1981) Adaptation problems with nursing home application for elderly persons: an application of the Roy adaptation nursing model. *Journal of Advanced Nursing*, **6**, 363–8.

Fawcett, J. (1981) Needs of caesarean birth parents. *Journal of Obstetric, Gynaecologic and Neonatal Nursing*, **10**, 372–6.

Fawcett, J. (1990) Conceptual models and nursing practice: the reciprocal relationship. *Journal of Advanced Nursing*, **17**, 224–8.

Fawcett, J. and Tulman, L. (1990) Building a programme of research from the Roy Adaptation Model of Nursing. *Journal of Advanced Nursing*, **15**, 720–25.

Fawcett, J., Pollio, N., Tully, A. *et al.* (1993) Effects of information on adaptation to Caesarean birth. *Nursing Research*, **42**(1), 49–53.

Helson, H. (1964) *Adaptation Level Theory*, Harper and Row, New York.

Hollingshead, A.B. (1978) Four factor index of social status. Department of Sociology, Yale University (unpublished).

Kaplan DeNour, A. (1982) Social adjustment of chronic dialysis patients. *American Journal of Psychiatry*, **139**, 97–100.

Kobasa, S.C. (1979) Stressful life events, personality, and health: an inquiry into hardiness. *Journal of Personality and Social Psychology*, **37**(1), 1–11.

Leech, J.E. (1982) Psychosocial and physiological needs of patients with arterial occlusive disease during the preoperative phase of hospitalization. *Heart and Lung*, **11**(5), 442–9.

Miller, J.F. and Hellenbrand, D. (1981) An eclectic approach to practice. *American Journal of Nursing*, July, 1339–43.

Milton, A.S. (1976) Modern views on the pathogenesis of fever and the mode of action of antipyretic drugs. *Journal of Pharmacological Pharmacology*, **28** (Suppl. 4), 393–9.

Morrow, R., Chiarello, J. and Derogatis, R. (1978) A new scale for assessing patient's psychosocial adjustment to medical illness. *Psychological Medicine*, **8**, 605–10.

Norman, S. (1979) Diagnostic categories for the patient with a right hemisphere lesion. *American Journal of Nursing*, December, 2126–30.

Nyqvist, K.H. and Sjoden, P-O. (1993) Advice concerning breastfeeding from mothers of infants admitted to a neonatal intensive care unit: the Roy adaptation model as a conceptual structure. *Journal of Advanced Nursing*, **18**, 54–63.

Oppenheim, A.N. (1992) *Questionnaire Design, Interviewing and Attitude Measurement*, Pinter, London.

Pollock, S.E. (1986) Human response to chronic illness: physiologic and psychosocial adaptation. *Nursing Research*, **35**(2), 90–5.

Popham, W.J. (1978) *Criterion-referenced Measurement*, Prentice Hall, Englewood Cliffs, NJ.

Randell, B., Tedrow, M. and VanLandingham, J. (1982) *The Roy Conceptual Model Made Practical*, C.V. Mosby, St Louis.

Riehl, J.P. and Roy, C. (1977) *Conceptual Models for Nursing Practice*, Appleton-Century-Crofts, Norwalk, OH.

Riehl, J.P. and Roy, C. (1980) *Conceptual Models for Nursing Practice*, 2nd edn, Appleton-Century-Crofts, Norwalk, OH.

Roberts, J. (1980) Alternative positions for childbirth. Part 2: Second stage of labour. *Journal of Nurse-Midwifery*, **25**, 13–19.

Rosendorff, C. (1976) Neurochemistry of fever. *South African Journal of Medical Science*, 41–8.

Rotter, J.B. (1975) Some problems and misconceptions related to the construct of internal versus external locus of control of reinforcement. *Journal of Consulting and Clinical Psychology*, **43**, 56–67.

Roy, C. (1970) Adaptation: a conceptual framework for nursing. *Nursing Outlook*, **18**, 42–5.

Roy, C. (1971) Adaptation: a basis for nursing practice. *Nursing Outlook*, April, 154–7.

Roy, C. (1976) *Introduction to Nursing: An Adaptation Model*, Prentice Hall, Englewood Cliffs, NJ.

Roy, C. (1984) *Introduction to Nursing: An Adaptation Model*, 2nd edn, Prentice Hall, Englewood Cliffs, NJ.

Roy, S.C. and Andrew, H.A. (1991) *The Roy Adaptation Model. The Definitive Statement*, Appleton & Lange, Norwalk, CT.

Roy, C. and Roberts, S. (1981) *Theory Construction in Nursing: An Adaptation Model*, Prentice Hall, Englewood Cliffs, NJ.

Secord, P.F. and Jourard, S.M. (1953) The appraisal of body cathexis: body cathexis and the self. *Journal of Consulting Psychology*, **17**, 343.

Shannahan, M.D. and Cottrell, B.H. (1985) Effect of the birth chair on duration of second stage labor, fetal outcome, and maternal blood loss. *Nursing Research*, **34**(2), 89–92.

Silverman, D. (1993) *Interpreting Qualitative Data: Methods for Analysing Text, Talk and Interaction*, Sage, London.

Tulman, L. and Fawcett, J. (1988) Return of functional ability after childbirth. *Nursing Research*, **37**, 77–81.

Tulman, L., Fawcett, J. and Weiss, M. (1993) The inventory of functional status – fathers. Development and psychometric testing. *Journal of Nurse-Midwifery*, **38** (September/October), 276–82.

Tulman, L., Fawcett, J., Groblewski, L. and Silverman, L. (1990) Changes in functional status after childbirth. *Nursing Research*, **39**, 70–5.

Weiss, M. (1991) The relationship between marital interdependence and adaptation to parenthood in primiparous couples. *Dissertation Abstracts International*, **51**, 3783B.

FURTHER READING

Aggleton, P. and Chalmers, H. (1986) *Nursing Models and the Nursing Process*, Macmillan, London.

Chapman, C.M. (1985) *Theory of Nursing: Practical Application*, Harper and Row, London.

Chinn, P.L. and Jacobs, M.K. (1987) *Theory and Nursing*, C.V. Mosby, St Louis.

Duldt, B.W. and Giffin, K. (1985) *Theoretical Perspectives for Nursing*, Little Brown and Co., London.

Fawcett, J. (1984) *Analysis and Evaluation of Conceptual Models of Nursing*, F.A. Davis, Philadelphia.

Fitzpatrick, J.J. and Whall, A.L. (1983) *Conceptual Models of Nursing: Analysis and Application*, Prentice Hall, Englewood Cliffs, NJ.

George, J.B. (ed.) (1985) *Nursing Theories: A Basis for Professional Nursing Practice*, 2nd edn, Prentice Hall, Englewood Cliffs, NJ.

Griffith-Kennedy, J.W. and Christensen, P.J. (1986) *Nursing Process: Application of Theories, Frameworks and Models*, C.V. Mosby, St Louis.

Kershaw, B. and Salvage, J. (1986) *Models for Nursing*, John Wiley, Chichester.

Lutjens, L.R. (1991) *Callista Roy: An Adaptation Model*, Notes on Nursing Series, Sage, Newbury Park, CA.

Marriner, A. (1986) *Nursing Theorists and their Work*, C.V. Mosby, St Louis.

Parse, R.R. (1987) *Nursing Science*, W.B. Saunders, New York.

Rambo, B.J. (1984) *Adaptation Nursing: Assessment and Intervention*, W.B. Saunders, London.

Riehl, J.P. and Roy, C. (1980) *Conceptual Models for Nursing Practice*, 2nd edn, Appleton-Century-Crofts, Norwalk, OH.

Orem's model of self-care

4

Table of chapter contents

Orem's self-care model

Topic researched	Model components	Results
Self-care in diabetic patients	Assessment of therapeutic self-care demand	Literature search of physiological factors
Self-care in diabetic patients	Assessment of therapeutic self-care demand	Identification of patients' self-care demands
Self-care in children	Ability to self-care	Identification of self-care ability
Self-care in the elderly living at home	Assessment of therapeutic self-care demands	Identification of self-care demands
Self-care in Alzheimer-type dementia	Assessment of therapeutic self-care demand	Identification of self-care deficits
Teaching children to self-care	The nurse as educator/developer	Children can be taught to be responsible for their own health
Teaching patients following a myocardial infarction	The nurse as teacher	Inconclusive results of teaching on anxiety reduction
Teaching patients about their chemotherapy drugs	The nurse as teacher	Cancer patients can learn about their chemotherapy drugs
Teaching post-operative pulmonary patients	Teaching the patient to self-care	Patients can learn therapeutic activities, but do not stop harmful activities
Teaching and supporting hypertensive patients	The nurse as teacher and supporter	Literature search of issues and problems
Teaching elderly patients	The nurse as teacher	Factors in the nurse affecting patient compliance
Teaching self-care in the mentally ill:	The nurse as teacher	Improvement in social competence only

Topic researched	Model components	Results
1. Social dramatics		
2. Behaviour modification	The nurse as teacher/ guider	Improvements in self-care
Nursing action to support	The nurse as supporter	Literature search
Quality of care for the elderly	Assessment of Sisters as self-care agents; assessment of patients' self-care ability	Link between Sisters' self-care agency and patients' self-care ability
Quality of care in the community	Assessment of nurses' self-care agency through documentation	Inconclusive results
The nurse as a self-care agent in breast self-examination	The nurse as a self-care agent	Nurses need to become self-care agents
Translating a self-care assessment tool into Norwegian	Assessment of self-care agency	Tool valid and reliable in Norwegian
Translating a self-care assessment tool into Dutch	Assessment of self-care agency	Tool valid and reliable in Dutch
Assessment of self-care abilities and deficits in patients with mitral valve prolapse	Assessment through to nursing intervention	Self-care deficits and changes in body structure and function found. Nursing inter-vention discussed
The fit of nursing in China with Orem's model	Philosophy of Orem's model	The completeness, practicality and feasibility of introducing Orem's model to a Chinese culture considered
Self-care behaviours in patients with cancer undergoing chemotherapy	Self-care deficits	Nausea, vomiting and tiredness are frequent amongst these patients

THE AUTHOR

Dorothea Orem graduated in 1939 with a BSc in Nursing, and obtained a Master's degree in Nursing Science in 1945, both from the Catholic University of America. From 1945 to 1948 she was Director of the Providence Hospital School of Nursing in Detroit and Director of the Nursing Service in this hospital. From 1949 to 1957 she was a Nurse Consultant to the Division of Health and Institutional Service, Indiana State Board of Health; from 1957 to 1960 she was the Curriculum

Consultant in the Office of Education, United States Department of Health, Education and Welfare in Washington, DC.

From 1959 to 1970 she held the post of Assistant Professor of Nursing Education at the Catholic University of America. During this time she also served as Acting Dean of the School of Nursing, and as Associate Professor. In 1970 she resigned her post to set up the consulting firm of Orem and Shields.

THE MODEL

The development of Orem's model began in 1973 with the setting up of the Nursing Development Conference Group of which Dorothea Orem was the Chairperson. Various volumes of her model have been published (Orem, 1971, 1980, 1985), the second edition being the most frequently cited. Practice-based research using the model also started to gather momentum following this publication. A brief description of the model follows, with an indication of the changes that have occurred with the publication of further volumes.

SUMMARY OF THE OREM MODEL OF SELF-CARE

The basic premise of Orem's first edition (1971) is stated at the beginning of her first chapter:

> Nursing has as its special concern man's need for self-care action and the provision and management of it on a continuous basis in order to sustain life and health, recover from disease or injury, and cope with their effects.

> (pp. 1–2)

The individual sustains his or her own health through their own ability to do so; this involves actions which are based on ability and skills to be able to start and to sustain self-care, the knowledge and understanding of these actions and how they relate to health and disease. The individual's ability for self-care will depend on his or her level of maturity, depth of knowledge, life experiences, thought patterns and bodily, as well as mental, health state. This is what Orem describes as the therapeutic self-care demand.

Orem identifies two kinds of therapeutic self-care demand categories. The first is **universal self-care**, i.e. the action an individual will take in order to maintain basic human needs, which consist of six subcategories.

- Air, food and water: these are vital to the continuation of life, growth, development and repair of body tissue.
- Excretion: as life continues the body processes food and oxygen and produces waste materials that need to be excreted.

- Activity and rest: certain levels of activity and rest are required for optimal functioning.
- Solitude and social interaction: normal human development requires periods of both being alone and being with others.
- Hazards to life and well-being: avoidance of situations or conditions which threaten or endanger life or well-being of the individual or of the group.
- Being normal: the effort by the individual to conform to what is currently considered to be normal, in lifestyle and cultural beliefs and practices. The ability of the individual to carry these out will depend on age, developmental state, life experience, sociocultural orientation, state of health and the individual's available resources.

The second therapeutic self-care demand category identified by Orem is **health deviation self-care**; this is when changes occur to the individual in his or her body structure, physical functioning, changes in behaviour or changes in activities of daily living. As a result of one or more of these the individual will make added demands. Health deviation may be one of two forms: derived from disease or injury; or derived from medical intervention, such as surgical procedures.

Therefore when there is a self-care deviation, either the individual will be able to make up for the extra amount of self-care needed or, if unable to do this, some kind of intervention will be necessary; this is where the role of the nurse is indicated. The individual's ability to carry out his or her own self-care depends on the amount of knowledge, skills, motivation and orientation he or she possesses. As Orem (1971) says:

> Available resources may affect the use of self-care techniques. Interests and motives are also determining factors. Individuals and families may adapt themselves to chronic ill health rather than learn about therapeutic measures of care.
>
> (pp. 19–20)

When an individual is unable to carry out self-care the intervention of the nurse will be to compensate wholly for the self-care deficit; to compensate partly for some part of the self-care deficit; or to educate and develop the patient in order for him or her to achieve self-care. Therefore the patient must be willing to come to terms with illness or disability and be willing to improve the condition or he or she will be an ineffective patient.

Orem used the nursing process with her model, organized around the following.

- Determining why the person needs nursing – assessing the therapeutic self-care demand, the ability of the person to self-care now and in the future, and the deficit of the person to self-care in relation to their self-care demands.

- Nursing intervention should then be planned around the therapeutic self-care demand, which will include the patient's abilities to self-care, and the role of the nurse as wholly compensatory, partly compensatory or educative/developmental.
- The nurse carries out this plan according to the five identified self-care requirements and limitations of the individual: acting for; teaching; guiding; supporting; and encouraging development.

In the second edition of her model Orem (1980) restates the need for nursing adults as:

> the absence of the ability to maintain continuously that amount and quality of self-care which is therapeutic in sustaining life and health, in recovering from disease or injury, or in coping with their effects. With children, the condition remains as the inability of the parent (or guardian) to maintain continuously for the child the amount and quality of care that is therapeutic.
>
> (p. 7)

Nursing, therefore, remains as a complementary relationship to the patient.

In this edition the model has not changed in its essential features, but the explanation of the assumptions of the model have been strengthened. Also the term 'self-care requirement' has now become 'self-care requisite' as Orem feels this more clearly specifies the nature of the concept.

Increased emphasis is given to self-care action being either internal or external. Self-care action can be detected by observation or by questioning. External self-care actions are knowledge seeking, assistance and resource seeking, expressive interpersonal factors and control of external factors. Internal self-care actions are resources used to control internal processes and thoughts and feelings to regulate internal factors.

In her third edition Orem (1985) states the difference from previous editions as being ' ... better organisation and continued development of the subject matter ... ' (p. vii). Again, essentially there is no change in the model. Two minor amendments are in the analysis of self-care agency (p. 124), and in the technologies used in nursing which are now organized as two categories, rather than eight factors, although they remain essentially unchanged (p. 146).

A fourth edition of Orem's model was published in 1991. Again there is essentially no change in the model, it is merely further refined. However, the use of language is no clearer than in previous editions, which has been a constant criticism of Orem's writing. Take for example the following sentence in one of her chapters called 'A general theory':

'Insights when formulated as concepts and expressed verbally or in writing constitute static representations of situational features and relationships' (p. 57). The majority of the book is written in this style. This does not encourage the general reader of nursing, who finds the concept of self-care important, to read on. However, it is not only the use of language that seems to be a problem, it is also the writing style. Take another example from the same chapter when Orem talks about the central idea of her theory:

> Within the context of day-to-day living in social groups and their time–place localization, mature and maturing persons perform learned actions and sequences of actions directed toward themselves or toward environmental features known or assumed to meet identified requisites for controlling factors that either promote or adversely affect or interfere with ongoing regulation of their functioning or development in order to contribute to continuance of life, self-maintenance, and personal health and well-being.
>
> (p. 69)

All this is one sentence. It is perhaps no wonder then that some students of nursing feel they have to try to use this sort of language in their written work. Could we make a plea for plain, well-written English for this important work?

To date research based on this model has had two major themes: to investigate the types of self-care problems (or 'deficits') that different patient groups will seek nursing help to alleviate; and to investigate the effectiveness of the nurse as an educator of different patient groups. This second theme explores Orem's method by which nurses aid patients in acquiring or maintaining self-care abilities through giving knowledge of health behaviours. Therefore different methods of providing patients with knowledge, and assessing compliance with that knowledge, become the crucial issues here.

This chapter contains sections which investigate the identification of patients' problems of self-care and nursing action in attempting to promote self-care where deficits exist. Two other sections have been devised where research into particular aspects of nursing based on Orem's model have been undertaken: assessment of quality, and the nurse as a potential self-care practitioner who could stimulate health care behaviours in patients. The papers in both sections have elements that overlap, but they deal predominantly with issues pertaining to the section in which they are situated.

IDENTIFICATION OF SELF-CARE REQUISITES AND DEFICITS

Some types of health problems lend themselves more easily to self-care than others. Diabetes is one of these, therefore it is no great surprise to find studies which assess diabetic patients' abilities to self-care.

SELF-CARE IN DIABETIC PATIENTS

Studies of self-care deficits of diabetic patients form the basis of two studies. The first is a review of the literature, the second is an empirical study.

Donohue-Porter (1985), although not conducting her own research into the problems faced by diabetics, has summarized from the literature the nature of the patients' difficulties. She has also given advice on how the patients should deal with these problems. She states that infections of varying kinds in various sites are due to a number of different organisms. Infections are identified as the main health problem associated with diabetes.

- Where vulval or vaginal fungal infections occur in women, she suggests that patients should be taught careful reporting of symptoms and self-management of perineal hygiene, and to give accurate self-medication and avoid harsh douches.
- Immunization against influenza has been recommended for diabetic patients (Schoenbaum, 1982), particularly in view of the chronic nature of diabetes contributing to increased morbidity and mortality from influenza.
- Diabetics are predisposed to staphyloccocal colonization of the skin and nasopharynx, so good skin hygiene should be taught. Evidence does not show that diabetics are more prone to boils and carbuncles than non-diabetics (Wheat, 1980).
- Foot infections are one of the most common problems for diabetics and can frequently lead to amputation. As neuropathy will reduce or eliminate sensation, injury may result in an infection. Donohue-Porter suggests patient teaching should be directed towards: (i) daily examination of the feet, and she recommends that they should not be exposed to heat; (ii) wearing comfortable shoes and avoiding being barefoot; (iii) regular visits to the doctor and chiropodist; (iv) not puncturing the skin of the feet by attempting to correct minor ailments such as corns and callouses; (v) going to the doctor immediately if pain, redness or a feeling of warmth is experienced in the feet.
- Dental disease is high in diabetic patients: peridontal disease has been found to correlate positively with the duration of diabetes, the presence of complications and blood glucose levels above 200 mg/dl (Finestone and Boorujy, 1967). Donohue-Porter suggests that preventive dental care should be stressed to diabetic patients as well as the importance of regular dental check-ups.

From research studies Donohue-Porter suggests that the efforts of health care workers in the treatment of diabetic patients are directed towards reduction of hyperglycaemia. Avoiding hyperglycaemia has been shown to help minimize vascular and neurological complications. Maintaining normal glucose levels can be achieved by teaching patients to use blood glucose monitoring at home. They should be taught to take capillary blood from their fingertips, having previously washed their hands thoroughly with soap and water. Infection of these sites has been found to be a problem (Skyler, 1982). Another method is through a continuous subcutaneous insulin infusion system. Infection and abscess formation at the needle site have caused problems with this method. Avoidance is by hygiene involving thorough handwashing before the pump equipment is handled, and using 70% isopropyl alcohol as an antiseptic to prepare the insertion site. The needle should be secured with tape and covered with a sterile dressing. Donohue-Porter recommends changing the infusion site at least every 48–72 hours, and inspecting it daily, particularly in the case of unexplained fever, tenderness or pain at the site. In pregnant women, the complications of serious infection must be eliminated; Rivera-Alsina and Willis (1984) suggest that the use of povidine-iodine solution after isopropyl alcohol will reduce the risk of infection at the insertion site.

In addition to these areas, Donohue-Porter suggests that nurses should teach diabetic patients self-care, mainly of the skin. What is important is the use of mild soaps, complete drying of all skin folds, and the use of creams to prevent overdrying. Patients should report problems to their general practitioner. Patients should also be instructed how to handle their 'sick days', by:

- calling the doctor in cases of fever, infections, diarrhoea and/or vomiting;
- perhaps taking more insulin than usual;
- monitoring blood glucose levels at least every 4 hours;
- resting and drinking fluids (if unable to eat then drinking high carbohydrate fluids);
- in the case of persistent vomiting, when it is not possible to get to the general practitioner, going to the accident and emergency department of the local hospital.

Donohue-Porter advises that patients must realize the importance of keeping blood sugar levels as close to normal as possible, by self-monitoring blood glucose and by knowing its relationship to diet and exercise.

This paper gives a comprehensive account of possible self-care deficits of diabetics and the underlying causes of most of these. The health deviations of diabetics are seen to arise from the changes in the structure of the pancreas, where insulin is secreted, which causes changes in physical functioning, such as infections as a direct result of diabetes or medically induced, due to using equipment such as continuous infusion systems, and hyperglycaemia, which may eventually cause vascular and neurological changes and problems in body structure. Donohue-Porter recommends appropriate activity on the part of the patient to cope with these various deficits, and also suggests where the limits of the patient's self-care agency are reached and when medical advice should be sought.

The second study is empirical; it was carried out in an American diabetic clinic by Miller (1982). She aimed to assess the self-care needs and deficits of ambulatory patients with diabetes who visited the clinic periodically. The sample size was 65 patients, age range 22–85 years, 42 of whom were from a lower socio-economic group and 23 from a middle socio-economic group. Data were obtained from the patients through both a questionnaire and observation.

An initial visit by patients to the clinic involved the use of a tool by the researcher to assess the patients' and families' strengths and abilities to achieve their current state of health. The tool assessed several areas: growth and development; self-concept; normal health practices using Orem's (1980) universal self-care requisites; level of motivation and understanding; the functioning of the family; resource utilization and problem-solving ability; life change units in relation to stress during the last year; coping strategies; role mastery; and locus of control. Use of the tool involves questioning the patient and can be seen to involve both the patient's internal and external abilities.

At subsequent visits by the patients to the clinic, data collection was by participant observation. Data were concerned with the extent of demands on the individual due to his or her state of health, and the ability to meet these demands. The use of questioning and observation fulfils both of Orem's methods by which a nurse should obtain information.

The methodology used to group the self-care requisites was that of Glaser and Strauss (1967) and Stern (1980). Using this methodology 10 categories of self-care needs were identified; no new categories were found and each category had many examples. The categories identified were as follows.

- Acquiring skills to care for oneself. This included the patient's understanding of the diagnosis and the skills required in caring for themselves and managing their care, for example diet, insulin, injection technique, exercise, urine testing and hygiene. Miller found that deficits in self-care by patients were due to lack of knowledge, especially of dietary intake, and inability to monitor the signs of hypoglycaemia or hyperglycaemia, to examine the condition of the skin and to detect urinary tract infections. Lack of knowledge also meant that patients did not know which problems could be dealt with by themselves and which needed professional help.

- Patients needed to receive feedback on their self-care management after this had been learned. This was given by the nurse in the form of interpretation of laboratory results and weight checks. The most frequent deficits concerned diet, and included: the patient's definition of good mothering involving giving large amounts of food to her family; inability to make food exchanges particularly with some specific foods; and the definition by some ethnic minority women of obesity as being sexually attractive and keeping them healthy. The nurse found it necessary to review food intake with patients in terms of type, amount and mood states when eating, and also the types of reinforcers used by patients. Patients' problem-solving strategies when hypoglycaemic were also evaluated.

- Patients needed help to discover their abilities and coping strategies in order to self-care in such areas as socializing ability, having a supportive family, religious beliefs and the ability to get a new job. Their internal resources needed to be discovered and used in creative activities, as a form of emotion release. Financial planning was often found to be a problem with this group, who could only afford insufficient and inadequate food. Leisure time as a resource was discussed with the patients who were encouraged to develop positive use of their time.

- While coming to terms with being a diabetic, feelings of self-esteem were challenged, sometimes due to loss of a job, a decrease in energy socially, or inability to travel or be involved in sporting activities. Patients needed help in overcoming these changes and acquiring new and useful activities or development of existing activities.

- Patients experienced grieving over losses such as physical functioning, eyesight, etc., and frustration with the chronic nature of the disease. Some needed to share resentment and anger, others to receive encouragement to continue with the self-care routine.

- Patients needed help to continue to evaluate their health care through monitoring their vital signs and physical examination. New concerns, such as vaginal itching and perineal abscesses, were shared with the nurse. Patients were also helped to inform the doctors of deficits that needed medical help.

- Patients needed help to alleviate physical discomforts such as pain, in preventing muscular atrophy, in identifying signs of hypoglycaemia, in improving hygiene and in decreasing the pain from abscesses. They also needed to alleviate mental worries such as those causing insomnia and fears that had arisen due to diabetic problems that affected friends and acquaintances and caused renewed anxiety to the patients. They also needed to discuss the relationship between mood and blood sugar levels.

- Services from other agencies were requested and consulted, for example dietitians, social services and pharmacists.
- Patients were encouraged to comment on health care services and to feel that they could alter the service accordingly. Help was also needed to encourage patients to consider their goals for each visit to the clinic.
- Self-care needs were also in the maintenance of family solidarity, particularly in the light of problems such as adolescent non-adherence to diet and insulin regimen. Patients in such cases needed help in balancing dependence and independence.

Miller accepts that the needs and deficits identified by her may be those from a predominantly lower socio-economic class, and a wider range may demonstrate other needs. She also states that these needs could be relevant to all ambulatory patients with chronic health problems.

This article shows the self-care requisites and deficits of these patients very clearly. However, there is no analysis of the motivation to be self-caring, therefore one is left wondering whether the nurse is encouraging a dependent role, rather than encouraging self-care. However, the internal and external resources of the patients and their relatives appear to receive a thorough analysis using Orem's model as a basis. Therefore this study fills some of the gaps left by Donohue-Porter's review of the literature.

The research method is clearly useful for this type of analysis, but the author gives no consideration to reactivity, therefore her effect on the patients she observes and interviews is not considered. Also no direct quotations from conversations are given, leaving the reader with the researcher's interpretation but without evidence. However, this may be because of the specified length of the article to meet journal requirements.

Although the first of these papers, by Donohue-Porter, discusses diabetic patients' self-care deficits and the nurse's role in teaching the patient to overcome these, it is based on a literature search. Therefore we are not able to assess the effectiveness of this teaching on patients with diabetes. However, the literature search is very thorough, so would form the basis of a good empirical study.

The second study, by Miller, is a descriptive study. It collects data from diabetic patients who attend a clinic. Therefore the study is theory led. While the data are gathered by different methods, there is no attempt to link patients' self-care deficits, of which there are plenty, with planning or nursing actions to promote self-care. Orem's model is clearly relevant for identification of these patients' self-care deficits, but we do not know from this study how adequately it will deal with helping these patients to become more self-caring.

Both these studies were conducted in the USA.

SELF-CARE IN CHILDREN

Other studies in this section investigate a wide variety of self-care abilities
and deficits. Some of them, as the following study shows, look at the
potential for self-care in children, showing the level of understanding of
self-care in young children and the influence of parents in promoting children's self-care.

Lasky and Eichelberger (1985) investigated the views and self-care
behaviours of young children, the major questions of the research being:

- what is the extent of the concepts of health in children aged 4–6 years;
- what are their self-care practices;
- what is their level of dependence or independence in decisions and
  actions about self-care?

The sample was 75 children from 3½ to 12 years from separate families:
there were 40 girls and 35 boys. Their mean age was 4 years 11 months
and their mean mental age was 6 years 11 months. The socio-economic
levels of the families ranged from semiskilled to professional. The
researchers suggest that this was possibly not a representative sample as
there was a high level of education due to the two major employers being
a university and the state government.

The method used was to visit the families at home on two occasions.
On the first occasion the child was given a Peabody Picture Vocabulary
test (Dunn, 1965); at the second visit the children were asked to respond
to health vignettes showing children eating vegetables, exercising and
cleaning their teeth. Parents were also interviewed about how they
encouraged health activities in their children.

The children were asked to view the vignettes, which were described
by the researcher, then asked if this activity would make them healthy. A
subsequent question asked these children what was the best reason that
the activity kept them healthy; additional prompts of asking for a guess
were given if necessary.

Ten self-care items were chosen by the researcher with reference to
developmental literature. Each of them was divided into decision and
action. Parents were asked to rate each item according to whether the
activity was child-initiated and performed independently, or if it was a
shared decision and carried out between the child and the parents.

Results from viewing the vignettes showed that the majority of children (67%) had an understanding of health: 65% gave a sensible answer
to why they should eat vegetables; 53% were able to give a reasonable
answer to why exercise keeps one healthy; and 83% were able to say why
cleaning their teeth keeps them healthy.

Regarding parental responses to reasons for their children carrying out
these activities, 152 responses concerning eating vegetables were given

with 47% of parents giving two reasons, mostly related to healthy body growth and to balanced nutrition. Parents gave 160 reasons for exercising, the most frequent being health promotion and illness prevention. Generally similar reasons were given for cleaning teeth.

Results showed that young children can indeed understand health promotion and how this relates to their own behaviours. They were frequently able to manage toileting independently, but managed combing their hair least well; eating activities and handwashing were the most shared activities between parents and children.

This study shows the level of knowledge of self-care agency and dependence of children. It also shows the beliefs and attitudes of the parents about healthy behaviours and how these may influence the children. However, what is not shown is the extent of the children's knowledge gained from outside the home, for example from school. The study was conducted in the USA; it could usefully be replicated in Great Britain.

This study is not based directly on Orem's model, although the method and results help to develop her model. The results also do not deny that Orem's model is useful for understanding these children's behaviours. The study is descriptive, as we understand better from it how these children view health behaviours and how they are helped to carry them out. We also are given evidence of which behaviours they are able to carry out for themselves and which they need help with at these ages.

SELF-CARE IN THE ELDERLY

At the opposite end of the age spectrum, one study using an action research approach investigated the type of problems faced by the elderly living independently. It also looked at how the nurse can promote self-care in such a situation.

Neufeld and Hobbs (1985) investigated self-care abilities in the elderly in a high-rise block. The study was conducted in a small prairie city in Canada with a population of which 9.6% were over the age of 65 years.

The high-rise building accommodates the well elderly, and the aim of the residents and administrators is to promote independence. It houses 223 residents of whom 195 are women and 28 are men, with a mean age of 80 years. There is an attached nursing home and a range of support services including provision of meals and specialist advice. The authors set up a health counselling service and informed all residents by letter of the opportunity to discuss specific health issues with a registered nurse. Half-day sessions were set up which, over 18 months, were attended by 26.4% of the residents, the majority on only one occasion.

Self-care concerns brought by the residents included: requests to check blood pressure (the most frequent); problems of stress related to moving house; isolation; difficulty in getting glasses that fit well and hearing aids; dental and foot problems. The authors suggest that the frequent requests for blood pressure recordings were due to the public concern over hypertension; also taking blood pressure is consistent with the public image of the nurse. This may also indicate an appropriate initial response to the letter from the researchers which is 'safe' and allows for further matters to be raised.

In some instances the stress related to moving house was associated with bereavement, i.e. death of a spouse, which made the move necessary. Homogeneity of the residents centred around church membership, which also made for isolation causing stress amongst those who were not church members.

Some of the other issues relating to self-care requisites were: diet, in cases of constipation, or to achieve weight loss; help to improve mobility; isolation; and the need for aids to prevent falls. Other concerns were bereavement and anticipatory grieving, or the death of another resident which was a frequent occurrence in this age group.

Questions relating to taking medications also arose. Teaching the residents about drug regimens, the actions and interactions and side effects of drugs was needed and was given by the nurse.

Self-care concerns were in the nature of coping with chronic diseases such as diabetes, arthritis and cardiovascular problems, confusion, accidents at home, depression and hopelessness. Patients also requested help with information on discharge from hospital, on making the best of visits to the doctor and for skin problems.

The researchers initiated patient teaching in one-to-one and group situations and although no formal evaluation had been conducted, they claim effectiveness due to the residents continuing to attend and to refer others. However, 26.4% attending in 18 months is not a very high level of attendance.

This study is based on Orem's model, as was the service to the elderly people. It shows that Orem's model is effective in identifying self-care agency in the group of elderly people and that all the universal self-care requisites are appropriate for identifying the abilities and needs of this group, however it does not show whether these are internal or external. The study also shows where self-care deficits exist or have the potential to exist, but the authors do not comment on the usefulness of the model, nor where its limitations lay. Therefore problematization of the model with these patients was not evident.

The research design, i.e. action research, allowed us to see how the identification of self-care agency and deficits could be developed into nursing interventions. However, as the model was not problematized, the level of success of nursing interventions is not known from the paper.

Action research can give some valuable results, as these authors have shown; however, the problems found in North America, although suggestive of general problems of self-care in this age group, would probably have a different emphasis if investigated in Great Britain, due to the differences in health care provision and culture. A formal evaluation which involved the users' responses would also give valuable information.

SELF-CARE IN DEMENTIA

A study that assesses the abilities of patients with Alzheimer's disease forms part of this section on assessment of the individual to self-care. It shows the effect of progress of the disease on the ability to self-care and also how this ability will vary from day to day. It also shows the influence that the nurse has on the patients' abilities to self-care. Moreover, this study, conducted in Sweden, shows the acceptability of Orem's model outside North America.

Sandman *et al.* (1986) investigated the self-care deficits in the ability of patients with Alzheimer's disease to carry out morning care. The study considered the concrete problems associated with performing morning care by these patients, which involved not only a series of actions, but also how these actions were combined, or not, into a meaningful series of activities. Morning care was seen to consist of washing, showering, combing hair, brushing teeth, shaving and dressing.

The assumptions of the study are that the nurse will compensate for the patient's deficits in performing morning care, but that care should be as independent as possible. Orem's framework was used to guide analysis of the behaviours of the patient and the nurse during morning care.

Five hospitalized patients were included in the study, two men and three women, aged 54–76 years. The patients represented different stages of the disease, from ambulatory to totally dependent; none was orientated in time or place.

Four observers watched the procedures of morning care using an unstructured technique on six occasions for each patient. Two independent observers collected the data. Analysis was through categorization using the method developed by Glaser (1978). From this 10 categories were developed describing the self-care abilities of the patients.

- Motivation to participate in and perform the actions – this was shown by the patients' abilities to follow suggestions or actively to resist or avoid the activity.
- Recognition or understanding of one's own body, as shown by how easy an activity was to perform depending on the part of the body concerned; also whether clothing was used appropriately.

- Having the sensorimotor functions to perform actions. Increasing difficulties were seen with motor functioning as the disease progressed.
- Understanding the purpose of each subsystem, examples included hand-drying without washing, and the general inability of the patients to proceed from one action to another.
- The patient's ability to recognize and understand the objects used during morning care, for example clothing and washing equipment.
- Being able to perform the necessary actions needed in an activity. This often depended on the simplicity of the action, for example wiping the stomach, or a complicated action such as doing up buttons.
- Being able to combine actions into a sequence to achieve an activity, for example putting on a pullover and then pulling it down, or putting on a shoe and then tying the laces.
- Being able to combine the activities such as washing, dressing and combing their hair (this was not possible for any of the patients studied).
- Having an understanding of how much time was needed to complete an activity. Patients were not able to refer to the amount of time necessary.
- Understanding the quality of their actions, such as if their hands were clean after washing them. Patients showed varying abilities unrelated to the progression of their disease.

In the patients who were totally dependent on the nurse two further categories were found.

- The ability to communicate, including crying, smiling and the ability to initiate communication.
- Recognition and understanding of the function of the nurse, which included not accepting help offered as well as asking for permission to do certain things.

Sandman *et al.* found that some activities were obviously easier to perform than others; for example, washing was easier than dressing, the former being completed on 55% of occasions after suggestions or instruction, the latter on only 5% of occasions. The reliability of the rating between each observer was 88%.

The authors state that using this system of classification of abilities it is possible to assess which patients have which skills deficits, but that these will vary from day to day. Motivation and understanding by the patients was influenced by emotional factors, such as the nurse talking in a calm and friendly manner which encouraged the patients, whereas trying to hurry or ruffling the patients caused their behaviour to deteriorate.

The researchers found that the most striking feature was the inability of the patients to undertake a sequence of actions, and to understand the use of the objects involved. The goal of nursing using a self-care framework should therefore be to compensate for this fragmentation in the patients' abilities.

The authors feel that nurses must understand the interpretation patients make of situations and subunits of activities; also the effects on the patients of different nursing activities. Therefore, nurses must 'be aware that the patient's highest level of performance is to a large extent dependent on the nurse–patient interaction' (p. 337).

Using the 122-item categorization, the authors suggest that patient assessment proceeds from macro- to micro-levels of self-care abilities and sequences of abilities. Having assessed the patient's abilities, the demands made on him or her should be assessed. Too heavy a demand will cause stress to the patient leading to deterioration in functioning, whilst too light a demand will create learned helplessness.

This study shows clearly both the self-care abilities and the deficits of patients with Alzheimer's dementia, and also the progressive nature of deterioration in self-care due to the fragmentation of actions. Using Orem's framework, self-care deficits in these patients are observed predominantly as changes in their behaviour and activities of living. Therefore, as the study is theory led, Orem's model is seen to be useful for helping to identify these abilities and deficits.

The research was impressive for its methodology and application to the practical problems of nursing these kinds of patients. However, no mention is made of exhaustion of categories, or of filling the existing categories which would leave room for further similar exploration.

The study is also explanatory, as the activities of the nurse are seen as either helping the patient to become more self-caring, or hindering this process. As the study was carried out in the normal environment of the patients and in a setting which allowed nursing care to be studied, it is a valuable contribution to the literature in its support of the model and in its addition to nursing knowledge of patients with Alzheimer's dementia.

CONCLUSIONS

The papers included in this section of identification of self-care requisites and deficits show strong support for Orem's model being able to identify self-care in those groups studied. The studies were the following.

- A literature search of self-care in diabetic patients. This paper also included a search of nursing activities to help these patients to be more effective in self-care.
- A descriptive study of diabetic patients' self-care deficits.
- A study of the self-care abilities of young children and the help their parents give them to promote their health and self-care.

- An action research study of the self-care deficits of the elderly living in a high-rise block for the elderly.
- An observational study of morning care of patients with dementia. The researchers also observed the way the nurse can help or hinder the patients' self-care.

A wide variety of methods were used in these studies. That the studies were conducted in both North America and Europe shows the wide acceptance of this model in practice.

No studies were found which showed planning to develop the patients' self-care abilities, therefore the next section will deal with nursing intervention.

NURSING ACTIONS TO PROMOTE SELF-CARE

In this section the ways that nursing care can be carried out according to Orem's model are examined. Orem calls these 'helping methods' or 'methods of assistance'. Many of the studies investigate the method of instruction given to patients or groups of patients and the relationship of this teaching to some measure of outcome; most frequently the effect of structured versus unstructured teaching is examined. A variety of settings and conditions are studied. As well as patient teaching, some studies in the psychiatric field investigate the effects of social skills training.

TEACHING THE CHILD

A single study was found which examined how children can be taught to take responsibility for their own self-care, and also assesses the effectiveness of this teaching.

Blazek and McClellan (1983) claim that little research has been conducted to determine the factors that affect the child's ability to self-care. Their study focuses on the difference in locus of control of children who were instructed in self-care, measured against those who did not receive such instruction.

The researchers randomly selected 42 fifth grade children attending an upper middle class, mixed sex school in south-western USA. The children were randomly assigned to either the experimental or the control group.

The study aimed to make the experimental children aware that they could actively participate in their health care, and so become responsible for their own health. These children attended three 40 minute, consecutive classroom sessions that emphasized their responsibility for their own health. As part of the sessions they also watched film strips with an associated manual that emphasized the importance of self-care. This aimed to teach the children how to ask questions, make decisions and record facts in a variety of health areas such as nutrition, exercise and daily health habits.

The children in the control group participated in the usual method of health education in the school. This consisted of group discussion utilizing films on first aid with subsequent discussion initiated by the children, ranging over any area of health.

The instructor in both groups was a student nurse working with a school nurse.

Measurements of locus of control used the Children's Health Locus of Control Questionnaire (Parcel and Meyer, 1978), designed to measure the extent of a child's view of health outcomes as being a result of his or her own actions. Questionnaires were administered immediately before and after both groups were held.

Results showed that the main gain score between pre-health and post-health sessions for the experimental group was +0.9286 and for the control group was +0.3333. A t-test showed a significant difference between the groups at less than 0.05 level.

The authors claim that participation in self-care instruction can improve a child's sense of responsibility for her or his own health. Moreover, they claim that lengthy and expensive classes are not necessary for this.

This study uses Orem's (1980) edition, where she states, 'Teaching another is a valid method of helping a person ... who needs instruction in order to develop knowledge or particular skills' (p. 67). The study is theory led and uses the model as intended by Orem, although there is no assessment of the children's prior knowledge. The results are impressive in showing the difference between the teaching methods in achieving a sense of responsibility by the children for their own health. Therefore the study shows a cause and effect; the cause being the teaching and the effect being the difference in the children's sense of responsibility for their own self-care.

The problems that are not addressed in this study are the permanence of the effects, and the possible differences in the effects of the variable length of the teaching sessions between the two groups.

TEACHING PATIENTS WITH MYOCARDIAL INFARCTION

A group of patients known to have high levels of anxiety are those who have experienced a myocardial infarction. As giving information to patients has been shown to reduce anxiety, the following study aimed to demonstrate this effect.

Toth (1980) investigated the effects of structured versus unstructured patient teaching following myocardial infarction; she related this to anxiety reduction at the time of transferring the patient from the coronary care unit (CCU) to a high dependency area. This transfer is known to cause anxiety to patients.

Toth measured the level of the patients' anxiety in three ways: by the IPAT Anxiety Scale (Krug, Scheier and Cattell, 1976), by measures of increase in heart rate and by measures of increase in systolic blood pressure.

The study was conducted in a large university hospital in Washington DC. This hospital had an eight-bed CCU and an 18-bed progressive coronary care unit (PCCU) to which patients were transferred from the CCU. The PCCU had telemetry with an ECG printout at the nurses' station.

Patients were divided into an experimental and a control group according to their admission dates to the CCU. The control group were the first patients to be admitted. They consisted of 10 patients who fulfilled the following criteria: a diagnosis of myocardial infarction; direct admission as an emergency; under 65 years of age; and English speaking.

Fourteen days was allowed to elapse following discharge from hospital of all the patients in the control group before the experimental group patients were chosen. This group also consisted of 10 patients who met the same criteria for inclusion as the control group. Table 4.1 shows the demographic details of both these groups of patients.

Table 4.1 Distribution of demographic details of patients in experimental and control groups in Toth's (1980) study

	Experimental group (n = 10)	Control group (n = 10)
Male	10	8
Female	–	2
Age range (years)	39–50	38–62
Mean age (years)	44.3	52.3
Length of stay in CCU (days)	3–10	3–8
Mean stay in CCU (days)	4	4.1
Skill level		
Professional	7	5
Skilled	3	5
Ethnic origin		
White	8	8
Black	2	2

The control group patients received instruction about their current care. They were all asked if they had any questions and if so their questions were answered. They were also given time to express their feelings. This involved the researcher seeing all the patients in the group for 20 minutes each day in the CCU.

The procedure for the experimental group patients was directly related to transfer from the CCU to the PCCU, and the information was structured. The investigator used a printed checklist which was ticked when patients had demonstrated knowledge in each area; this was assessed by repetition of the content to the researcher. The areas covered in the structured information are shown in Table 4.2. The experimental group patients also had their questions answered. Toth spent the same amount of time with these patients as with those in the control group and all teaching was completed before the patients were transferred to the PCCU.

Table 4.2 Structured teaching given to experimental group in CCU to prepare for transfer to PCCU in Toth's (1980) study

Length of stay in CCU
Length of hospitalization
Time of decision to transfer from CCU
Timing and procedure on transfer from CCU
Transfer as indication of progress
Location of PCCU
Doctors responsible for patients in PCCU
Type of medical care in PCCU
Availability of doctors in PCCU
Nurses in PCCU
Structure and facilities in PCCU
Nurse training for working in PCCU
Monitoring by telemetry
Anxiety and depression post-transfer to PCCU is normal
Medication after transfer to PCCU
Importance of continued rest in PCCU
Levels of activity in PCCU and afterwards (patients also given handout)
Symptoms to report to PCCU nurse
Visiting times in PCCU
Education on PCCU will be given

The patients' level of anxiety was assessed in three ways.

- The IPAT Anxiety Scale was used on the day of transfer to the PCCU.
- The researcher measured the systolic blood pressure of the patients when they were transferred to the PCCU, using the same equipment for all patients. Readings of systolic blood pressure from the previous day and the day of transfer were taken from the patients' records.
- Heart rate was taken from the ECG monitor on three occasions: the day of transfer, the day before transfer and at the time of transfer.

The results showed that there was no significant difference between the experimental and the control groups in anxiety on the day of transfer from the CCU as measured by the IPAT Anxiety Scale. Systolic blood pressure and heart rate measured on the day when the patients were transferred from the CCU showed a statistically significant decrease ($p < 0.05$) in anxiety for the experimental group compared with the control group.

Toth comments that measuring anxiety by questionnaire has been shown to be unreliable, although changes have been shown to occur with other measures of anxiety (Buros, 1972; Foster, 1974). She suggests several possible reasons for her findings: she did not carry out a pre-test, so a change in anxiety levels on transfer from CCU might not be demonstrated by a questionnaire; there was a possibility that questions were answered so as to please the researcher, particularly as previous teaching allowed the patients to know what was an appropriate response. She therefore concludes that physiological measures of anxiety are more sensitive to change than psychological measures.

This study has a number of problems. First, the sample size was small. This is often a problem, with a limited number of people available with any condition at one time. Second, a pre-test/post-test anxiety rating needs to be included to show the full effects of structured teaching. Third, the gender balance in the groups was highly biased towards men.

Toth's study was directly based on Orem's model. The condition of the patients was therefore problematized by the model. Toth showed that Orem's model was appropriate for these patients, as following a myocardial infarction they will have increased demands for self-care which are going to involve them learning to cope with levels of stress. As the study used a cause and effect design, the cause of the patients' anxiety being the myocardial infarction and the effect being the hypothesized reduction in anxiety, it became possible to assess the effectiveness of teaching patients in order to reduce their anxiety. Anxiety reduction would allow promotion of self-care.

However, this study does not show that teaching patients is a valid method of promoting self-care, as no indication is given of the levels of anxiety on admission to the CCU, and how or whether teaching relieves this. So in this study there is no indication of the relationship between giving patients information and their ability to cope with the stress of their illness or situation. Also differences between the teaching methods have not shown conclusively that either is superior in lessening anxiety. Further studies are needed in this area to give more conclusive results.

Toth's study does not show support for Orem's model, as teaching as a method of prompting self-care is not seen to be effective in reducing anxiety in this group of patients.

TEACHING ABOUT DRUG USE

Patients who are receiving drug therapy with known side effects could potentially be taught to know about these side effects and could also be taught remedial self-care when the side effects occur.

This aspect of patient teaching was investigated by Dodd (1984a) who questioned the relationship between giving patients structured knowledge and their ability to self-care. The study was designed to select different types of information that could be given to patients: information on drugs; information on how to manage their side effects; and the combination of these two types of information. The results of gaining this information on the patient would be used to assess: (i) the patients' knowledge of chemotherapy; (ii) the patients' self-care behaviours; and (iii) the patients' general state of well-being.

Dodd tested three hypotheses.

1. Patients receiving drug information alone or in combination with other information will respond more accurately to the Chemotherapy Knowledge Questionnaire than patients not receiving the information.
2. Patients receiving information on the management of side effects of drugs, alone or in combination with other information will report more self-care behaviours than those not receiving the information.
3. Patients receiving a combination of the above two types of information will demonstrate as much knowledge of drugs, and use as many self-care behaviours as those in the other two groups, but in addition will report a more positive state of well-being than those in the single knowledge groups.

(p. 45)

All subjects fulfilled the criteria of being aged 18 or over, being able to understand English, currently receiving chemotherapy and having done so for the last 2 weeks, having a life expectancy of at least 9 weeks and not having been hospitalized for more than 50% of the time during the pre-intervention and post-intervention stages of the study. This last criterion was felt to be important due to the possible learning of self-care behaviours when in hospital.

Of the 56 patients who were selected as fulfilling these criteria, 48 completed the study, the remainder being lost due to morbidity or mortality. The 48 patients were randomly assigned in equal numbers to one of four groups, identified in the three hypotheses, and a control group. Assessment of the knowledge and behaviours of the patients in the four groups was made on two occasions – before and after giving structured knowledge. The time interval between the two assessments was between 4 and 9 weeks.

Knowledge of chemotherapy was assessed using the Chemotherapy Knowledge Questionnaire (Dodd and Mood, 1981), which has 23 items. Patients were asked to indicate from a list of 27 drugs which ones they were receiving; a further category asked them to name any other drugs they were receiving that were not on the list. Items also included a list of

44 possible side effects and asked patients to indicate those that they had been told could result from their drugs. This resulted in a knowledge score for each patient on drug accuracy and potential side effects.

The Self-Behaviours Questionnaire asked patients to indicate on a 5-point scale the severity of any side effects. Where these had occurred the patient was asked to specify what action they had taken to alleviate them, and also to rate on a 5-point scale how effective the action had been. Patients were also asked how they knew of the self-care behaviour. Reliability was assessed by test–retest methods with the control group.

The Profile of Mood States Questionnaire was used successfully by Weisman and Worden (1975) in studies of cancer patients; its validity and reliability had been established by McNair, Lorr and Droppleman (1971). The questionnaire consisted of 65 items each with a 5-point rating scale.

Patients in the first group (drug information) were given the names of their chemotherapeutic drugs and the potential side effects. Written information, developed from pharmaceutical literature, was also given and the investigator discussed this with the patients.

Patients in the second group (information and the management of side effects) received a booklet which described 44 side effects of chemotherapy and how to manage them. This was developed from a review of the oncology literature. The investigator discussed this in general with the patients, not specifically relating it to their treatment.

The third group of patients (drug information and information about the management of side effects) received both written and verbal information as given to the first two groups.

Patients in the control group spent an equal amount of time with the investigator but discussed general issues and specific matters at the patients' request; for this group there was no systematic review of drugs, side effects or the management of side effects.

All initial interviews and information giving were conducted by the investigator. Nurse interviewers who had been instructed by the investigator carried out the second and subsequent interviews with the patients.

Analysis was by a 2×2 design analysis of covariance. The first hypothesis was confirmed with $p < 0.01$. It showed that patients receiving drug information and knowledge about side effects had significantly greater knowledge than the control group. However, when the accuracy of the patients' knowledge was corrected for guessing the significant difference disappeared.

The second hypothesis showed a significant difference ($p < 0.01$) between the experimental and the control groups in knowledge of the management of side effects.

The third hypothesis showed a higher score on both knowledge of drugs and side effects after information had been given. This was also shown in the patients' knowledge of the measurement of side effects;

these differences were the same as for the single information groups. However, the combination of knowledge made no difference when measured by the Profile of Mood States Questionnaire. The retention of information by patients was found to support previous studies carried out by Dodd and Mood (1981) and by Muss *et al.* (1979).

Orem's model is not central to this paper, although the hypotheses can be shown to support Orem's concepts that self-care behaviours can be learned and that patients are able to care for themselves more effectively when given specific information. Dodd (1984a) reported that some of the patients in the study also 'acted promptly before side effects had become persistent' (p. 49). However, patients were only shown to improve their knowledge in the area where they received specific information. Thus a link between knowledge and an improvement in mood state was not demonstrated and further work on this is needed.

Compared to Toth's study above, Dodd's study does support Orem's claim that teaching is a valid method of helping patients to achieve more effective self-care, although teaching does have to be very specific. According to Dodd's study patients cannot be expected to generalize or to make links between different pieces of information, unless the link is made for them by the teacher.

This study is again a cause and effect design, the cause being the results and side effects of chemotherapy drugs, and the effects being the patients' knowledge of their drugs and how to cope with their side effects. Therefore, in this study, teaching as one of Orem's nursing actions to promote self-care is seen to be effective.

TEACHING SELF-CARE POST-OPERATIVELY

Recovery from extensive surgery can be a problem for patients if they are not given specific instructions on the types of behaviours to adopt to prevent complications. This can be especially the case during the period following discharge from hospital.

Goodwin (1979) investigated the effects of a programmed instruction booklet on patient recovery following pulmonary surgery. She designed the booklet to give to post-operative lobectomy and pneumonectomy patients. It was compiled with reference to Vicary's (1974) work which showed that these patients need support and information to overcome the illness crisis. Other sources of information in compiling the booklet were interviews with surgeons and clinical nurse specialists, and also with patients who had had this type of surgery:

> These discussions included the surgical procedure and effects, recommendations for self-care during recovery, problems and concerns experienced by patients and what patients and family

members said they wished they had known, and thought other patients should be told.

(p.30)

The aim of the booklet was to give patients knowledge of their surgery and its effects, what to expect during recovery and how to care for themselves, including knowing when to involve others as a problem arose. Learning occurred through relating the information to specific objectives, which allowed the patient to discriminate between the effects of surgery and expected recovery, and problems.

Evaluation of the effectiveness of the booklet involved 26 patients from three hospitals in a midwestern American city. They were all over 21 years of age, were mentally competent and able to speak, read and write English. The design of the study needed subjects to be as similar as possible in diagnosis and prognosis, therefore eligibility was through confirmed bronchiogenic carcinoma without metastases beyond the mediastinal nodes. Subjects were recruited 6 days after surgery.

Subjects were randomly assigned to experimental or control groups; these groups were shown not to be significantly different in the incidence of chronic lung disease, their sex composition, the patients' smoking history, type of surgery, the hospital where patients were treated, or the patients' length of in-patient stay. Marginally significant differences were found between the groups in the patients' age and education, the experimental group being younger and better educated.

The investigator saw all subjects. She told them that she was interested in how people got on after their particular operation, but the booklet was mentioned only to those patients in the experimental group. All other patient care continued as usual during the study.

Evaluation of the booklet was conducted by a 36-item written test administered on two occasions, the first near the time of patient discharge from hospital and the second at the patient's first visit to the out-patient department, an average of 30 days later. The test asked patients for physiological knowledge of respiration, to name their operation and to show on a diagram what had been removed, to identify irritant substances to the air passages, to discriminate between expected and unexpected effects of surgery, and to describe appropriate activities after 6 weeks at home.

The effects of the information on the recovery process were assessed through physical measures at the first visit to the out-patient department. These included respiratory rate, rhythm, sounds and diaphragm movement, chest expansion, scapula–spine distance and head rotation and arm movements. These measures had previously been shown to be valid and reliable.

Results showed that patients in the experimental group had more knowledge on both test occasions than patients in the control group.

However, no significant differences were found in patients abstaining from harmful activities mentioned in the booklet, including smoking. Despite this the experimental group was found to perform statistically more therapeutic activities than the control group. Significant differences were found with the experimental group in measures of recovery of respiratory function – this was also corroborated by their report of less frequent and less severe coughing than the control group – but with other symptoms there was no significant difference in severity between the groups. However, the experimental group reported marginally less worry. No significant differences were found between groups in ranges of movement of the head and upper limbs. A surprising finding was that posture in the control group was better than in the experimental group as measured by the scapula–spine distance. The researcher could give no explanation for this finding.

This study shows how patient teaching can give patients information, but that teaching is not necessarily a valid method of helping a patient to become more self-caring. Teaching patients after pulmonary surgery did improve their self-care in some areas, for example in resting with their feet supported after meals, lying down in the afternoons, walking daily and getting up from a sitting position every hour to walk around. However, teaching had no effect on harmful habits such as giving up smoking, lifting heavy weights, driving a car and sitting with their feet unsupported for prolonged periods. Therefore Orem's assumption that teaching is always a valid method of helping has been questioned here. The relationship between patient teaching and the willingness and ability of patients to self-care evidently needs further investigation. Using Orem's assumptions, it may be that the patients in this study were unable to come to terms with their illness or level of disability, and unwilling to improve their condition apart from in the areas where improvement was actually seen. If this is the case then Orem's model is clearly unsatisfactory for all problems faced by these patients.

This appears to be a well-controlled study which uses a cause and effect design. However, the assessments of the patients' self-care at home were not conducted in their homes but were conducted in the out-patient department using measures to indicate the patients' self-care at home. These indicators themselves may have been part of the problem of the lack of support for teaching as an effective self-care method. The article based on the study would have been improved by showing some diagrams from the booklet and giving examples of the questions used in the evaluation.

Results from these three studies investigating different aspects of Orem's method of helping through teaching have shown mixed results. In structured versus unstructured patient teaching there was a tendency for structured teaching to be more effective than unstructured teaching, whether the instruction was given in a verbal or booklet form. There is also evidence that giving information does lead to improved abilities of patients to self-care in certain situations, although the information given to achieve this effect must be very specific. However, in other situations, particularly with harmful activities, structured patient teaching does not lead patients to modify their activities or behaviours. Also the long-term effects of teaching have not been shown in any of the studies.

Therefore, from these three empirical studies we cannot assume that Orem's method of teaching to promote self-care will necessarily be effective.

TEACHING HYPERTENSIVE PATIENTS

This study is a comprehensive review of the literature compiled to show the problems faced by patients suffering from hypertension, and the issues faced by the nurse in teaching and providing support for such patients. It shows clearly the nurses' role in assisting these patients to live with their chronic condition.

Heine (1981) assumes that successful work with hypertensive patients is based on three premises.

- The most favourable condition for blood pressure control is active patient participation.
- The nurses' role is to help patients to make decisions about their care, but ultimately patients are responsible for their own care.
- A critical element of successful long-term control is the patient–health care provider relationship.

Heine sees the nurses' role as educating and counselling patients in understanding and accepting the chronic nature of their disease. She says that nurses can assist by recognizing the patients' power and responsibility for performing self-care; also, providing, where possible, continuity of care and the use of verbal and written information to aid memory. She cautions that unless a good patient–health care provider relationship is established, successful implementation of other methods of assistance will prove difficult.

The nurse can help patients to make decisions through giving them information about alternatives and helping them to choose the alternative most appropriate to their lifestyle. The nurse can also help the patient to acquire the skills to carry out self-care.

Heine says that the first line of therapy is frequently the use of drugs as this is the least disruptive to an individual's lifestyle, but problems arise with adherence to the regimen, particularly when multiple medications are prescribed. Prescribing needs to consider the minimum number of doses per day, as this will decrease the time, energy and expenditure the patient has to make to adhere to the regimen. Assessment of the patient's daily routine will allow for tailoring the medications to fit this. Nurses can help the patient to keep medications in close proximity to where these routines are performed, so that taking them is part of the performance of the routine. An alternative approach is to ask the patient to keep a record, using a calendar or diary, of the medications taken and missed each day. With both these techniques, reviewing their effectiveness can be carried out in the out-patient department when problems and difficulties can be discussed, as can the importance of medications, their expected results and their side effects.

Nurses can also inform patients of other self-care measures such as weight reduction, a low sodium diet, regular exercise, stress reduction, alcohol regulation, stopping smoking and the relationship between these activities and the control of hypertension. Heine hoped that time spent in discussing these issues with patients would help them to modify their lifestyle, but she anticipated difficulty in achieving this as patients need continual reinforcement. She suggests two methods that may prove useful:

- contracting (Steckel and Swain, 1977), which involves the patient choosing the goal or goals and making a written agreement with the nurse which also states completion date when an appropriate reward may be negotiated on successful completion;
- self-help groups to deal with specific problems, such as Weight Watchers or Alcoholics Anonymous.

Heine considers supporting the patient as a major nursing function, as does Orem, particularly in helping the patient to adapt to chronic illness. Ackerman (1977) and Kockar and Daniels (1978) describe the five stages of progress in adapting to such illness:

1. shock and disbelief;
2. developing awareness;
3. reorganization;
4. resolution;
5. identity change.

Nurses' counselling and help should be consistent with these stages.

Social and emotional support for patients should involve the nurse in counselling and educating their family, so that they may help the patient to adhere to therapy. This will also reduce stress levels and facilitate coping which aids blood pressure reduction. She suggests the nurse should be an educator to help patients to understand the need for long-term treatment. As shown by previous studies in this section, knowledge in itself does not necessarily mean the patient will adhere to therapy. Heine suggests that other motivational strategies need to be built in, as most patients are asymptomatic on diagnosis, and therefore do not understand the reasons for, or the importance of their medication (Kockar, 1977; Watson, 1979; Himmelhoch, 1980; Ryan, 1980; Sackett, 1980; Todd, 1981). Patients may feel worse on medication than previously (Todd, 1981), and so discontinue their treatment. Patients can block information if it is too stressful, and the nurse needs continuous feedback from the patients to assess their individual levels of understanding. Education can include individual education tailored to the patient's needs, or group education which allows for peer support and sharing of ideas and problems; this latter strategy also saves nursing time. Other teaching methods include self-instruction books, tapes and slides.

Feedback to enhance the patients' adherence to therapy can be through self-monitoring of blood pressure (Sackett *et al.*, 1975; Grancio, 1979); also family members can be taught to take blood pressure readings to reinforce the patient's motivation and skills.

This paper shows some of the difficulties faced by nurses when helping patients to develop an effective range of internal and external self-care behaviours. Heine reviews the literature to develop the role of helping patients through Orem's methods of supporting another, both physically and psychologically, and teaching another. However, Orem's model is not developed uncritically in this paper; Heine shows the problems that nurses will have to overcome if supporting and teaching patients is to be an effective self-care action.

TEACHING ELDERLY WOMEN

Another important factor in patient teaching is knowing what will affect the patients' willingness or intention to comply with a plan of care. One such study has examined these variables in elderly women.

Chang *et al.* (1985) studied the effects of different variables on the intention by elderly women to adhere to a nursing plan designed for them. The study aimed to show the effects of different levels of technical, psycho-social and patient participation in nursing care on the intentions of elderly mobile women to comply with a nursing care plan. The authors make the point that as self-care aims to shift decision-making to the patient, it is therefore necessary that nurses recognize the interaction between patient characteristics and beliefs and their predisposition to satisfactory self-care.

There were three research questions for this study.

- What is the effect of high levels of technical quality and psychosocial care by the nurse, and participation by the patient on the intention to comply?
- Which interactions in the components of care are significant in the intention to comply?

- Which personal characteristics of the patients are significantly related to intentions to comply?

The method used a 2×2 experimental design using eight videotapes showing patient interactions with nurses; these were shown to patients in randomly chosen settings. Levels of high or low technical quality of care were experimental variables on the videotapes. High technical quality was defined as four correct medical histories and five correct physical examination items; low technical quality was one correct medical history, three irrelevant medical items and one correct physical examination.

Similarly, high and low levels of psychosocial care were built into the videotapes, high levels of care being four appropriately related cues given by the patient relevant to her illness or treatment, for example how it affected her daily living activities; low psychosocial care was shown as a lack of any cues of this nature. Patient participation similarly showed high or low levels: high levels showed active participation by the patient in planning the first five steps in the decision-making about her care at home; low participation showed the nurse directing the patient in her care. In all the videotapes the level of courtesy was held constant. Each videotape showed the same patient with chronic angina being treated by the same nurse in the same setting.

Scripts for the videos were viewed by a panel of five judges made up of nurse researchers and physicians who were asked to rate each component high or low. One hundred per cent agreement was achieved between them and with the investigators.

Experimental subjects were 268 women between the ages of 56 and 89 years, who had a mean age of 70.9 years with standard deviation 6.2 years. Their mean number of years of education was 11.4; their marital status was 28.4% married, 56% widowed and the remainder single or divorced.

Videotapes were randomly assigned to the sites where they were viewed and subjects were then asked to answer questions about their reactions to the videotapes. A typical question was 'If you were the patient in the videotape, would you cut down on your potatoes and bread as discussed with the nurse?' Answers were on a 5-point scale ranging from 'definitely would' to 'definitely would not'. In addition a question to determine how subjects rated their own health gave five alternatives, excellent, good, fair, poor or very poor.

Results showed that when an overall rating of patient characteristics was set against the levels of technical and psychosocial care and patient participation, no significant difference was found in the intention to comply. Taking the variables individually, patient participation in care was not found to be related to the intention to comply with a plan of care; this shows that the expectation by health workers that increased participation by patients will lead to compliance is ill-founded. However, Chang *et al.* suggest there may be a cohort effect, in that elderly women may expect to have their care planned by a health worker and not be actively involved in this stage. This comment throws into question the validity of Orem's model for this group of women.

Significant patient characteristics that were related to the intention to comply were pre-existing satisfaction with health care, being widowed, having a good social network and perceiving the health examination as important. The researchers suggest that the relationship between widowhood and a good social network could indicate that those who are widowed develop wider social networks which produce more likelihood that compliance will result. They suggest further work is needed in this area, but that nurses should bear in mind the strong impact of a supportive network in producing compliance.

In this study, based primarily on Orem's model, satisfaction with care and intention to comply are highly correlated, but the authors suggest that these two concepts may be different as their previous work (Chang *et al.*, 1982) has shown patient participation to be related to satisfaction with care.

This study fills some of the gaps in Orem's model related to the role of the nurse in helping the patient, and the effects of this help on the patient's self-care demands. The study suggests that elderly American women may not wish to participate in setting goals to improve their health. There is an indication that existing satisfaction with health care leads to increased likelihood of compliance. However, how the nurse presents the information to the patient, her accuracy and her caring approach do not seem to make any difference to whether this group of women are likely to comply with a nursing care plan. Therefore it seems that Orem's model may have limited use in attempting to improve self-care behaviours in this group of women, and the model is further undermined by this study.

The study has a good sample size and advocates further work in the area with more diverse samples. However, a shortfall of the study is trying to assess intention to comply through a group of women who are not actually participating, but merely observers of a video. It can be strongly argued that watching a video does not constitute the same situation as being a patient; this distancing has not been addressed in the study. Also participation in planning care has been shown elsewhere not to lead to increased compliance, but this is not mentioned by Chang *et al.* These aspects may make a considerable difference to their arguments.

TEACHING SELF-CARE FOR THE MENTALLY ILL

Two further studies in this section are concerned with patients who are mentally ill. The emphasis on education is evident, but strategies must obviously be different from those used with the physically ill.

Whetstone (1986) investigated the use of social dramatics as a nursing tool for developing social skills in chronic schizophrenic patients, where social isolation tends to be normal. Orem's self-care deficits show these patients to need skills in social competence, social interaction and promotion of normalcy. The research question was whether patients who undertook social dramatics with videotape feedback would demonstrate improved self-care social skills as measured by the Nurses Observation Scale for In-Patient Evaluation (NOSIE-30) (Honigfeld, 1974), compared with patients not exposed to such a programme.

The NOSIE-30 scale has 30 items which are factor-analytically derived. It has six factors: social competence, social interest, personal neatness, irritability, manifest psychosis and psychotic depression. It allows psychiatric assistants to observe behaviour and evaluate patients' strengths and weaknesses on a 4-point scale.

Social dramatics evolved out of the psychodrama techniques of Moreno (1946) as a technique for playing out roles. The technique Whetstone used involved two people playing out a social situation:

> ... during the interaction process, avoidance of psychopathology issues is discouraged; instead working with the positive ego strengths of the patient, emphasis is on cognitive understanding of the social deficits.

(p.69)

The study was conducted using a selection of patients from four wards in a state hospital in Missouri, USA. Twenty patients emerged as suitable; the criteria were being chronically mentally ill, aged between 22 and 55 years and meeting the criteria of schizophrenia according to the American Psychiatric Association's 1980 definition. The patients were randomly assigned to an experimental or control group. From the 10 patients in the experimental group, only five willingly consented to participate in the study: two males and three females with a mean age of 36.8 years and a mean hospital stay of 6.8 years, made up of repeat admissions. The control group was six males and four females, mean age 39.9 years and a mean length of hospitalization of 9.4 years.

Patients in the experimental group undertook social dramatics sessions on a weekly basis for 2 hours over a period of 8 weeks. Scenario examples used in the sessions were: 'share with the person next to you what you feel about seeing yourself on videotape'; and 'think about yourself as a room-mate. Tell the person next to you what you think is important for being a good room-mate. Describe some qualities for being a good room-mate.' Content validation of the scenario was assessed by an expert panel of psychiatric and mental health nurses.

The social dramatics sessions took place in a television studio which had a theatre atmosphere. It was in the hospital grounds. Scenarios were randomized; two patients were asked to perform them on stage for a minimum of 5 minutes.

Initially all the patients found this activity extremely difficult; they suffered shyness, embarrassment and self-consciousness and were extremely anxious and uncomfortable. The researcher needed to continually encourage and empathize with them, and cueing was initially necessary to provide a start for the patients and to give them ideas.

Following the 8-week experimental period 14 psychiatric attendants carried out an assessment within 2 weeks of the end of the period; they used the NOSIE-30 scale on all patients in both groups.

From this cause and effect design the findings showed a statistically significant positive increase ($p < 0.04$) in social competence in the experimental group using a Wilcoxon test for independent samples. Social dramatics with this group of patients is therefore of use in Orem's category of 'helping methods'. Although not mentioned directly by her, social dramatics could be seen as 'supporting another psychologically'. So this study helps, in some respects, to support Orem's nursing actions to promote self-care.

Reliability between the assessors was 60%. Patient behaviours not assessed by the NOSIE-30 such as social interest, personal neatness, irritability, manifest psychosis and psychotic depression showed no significant difference at the $p = 0.05$ level. Therefore social dramatics is not an effective method with these behaviours.

These findings in part agree with Underwood (1978), who also found subjects were still sloppy, impatient, irritable, hearing and seeing things and resistant to change. Whetstone says that the use of videotape captured subtle changes in socialization patterns over the experimental period, but feels that its use with the mentally ill needs further evaluation to overcome problems of usage, as conflicting evidence has been shown by previous studies (Edelson and Seidman, 1975; Griffiths and Gillingham, 1978). The NOSIE scale could be criticized as being insufficiently sensitive to pick up some of these changes seen on the video.

Whetstone also questioned the permanence of such improved skills in social competence. Larson (1982) found skills were evident after 3 months, as did Spencer, Gillespie and Ekisa (1983).

Whetstone also comments on the small sample size in the study, and feels this restricts the findings being generalized, but despite this he urges professionals to evaluate practice using practical methods.

The second study in this section on self-care in the mentally ill is by Blair (1985). He uses a case study of a single patient to show the effects of behaviour modification techniques. The subject was a 39-year-old male patient in a large psychiatric hospital. He had been hospitalized for a month and was unable to carry out basic hygiene requirements of shaving, bathing and changing his clothes. Blair claims he continually asked staff to carry out these tasks for him, although no physical impairment was evident. However, his past history showed that for over 10 years these activities had been carried out by his mother and lately his sister. His intelligence level in other ways was normal.

A behaviour modification programme was commenced, as planned discharge depended on his ability to undertake these functions. Specific behaviours were chosen for modification, the criteria being those which needed prompting on more than 3 days of the week in which the assessment was made. The behaviours were mouth-washing, shaving, face-washing and bathing.

The first 2 days of the programme involved teaching the patient the behaviours in detail. A token economy scheme was begun from the third day, which involved small monetary rewards and being accompanied by a staff member to the cafeteria to buy his favourite food and drink each time one of the activities was undertaken without prompting. In addition, bathing without prompting on 3 out of 4 days was rewarded with a long-distance telephone call to his sister.

During the first and second weeks of the treatment programme there was a reduction in prompting which achieved behaviours of up to 87% in mouth-washing, 73% in washing his face, 56% in shaving and 50% in bathing. However, there was regression in week 3 which Blair claims was due to new staff who did not know to reward the patient immediately on completion of the activities. Week 4 showed continued improvement over past weeks in face washing only; shaving showed no change and the other two activities showed an improvement over the regression in week 3 only. Premature transfer of the patient cut the programme short, but follow-up of the patient found him to need no more than 30% prompting to carry out the tasks.

Blair claims success has been demonstrated by the outcome of the programme. However, it is unclear from Orem (1980) whether behaviour modification is a valid method of guiding another. Of this category, Orem says (p. 64):

> Guiding another person considered as a method of assistance is valid in situations in which persons must (1) make choices – for example, choosing one course of action in preference to another – or (2) pursue a course of action, but not without direction or supervision.

Therefore it remains debatable whether behaviour modification using a token economy scheme is valid as a helping method when using Orem's model. It could be argued that the patient in the study is insufficiently able to make a choice between his actions, or that the direction or supervision was more than mere guidance. Disregarding the validity and moral objections to this type of nursing action, the study is an impressive record of changing behaviour, but with only one patient being involved replication is needed to show good reliability. Studies using this technique would also need to examine the permanence of the effects.

NURSING ACTION TO SUPPORT

The last paper in this section offers a more philosophical perspective to the third of the five 'helping methods' outlined by Orem (1980). She calls this method 'supporting another (physically or psychologically)' (p. 61).

Schoenhofer (1984) offers a definition and analysis of support as being a legitimate nursing action, in order to provide a framework for the structure and knowledge of support. She offers the *Oxford English Dictionary* (1961) definition of support as 'to strengthen the position of; to keep from falling or sinking; to sustain; to maintain in action or being; to provide the necessary matter for'.

She uses the work of Braimner (1973) who distinguishes support from false and/or inappropriate attempts to reassure. He says support ought to be the experience of feeling one is permitted to learn without having to walk before one can run. He identifies three sources of support as experiencing: warmth and acceptance in a relationship; direct help which produces stress reduction or environmental aid; and the temporary lifting of a major responsibility by a helper. Kyes and Hofling (1974) relate this to supportive psychotherapy as being an effective form of treatment during temporary stress, to allow the patient to regain his coping patterns and strategies.

Caplan (1974) says support will probably consist of three elements: significant others help to mobilize the individual's resources and so master the environment; share some of the tasks; and give practical help and cognitive guidance to help coping abilities:

> What we have in mind is not the propping up of someone who is in danger of falling down, but rather the augmentation of a person's strengths to facilitate his mastery of his environment.
>
> (p. 218)

This article is useful in identifying some of the literature on support which further elaborates Orem's concept and provides evidence of its validity where a self-care deficit occurs. Shoenhofer says in appropriate support:

> The patient must be capable of controlling and directing his own behaviour in the situation once he has received psychological, physical and material support.
>
> (p. 219)

To give support the nurse must understand and give appropriate assistance to the patient so that the latter may achieve his or her own goals. Nursing support is seen as a secondary activity, the primary activity being the patient's good.

Shoenhofer indicates how resources between the nurse and the patient should be organized:

> Support is a class of nursing assistance whereby resources of the nurses are added to resources of the client, such that the client in nursing is enabled to initiate and successfully carry out action to accomplish a desired health result.
>
> (p. 219)

She argues for support as being a deliberate form of action and therefore worthy of study in nursing. This paper develops Orem's notion of support and the nurses' role within it.

CONCLUSIONS

Eight studies have been found that developed and investigated how nurses can promote self-care. Most of these studies looked at the effects of teaching on different groups, therefore many of the studies in this section have been of a cause and effect design, in which teaching has been shown to have an effect on the groups studied.

However, in many of the studies, teaching has been a less than effective method of promoting self-care. It is unclear from the studies whether it is the method of teaching which is the problem, or the research design or the model, or a combination of all these. But what is clear is that these studies create a number of problems for Orem's model in which her helping method of teaching as a means of promoting self-care is questioned. It would seem from this that, despite persistence, the model may not be able to help the nurse to overcome some of these problems.

There were no studies which specifically investigated the evaluation of self-care, therefore the next section of this chapter passes on to two studies based on quality assurance in nursing using Orem's model.

ASSESSMENT OF QUALITY USING A SELF-CARE FRAMEWORK

The topical issue of assessing quality of care, with its professional and economic consequences, is discussed in this section. What is encouraging is that these studies are based on a model of nursing, which gives them a theoretical nursing base. Two studies are outlined, one British and one American. Both use Orem's model to provide the framework for the analysis of quality of care in nursing.

QUALITY OF CARE IN THE ELDERLY

The first study is well known; it attempted to show the relationship between the nurses' attitude to geriatric care and the effect this had on the care the patients received. As Orem's model was used in Great Britain this study also shows its growing acceptability as a model of practice in this country.

Kitson (1986) used the conceptual framework of the caring function of the nurse and the adoption by nurses of a positive approach to health problems in the elderly. In this study the goal of nursing was seen as optimal self-care for all patients. Orem's description of the nurses' modes of helping and the classification of patients into needing wholly compensatory, partly compensatory and educative/developmental care was used.

The goal of nursing was identified in three ways: the definition of geriatric nursing by the nurse; the amount of time spent on basic nursing care activities by the nurse; and the proportion of time spent in nursing as against other priorities.

The nurses' definitions of geriatric nursing were assessed using an instrument constructed by Kitson, the Therapeutic Nursing Function (TNF) Indicator, comprising 34 questions, which was administered to ward sisters. A ranking scale was used for each response.

> Examples of the type of response obtained to the question regarding a definition of geriatric nursing illustrates how responses were ranked ...
> Question. 'How would you describe nursing in a geriatric ward?'
> Answer (5 points awarded). 'Geriatric nursing involves ... having a genuine caring attitude, seeing patients as individuals, being progressive enough on the ward to make alterations, provide a therapeutic environment and ensure patient safety without overprotection'.
> Answer (1 point awarded). 'Geriatric nursing involves ... really hard work, real nursing.'
>
> (p. 136)

Ward sisters tested on the TNF instrument were found to fall into two groups: low scoring sisters were predominantly in the 40–45 age group, had worked on the same ward for more than 5 years and had few academic qualifications; sisters with a high score were predominantly aged between 31 and 40 years, had worked on their present ward for between 2 and 6 years and had educational levels from '0' levels to a diploma in nursing.

This understanding of nursing by the ward sister was then used to assess nursing care given on the respective wards. Assessment of nursing care was in terms of whether the patients were enabled to function at their optimal, preferred or chosen level. Participant observation was carried out on three wards to assess the patients' self-care activities; a total of 24 patients with a range of mobility levels were included.

The TNF matrix was used to assess self-care in nurse–patient interaction in three phases.

1. The initiation phase – four points were awarded if the nurse responded positively to the patient's request, one point if the nurse initiated the interaction without the knowledge or consent of the patient.
2. The process stage – this assessed the nurses' knowledge of the patients' self-care abilities and used their potential to aid mobility.
3. The outcome stage – this assessed the activity and the extent of the patients' ability to perform it, given appropriate equipment and assistance from the nurse. Points were scored for outcome if the patients' needs were anticipated and self-care was aided (four points), minimum points of one or two were given if self-care was limited or was unsuccessful.

The main activities assessed in this way were elimination, feeding, washing, dressing, undressing, exercising and communication.

Results showed that the wards where the sister had a high TNF score also had significantly higher scores on self-care when compared with scores from wards where the sister had a low TNF score, which showed corresponding low self-care scores. The exception was in the activity of exercise.

When the amount of time involved in these activities was compared, no significant difference was found between wards, taking into account other variables such as medical policies, paramedical involvement and environmental constraints. Differences in the time of activities were also not found despite the ward designs differing to a considerable extent.

It was therefore shown that the attitude of the ward sister was the one factor that significantly changed the care the patients received, from one of routinized care where patients were not able to use their potential for self-care, to individualized care where patients' self-care abilities were enhanced:

> It would seem, therefore, that staff performance and patient experiences are related to the ward sister's therapeutic awareness.
>
> (p. 141)

Good levels of validity and reliability were obtained for the TNF Indicator by pre-testing and piloting; a random selection of ward situations was also used. By outlining what constituted therapeutic activity prior to data collection, subjectivity was minimized. The TNF matrix was scaled according to Orem's concept of self-care; patients were also considered in terms of age, sex and dependency using Orem's levels of nursing activity. Kitson also considered her role in affecting the behaviours of those she observed; steps were taken to minimize this by discarding the first 8 hours of observation from each ward.

This study has developed some of Orem's concepts, and also helps to show the link between these concepts in the model. This is done first by assessing the level of belief of the sister in promoting self-care in her patients. Orem (1980) says that there are two main ways the nurse should behave in order to provide self-care for patients, i.e. social and interpersonal technologies and regulatory technologies:

> (1) technologies necessary for social and interpersonal (and multi-person) relations and (2) regulatory technologies. *Social and interpersonal technologies* include (1) communication adjusted to age and developmental state, to health state, and to sociocultural orientation; (2) bringing about and maintaining interpersonal, intra-group, or intergroup relations for coordination of effort; (3) bringing about and maintaining therapeutic relations in the light of psychosocial modes of functioning in health and disease; and (4) giving human assistance adapted to human needs and action abilities and limitations. *Regulatory technologies* include (1) maintaining and promoting life processes, (2) regulating psychophysiological modes of functioning in health and disease, (3) promoting human growth and development, and (4) regulating position and movement in space.
>
> (pp. 91–92)

Therefore the TNF Indicator has been developed to investigate these features of the sister.

The second way in which this study has developed a concept of Orem's model is by observing the practice of nurses with patients on several wards using the TNF matrix. As described by Kitson, the use of this matrix showed the level at which patients were encouraged to use their own abilities to self-care, or the level at which the nurse inhibited the patients' self-care agency.

One of the most impressive features of the study is that these two concepts are then shown to be related to each other, the belief of the sister being found to be directly related to the patient's level of self-care agency in the wards. This finding not only supports Orem's model in a wider context than any of the papers found so far, but also adds support to studies such as Orton (1981) and Fretwell (1982), which show the sister's influence as central in creating the ward environment.

This study evidently adopted a cause and effect design in which the model was central. The results show that the attitude of the ward sister to care of the elderly, particularly relating to self-care, crucially affected the nurses' willingness to help patients to be more self-caring. This helps to support the claims of Orem's model in the social and interpersonal technologies and in the regulatory technologies.

QUALITY OF CARE IN THE COMMUNITY

This study was more concerned with the economic factors of operating a nursing service. It considers whether some method of classifying patients will enable a more effective use of nursing time in the community.

In the North American community setting Sienkiewicz (1984) investigated the effects of a patient classification system which would allow some patients a higher weighting than others, so that the patients in the higher category were given more nursing time per visit. The effect of the classification system was then examined to show the quality of care given using Orem's framework, which was assessed through the use of nursing documentation following the visits.

The study was designed so that patients who made new calls were randomly selected until 50 were chosen. These patients were then randomly assigned to two groups, an experimental and a control group. The distribution in the experimental group of age, sex and geographical location was examined by Sienkiewicz and was found to be a normal distribution. Data substantiated in 1982 by MCOSS Nursing Service showed that double the amount of time was needed on an admission visit than on a return visit. Accordingly, a weighting of two was given to every patient in the experimental group, and a weighting of one for each patient in the control group. Nurses visiting the patients in the experimental group had twice the amount of time allotted for these visits by curtailing their caseload for the day. Nurses were not informed of any patient classification and all carried a workload of new patients and return visits.

The day following each visit to the new patients the nursing record was reviewed using an instrument developed for the study from the MCOSS written guidelines for use with the Problem Oriented Record System. Reliability and validity of this instrument were tested through a pilot study. Sienkiewicz considers that the quality of care which was shown in the record was a valid measure of patient care. The quality of documentation using the instrument allowed assessment of completeness of the nursing records which were given numerical ratings; above 60% of completeness was considered a high rating.

Raw scores showed more complete areas on the records of the experimental than the control group. However, a chi-squared test showed no statistically significant difference between the groups.

Thus the study results did not support our hypothesis that admission visits to classified patients (the experimental group) are of a higher quality than those made to unclassified (the control group) patients.

(p. 312)

Although this study claims to be based on Orem's model it is difficult to see how nursing can be assessed by using the nursing documentation alone. Orem clearly states that assessment of therapeutic self-care demand is through observation and questioning, so the quality and quantity of this cannot be assessed using the nursing records alone, as is assumed from this study.

The study also clearly has some difficulty in design; for example, no account is taken of the actual level of dependence of the patients, whether at new or return visits. This lack of control may mean that new patients were either very dependent and needing more than double the time allocation, or that their dependency was not sufficient to need twice the amount of time allotted to them. The latter discrepancy could mean that the nurse used her extra time for one of her return visits which she felt was more deserving. This may particularly be the case as the nurses who were looking after patients in the experimental group were not informed of the extra time given to them.

The question of whether quality of care can be assessed from records alone has not been dealt with adequately in this paper; there is mention of the different levels of ability of the nurses, but the study was not sensitive enough to detect these.

Sienkiewicz suggests that the development of a patient classification system for the community nursing service is essential in order to estimate nursing need for the service. However, the design of the study, which was descriptive, needs to be tightened to produce valid results. It is also not helpful that nurses were not observed in their natural environment, where they were assessing and treating patients, but measures were taken of the representation of their work by removing the records and studying them in a different environment.

This study does nothing to support or overturn Orem's model, mainly due to the research design.

CONCLUSION

These two very different studies had different aims and therefore different approaches to the investigation of quality. One showed very convincingly that the level of self-care orientation of the ward sister influences the care elderly patients receive. Where a positive self-care orientation was found elderly patients were able to use their self-care agency.

The other study failed to show a relationship between the amount of time spent by the nurse with new patients and the level of completeness of the nursing record. This study had considerable problems with design and did not elaborate Orem's model further.

THE NURSE AS A POTENTIAL SELF-CARE PRACTITIONER

This last section contains a single study which used Orem's (1980) model as its basis. Orem does not make a clear statement on the role of the nurse as a self-care practitioner, and therefore the effect of this on patients and clients, although she does say:

> Nursing agency is analogous to self-care agency in that both are abilities for specialized types of deliberate action. They differ in that nursing agency is developed and exercised for the benefit and well-being of others and self-care agency is developed and exercised for the benefit of well-being of oneself.
>
> (p. 88)

The results of the study are of considerable importance in their implications for initial nurse education as well as for post-registration education.

Edgar, Shamian and Patterson (1984) assumed that the concept of self-care should be the aim of nurses towards themselves, as well as in patient teaching. To this extent they expected that as nurses generally have more knowledge of health behaviours than non-nurses, they would practise self-care behaviours on themselves more frequently, would have more confidence to carry them out, would know the relationship to disease and would have a more positive attitude than non-nurses. The particular health behaviour investigated to explore the actions of nurses compared with non-nurses was breast self-examination.

Questionnaires with multiple choice questions were sent to 1900 hospital staff in a large Canadian general hospital, following personal contact by the researchers with each hospital department. This resulted in a 28% response rate. Items on the questionnaire measured the respondents' knowledge of how to carry out breast self-examination; the relationship of various signs and symptoms to breast cancer, including personal and family history; confidence in being able to carry out breast self-examination adequately; and the reasons for practising self-examination. Content and face validity were ensured by a pilot study on six staff nurses, 15 nursing co-ordinators and two non-nurses. Reliability was not assessed, but Stillman (1977) and Hirschfeld-Bartek (1982) had used most of the questions previously and had found them to be reliable.

Findings were that only 24% of the nurses and 21% of the non-nurses who responded to the questionnaire practised breast self-examination regularly. This varied considerably from other studies (e.g. Turnbull, 1977; Bayley *et al.*, 1980) who found that two-thirds of their postgraduate nurses practised regularly. Edgar, Shamian and Patterson accounted for these differences as being due to educational level. Nurses reported being significantly more confident than non-nurses in how to practise breast self-examination ($p < 0.05$). This seemed surprising in the light of their reported lack of practice; the authors attribute this difference to nurses feeling that an acceptable response is one of confidence, although anonymity of the respondents was assured. However, the results showed that nurses knew the method of carrying out breast self-examination better than non-nurses ($p < 0.05$), but the knowledge of signs and symptoms and predisposing factors to breast cancer was only slightly better in nurses than in non-nurses. The attitudes to breast self-examination showed no difference between the groups.

Commenting on the findings, the authors suggest that the level of educational preparation (non-degree level) may prevent these nurses from incorporating their own self-care behaviours into a system that will work for them. They believe that further success in patient teaching by nurses will only meet with success when nurses themselves become competent practitioners, and are also able to explore their own attitudes to cancer and their responsibility for self-care.

These findings contradict previous research, in that confidence here was not an incentive to practise. The link between attitudes, knowledge and confidence was unclear.

A difficulty with this study was the sample. No attempt was made to sample from any community except the hospital, nor was mention made of the representativeness of the sample. The 28% response rate was poor, but speculation on this was not made, nor were efforts made to follow up non-responders. It could be that the small response rate indicated apathy about the subject, therefore the results must be suspect and clearly liable to bias.

However, the point is well made that in order for nurses to have effective nursing agency they must be effective self-care agents. As Edgar, Shamian and Patterson argue, in order for the nurse to be convincing she must have appropriate attitudes to self-care and be sufficiently convinced of the benefit of self-care agency to know how to advise patients.

Due to the problems with this study, the results neither support nor refute Orem's model.

CONCLUSIONS ON THE USE OF THE MODEL TO 1990

Orem's model has generated a considerable amount of research in practice settings in a relatively short time, most of this since the publication of the second edition of her work in 1980. The research has been conducted in a variety of settings and considers a variety of issues raised by the model. Also impressive is the evident acceptability of the model to nurses working in a wide range of practice settings, and to nurses from a wide variety of cultures, both North American and European. Most of the work that comprises this chapter has used the model as intended by Orem, without finding it necessary to alter its components to 'fit' the practice settings; this is further evidence of the acceptability of the model. Also, many of the studies have used the model as central to their enquiry, showing that the questions raised by the model are useful in practice.

The studies found were in the areas of identification of self-care requisites in different groups. In this the model was seen as providing a very good basis for identifying self-care abilities and deficits. Other studies investigated nursing actions to promote self-care. In this area there were many problems, as the patient, according to the model, must be willing to promote his or her own self-care. Therefore it is no great surprise that in situations where it is difficult for patients to change their lifestyle, such as giving up smoking, promoting self-care by teaching the patient has been shown to be less effective. This tends to throw into doubt not only Orem's nursing actions to promote self-care, but also the validity of the model itself.

This chapter has also looked at standards of care and the nurse as a self-care agent. In the promotion of standards of care, a well-designed study from the UK has shown the effect of the ward sister in promoting self-care in elderly patients. The design of the study of a nurse as a potential self-care practitioner was flawed, so the results neither support nor overturn the model.

DEVELOPMENTS SINCE 1990

When conducting a literature search for the development of Orem's model since 1990 I was very struck by the continued international work on this model. Since 1990 Orem has published a further edition of her model (Orem, 1991), which I have discussed at the beginning of this chapter. In this section I will now analyse the papers since 1990 which have helped to develop and explain this model further.

The papers published since 1990 have been in the following areas.

- The testing of an assessment tool to measure self-care agency which had been translated from English into Norwegian and Dutch.
- The identification of self-care needs of patients with mitral valve prolapse.
- The ways in which Orem's model can help Chinese nurses to conceptualize nursing.

- The use of Orem's model in studies of self-care in patients with cancer who are undergoing chemotherapy and experiencing tiredness, nausea and vomiting.

Although not all of these papers are strictly research studies, they all show the potential use of the model in practice settings.

IDENTIFICATION OF SELF-CARE REQUISITES AND DEFICITS

CROSS-CULTURAL TESTING OF AN ASSESSMENT TOOL TO MEASURE SELF-CARE AGENCY

An assessment tool developed and validated in English by Evers (1989) was translated into both Norwegian and Dutch. This formed the basis of two papers that appeared in the literature in 1993. The tool assesses a person's ability to meet their own self-care needs (format A) and how another person rates that self-care ability (format B). The validation of the tool in both Norwegian and Dutch is analysed below.

Lorensen *et al.* (1993) translated the Appraisal of Self-Care Agency (ASA) scale (Evers, 1989) into Norwegian. This project was undertaken by a collaborative team from Norway, Belgium, USA and the Netherlands. The ASA scale is designed to assess whether a person can meet his or her own self-care needs.

Following translation into Norwegian both the A and B formats were administered in Oslo, Norway to convenience samples of elderly people. Format A was administered to a group of 40 elderly people in two geriatric rehabilitation units. Format B was administered to 40 nurses and 40 nursing assistants who cared for these patients. Therefore each patient had three sets of ratings completed on them: one completed by themselves, one by a nurse and one by a nursing auxiliary. This formed group 1.

Format A was also self-administered to a group of 40 elderly people who were living independently. Format B was not completed for this group. These patients formed group 2.

The results were analysed using Pearson's correlation coefficient between the nurses, the patients and the nursing auxiliaries in group 1. The correlation between the nurses and the nursing auxiliaries was 0.57 ($p = 0.00$). The correlation between the patients, the nurses and the nursing auxiliaries was 0.38 ($p = 0.025$). However, the nurses had a higher correlation with the patients depending on their level of education and length of experience. These findings suggest that experienced nurses who have higher levels of education have greater agreement with the patients of the latters' self-care abilities.

The internal consistency of the scales was tested using Cronbach's alpha: for Format A for both groups this was 0.77; for Format B, tested on nurses, the value was 0.82; and tested on nursing auxiliaries it was 0.88.

Therefore, testing the scale which had been translated into Norwegian found both Formats A and B to be valid and reliable. The scales were therefore able to differentiate between different patients' levels of self-care abilities and needs. However, there was no retranslation of the scales into English to check the sense and meaning of the Norwegian translation.

The authors recommend the tool as a means of promoting discussion between themselves and the patients about self-care abilities and needs for assistance. They also recommend that further cross-cultural testing of the tool be carried out.

The second study (Evers *et al.*, 1993) carried out further validity testing of the tool, this time in the Netherlands, by translating the ASA scale into Dutch. The team involved in this work came from Belgium, USA and the Netherlands. This paper indicates that the scale has already been translated into seven different languages.

This study, as well as testing the meaning of the translated version of the scale, also tested its validity with elderly people.

Once Formats A and B had been translated into Dutch, a retranslation, by professional translators who were unfamiliar with the original, was undertaken. The researchers found that a number of words and phrases were ambiguous when retranslated.

Finally, three unilingual English speakers were asked to rate the accuracy and quality of the grammar of the original and the retranslated version. When the agreement of at least two of the raters was used as the criterion, only 4% of the items showed no agreement, while 47% of the translation was judged to be worse, 32% comparable and 17% was considered better. The researchers therefore concluded that the Dutch ASA scale was fully comparable with the English version with the exception of one item.

The validity of the ASA Format A was tested on 130 elderly people over 65 years of age. Forty of these were elderly patients in a nursing home, 30 were residents in a 'personalized care facility' (p. 338), 30 were residents in 'a service flat' (p. 338) and 30 were elderly people who lived independently. All were randomly selected using a random digit table.

This was an important test of validity, as these elderly were known to have different levels of self-care ability, which differed depending on where they lived.

The results showed the following.

- Those living independently had a higher self-care ability than those living in service flats (one-tailed t-tests, $p = 0.001$).
- The residents of the service flats had higher self-care scores than those in the personalized care facility (one-tailed t-tests, $p = 0.008$).
- However, residents of the personalized care facility did not have a significantly higher level of self-care ($p > 0.05$) than those in the nursing home.

- The service flat residents had a higher self-care ability than the residents of the nursing home (*t*-test, $p = 0.001$).
- The nursing home residents had a statistically lower level of self-care than those in the community (*t*-test, $p = 0.001$).
- Those living in the community had a significantly higher level of self-care than those living in the personalized care facility (*t*-test, $p = 0.001$).

The researchers claim that the proven validity of this scale in Dutch, through testing on four groups of elderly people, shows that Orem's self-care deficit theory can be tested in a Dutch setting; also that the ASA instrument is valid and can therefore be used to measure self-care agency in the Netherlands.

It is interesting to note the widespread translation that this scale has received. However, it cannot be assumed from this that the notion of self-care, as proposed by Orem, is equally widespread, as this assumes a similar social construction of self-care. The scale may just be a useful measure outwith the use of Orem's model.

However, the translation of the scales was rigorously carried out both for validity and reliability using mathematical indices of correlation. This study did not test for cause and effect, therefore variables in Orem's model were not being tested. However, the fit of the model with the nurses and the elderly people on which the tool was tested was evidently good. Therefore, a translation of Orem's assessment and the concepts of self-care as proposed by Orem, using this assessment tool, can be said to be valid and reliable in the situation in which it was tested and by those involved in the ratings.

THE EFFECTS OF MITRAL VALVE PROLAPSE

This paper does not only deal with the identification of self-care abilities and deficits, it also briefly considers the ways nurses can help patients with the condition of mitral valve prolapse. However, no evaluation of the effectiveness of nursing intervention is carried out. The study is based firmly on Orem's (1991) model and was conducted in both Ohio and Virginia, USA.

Utz and Ramos (1993) saw Orem's model as highly relevant to people with mitral valve prolapse for two reasons; first, the person's perception of their condition is important in assessment of their self-care abilities and needs; and second, assessment also covers the patient's knowledge of their condition, which is often not provided by their doctors. Doctors often believe the condition to be benign, but in the experience of the researchers, people often suffer worrying symptoms as a result of it.

The study of people with symptomatic mitral valve prolapse had a number of stages. Stage 1 was the analysis of 124 patients' medical records. The most frequent finding from this stage was the prescription of prophylactic antibiotics and beta-blockers. However, data on patients' therapeutic self-care demands were incomplete, so that Orem's framework could not be used.

Stage 2 involved interviewing patients with symptoms. Twenty people, who were located through their medical records, agreed to be interviewed; however, we are not told how many patients were initially approached. A semi-structured interview guide was developed based on Orem's six categories of health deviation self-care. This used Spradley's (1979) ethnographic method.

Analysis of the data from the interviews found that patients expressed concerns in all six of the health deviation self-care requisites. Patients nearly always asked for an explanation of their symptoms and also wanted to let health professionals know just how serious they perceived their symptoms to be and how it had changed their lives. They also frequently looked for help to prevent further problems with their health.

From this stage of the study researchers were able to identify those suffering from mitral valve prolapse as having:

- patterns of help-seeking;
- perceived needs for help;
- levels of understanding about their condition;
- individual success with the management of symptoms.

The researchers therefore saw a real need for nursing services for these patients. This led to their looking for other nurses working in a similar field, to assess whether they saw these patients' needs as similar. However, we are not told what the outcome of this stage was.

The third phase of the study involved investigating changes in the patients' body image with the diagnosis of mitral valve prolapse. The data from the previous interviews were analysed for evidence of changes in body image. Utz and Ramos found that 19 of the 20 people with mitral valve prolapse had concerns that reflected changes in body structure and function associated with the condition. This shows the link between two of the stages of assessment – assessment of self-care deficits and how this is linked to changes in body structure and function. This completes the assessment phases of the study.

The fourth phase of the study looked at nurses' perceptions of the problems that patients with mitral valve prolapse most frequently had, and the kind of nursing help that was most commonly given. A mail questionnaire was produced as a pilot study and sent to 84 nurses in the USA who were known to work in the area of cardiac nursing. A 42% response rate was achieved; however we are not told if efforts to increase the response rate were made. Responses showed that Orem's model was highly appropriate for these patients, as nurses predominantly taught the patients about their condition, supported and guided them on the types of self-care actions to take and sometimes acted for or did things for the patients. Many of the respondents indicated their frustrations with medicine by diagnosing the condition and then dismissing it as unimportant. However, the sample size and the response rate limits the credibility of the results.

The final stage of the study involved the design and validation of a questionnaire asking about the lived experience of mitral valve prolapse, for example the experience of symptoms and the seriousness of mitral valve prolapse as a health problem. This was based on Orem's health deviation self-care requisites. The questionnaire also asked about perceptions of treatment for the condition. Validation was carried out to test the construct validity of the items and also the external validity of the tool.

The questionnaires were sent by mail to 132 people with symptomatic mitral valve prolapse who were found through a medical record review from one large centre. The response rate was very poor; only 38 were returned (29%). We are not told if any follow-up was conducted to try to increase the response rate, or if this level of response was after follow-up. This throws some doubt on the validity of the questionnaire and its attractiveness to the respondents. If, as we are led to believe from the previous stages of the study, people with mitral valve prolapse are acutely concerned by their symptoms, then one might expect a much higher rate of response to something that interests and is important to them. This level of response casts some doubt on the validity of the findings of the previous stages of the study. If the previous findings are valid, all one can think is that either the questionnaire did not ask the kind of questions that the recipients found relevant (problems of validity) or it was so poorly constructed, or so lengthy, to deter them from replying.

However, the researchers increased their response rate by advertising in local newspapers. The advertisement said that there was a mitral valve prolapse support group being set up and an open evening was being held. At this evening the research instrument was given out to be completed at home and returned. Thirty-eight questionnaires were returned, but we are not told the original number handed out, so the response rate cannot be calculated. However, this was a self-selecting group, unlike those who received the questionnaire through the post, so maybe the experience of mitral valve prolapse is very variable. According to the article there was much appreciation expressed by those who attended the group 'for the opportunity to "tell their stories"' (pp. 749–750). This statement makes it even more surprising that the response to the mail questionnaire was so poor.

The returned questionnaires, both mail and from the support group, indicated that the self-care deficits of those with mitral valve prolapse led to them seeking help for such symptoms as chest pain, palpitations, shortness of breath, syncope, fatigue and tingling and numbness in their extremities. Moreover, medically prescribed treatments, such as taking medication, were often experienced as ineffective or gave troublesome side effects. Respondents also indicated a dramatic impact on their daily lives.

This study has clearly demonstrated the severe effect that mitral valve prolapse has on some people with the condition. It also shows how Orem's model can help these people to identify their health needs (therapeutic self-care demands) and their deficiencies in self-care (self-care deficits). Although many problems for these patients are clearly shown, what is less clearly shown is the effectiveness of nursing actions in helping them to meet their self-care demands (self-care agency), although the forms of helping advocated by Orem are evidently appropriate with these people.

A worrying aspect of the paper is the possible extent of attributing pathological symptoms of mitral valve prolapse to all those with the diagnosis. This can most easily be queried as a result of the return rate from the questionnaire which was sent to unsolicited people.

Many different research strategies were used to deal with the questions that the researchers asked. Both structured questionnaires sent through the post and interviewing patients using an ethnographic approach (Spradley, 1989) were used. All these methods are consistent with Orem's model and help to develop an understanding of the model in use in practice. The results from the methods give a clear picture of the worrying symptoms of some patients diagnosed as having mitral valve prolapse. The results also help to confirm the appropriateness of Orem's model in assessment of these patients' self-care deficits, as her model was central to the research design.

However, the study was mainly descriptive, with the link between assessment and nursing actions to promote self-care not being developed. Therefore the effectiveness of nursing actions is not dealt with in this work.

THE WAYS IN WHICH OREM'S MODEL CAN HELP CHINESE NURSES TO CONCEPTUALIZE NURSING

This paper, written by one North American author and one Chinese author, looks at the developments in Chinese nursing. It appears that in China nurse leaders are very keen to improve nursing education as one way of dealing with the tremendous shortage of nurses. The authors consider a model of nursing as one way of making these improvements.

Morales-Mann and Jiang (1993) consider Orem's model and its fit with Chinese nursing and Chinese culture. They assess the fit along the lines of the model's completeness, compatibility, practicality and feasibility. Their analysis gives us some insight into Chinese nursing, its roots and its aspirations.

At the time of writing the paper Chinese nursing was at the technical level, mainly limited to the hospital setting which involved observation and reporting of the patient's situation and the administration of drugs and treatments. In this role nurses provided the care with doctors making most of the decisions.

According to the authors, despite the present level of nursing in China, Orem's view of nursing is very similar to that of Chinese nurses. This is particularly so as nursing and medicine work closely together in China; due to nursing shortages, doctors and nurses often have the same function. Therefore, both Chinese nurses and Orem's model see nursing as comfort and relief of sickness, promotion of health and disease prevention. Furthermore, Orem does not reject medicine but incorporates it into nursing. Therefore, as far as compatibility is concerned, the emphasis by Orem on self-care in order to maintain and promote health is entirely compatible with Chinese goals for nursing. However, because the Chinese, and therefore by implication Chinese nursing, stress the importance of the individual's harmonious relationship with the environment as promoting health, this finds less compatibility with Orem, as her definition of the environment is somewhat limited.

Looking at completeness, Morales-Mann and Jiang consider that Orem's theory is well defined, as are its interrelationships, including the nursing process and the role of the nurse. All this would help the Chinese nurse. However, the environment is not well defined, but its components, such as factors and conditions in the environment, have been well described by Orem. Also less clearly defined is the relationship between the nurse and the well person (Meleis, 1991); this is important for Chinese nurses who want to develop community nursing, which would include health promotion and illness prevention.

The practicality of Orem's model for Chinese nurses is considered first in relation to use of language, and second as a system of nursing care. The language of Orem's model is known only to a few nurses in China, mainly those involved in education. However, Orem's concepts of the sick and the aim of promoting self-care is similar to the medical model, involving pathophysiology, so would ease the transition to Orem's concepts. Furthermore, Chinese nursing is currently organized through classifying patients into three levels of care – those needing constant care, those needing less care and those with an increased independence – each of which is described in the Chinese system. As this is similar to Orem's system of nursing care it will increase the model's level of acceptability and credibility.

Feasibility of the model will depend, according to Morales-Mann and Jiang, on the openness and readiness for the application of the theory. In China there were, when the study was undertaken, some pockets of interest and some nurses with knowledge of the model. If more general acceptability were to occur then increased familiarity with the model would be important; this could occur in a number of ways, including workshops, study abroad and setting up pilot schemes.

It therefore appears to Morales-Mann and Jiang that there is a good level of compatibility between Orem's theory and Chinese nursing, with limitations in the area of the environment. The completeness of Orem's model is deficient in her emphasis on the ill, rather than the well person. Practicality is enhanced by Orem's classification of nursing into three systems of nursing care which are similar to the Chinese system. The feasibility of the model will depend not only on the readiness of Chinese nurses to accept the model, but also on the amount and access of resources to promote its implementation.

However, although the concepts of compatibility, completeness, practicality and feasibility have been chosen by the authors, they question whether these are entirely appropriate given the very different cultures of North America and China. I would endorse this, although it is very useful to see a comparison of the model from two different cultural perspectives. What the authors of this paper have probably underplayed, among other factors, is the difference in the social construction of self-care and other key concepts in Orem's model between the different cultures.

What this paper does show, however, is the push for models generated in a North American setting to be tried out and understood in other, very different cultures. But will this negatively affect the culture into which the model is being introduced by changing that culture to look more like a Western culture? And why is a Western culture so much better?

A REVIEW OF THE STUDIES OF SELF-CARE IN PATIENTS WITH CANCER

This paper summarizes the literature in a discrete area of nursing practice, but it also makes a considerable contribution to the knowledge gained to date in the use and appropriateness of Orem's model. It therefore provides an excellent summary of the model for a certain group of patients.

Richardson (1992) first outlines Orem's model, then analyses its use in a number of research studies with cancer patients who are receiving chemotherapy. The self-care behaviours of these patients are examined as a result of chemotherapy-induced nausea and vomiting. However, as Richardson says, there is no attempt on her part to test the assumptions and propositions within the model.

Discussing a study by Fernsler (1988), Richardson comments that 'Patients generally reported more self-care deficits than did nurses' in the physical side effects of therapy, but nurses perceived more side effects in psychosocial problems. Therefore nurses did not perceive the level of problems that the patients had, particularly with activity and rest. The disparity between nurses and patients is made very clear in this study. Kubricht (1984) also found, through the use of open-ended interviews with 30 patients, that they experienced changes in all the universal self-care requisites. Assessment of the therapeutic self-care demand showed that nursing was certainly needed to help alleviate some of the effects of treatment, however what this care was and its effectiveness were not given.

Rhodes, Watson and Hanson (1988) interviewed 20 patients by telephone about their symptoms and self-care. They found that tiredness and weakness were the main problems to self-care which affected their planning and scheduling of activities and their work. Patients decreased non-essential activities and they were increasingly dependent on others. Further, Hanucharurnkul (1989) found that socio-economic level and the amount of social support were directly related to self-care.

The work of Dodd receives special note in this paper. Some of the papers by Dodd (e.g. Dodd and Mood, 1981; Dodd, 1984a, b) are discussed earlier in this chapter. Her later studies (Dodd, 1987, 1988), according to Richardson, have moved from identification of self-care agency and deficits in patients taking chemotherapy for cancer, to teaching the patients self-care behaviours. She says that although there are a large number of side effects to chemotherapy experienced by the patients, their number of self-care behaviours are limited. Dodd attributed this to the lack of information given by health professionals and the lack of knowledge of the patients themselves of how to cope with the problems they experienced. She indicates a strong need for health professionals to give information to patients to help them to prevent these side effects.

Later work by Musci and Dodd (1990), in a longitudinal study, emphasized the role of the family in helping self-care by the patient. Dodd's earlier work was corroborated by the finding that neither the families' nor the patients' mood nor the families' coping strategies were associated with the management of the side effects. The more severe the side effects the more the sufferer risked diminishing self-care over a period of time.

Further work which supported the findings of Dodd (1984c) was by Li-Hua Lo (1990). She found that in order to deal with nausea and vomiting, patients were taking over-the-counter and prescribed anti-emetics, eating foods which are well known to be easily tolerated, drinking carbonated drinks, eating crackers and resting. Richardson (1989) asked patients to keep diaries of self-care behaviours during a 5-day period. She found that they took anti-emetic tablets, changed their diet and fluid intake, regulated their activity and rest patterns and wore acupressure bands. Tierney, Taylor and Closs (1989) also looked into the most prevalent side effects of chemotherapy. They similarly found that nausea and vomiting were frequently reported, followed by tiredness.

However, they found that in many cases no actions were taken by the patients, who often felt that they had to put up with it.

From the review of these studies we can see that nausea, vomiting and tiredness are very frequent occurrences in chemotherapy. Although patients do take self-care measures, they frequently try to ignore the symptoms. It seems that nurses can help these patients to develop their self-care behaviours by giving information. Richardson (1992) sums up her literature review in this area by saying that research needs to develop the relationship between patients' abilities and motivation to undertake effective self-care in relation to side effects. She also feels that nursing as well as pharmacological intervention and its effectiveness in helping patients needs to be shown.

This paper adds to our understanding of the self-care deficits of cancer patients, however it neither supports nor overturns Orem's model and its concepts.

Four other studies were found since 1990 in the popular nursing literature. All of them are from the UK. These are included as they give some indication of the general acceptability of the model in different environments where nurses work. However, they do not investigate these situations in a systematic fashion. MacDonald (1991) considers Orem's model in rehabilitating a patient with a long history of mental illness who is being housed in a hostel in Edinburgh. He finds the model very appropriate. He says that psychiatric patients have needs in the areas of money handling, learning to use public and community facilities and they also need to build up their self-esteem and self-confidence. MacDonald found that Orem's terminology helped not only the patients, but also the nurses and 'made the plans easier to follow for everyone involved' (p. 42). This is surprising as a new language must have had to be used by everyone concerned. A worrying feature of the paper is the lack of confidentiality, as the exact location of the hostel is given as well as the patient's name and a great deal of his past medical history. However, the paper shows the acceptability of the model in psychiatric rehabilitation settings in the UK.

Weir (1993) finds Orem's model totally appropriate in theatre. Lacey (1993) applied Orem's model to a psychiatric nursing setting, through a review of the literature. Many of the concepts of the model are criticized by Lacey, such as how differences in cultural and socio-economic status of individuals can have implications for taking responsibility for their own health. Some settings, such as nursing homes, felt more comfortable if the patients were dependent on staff, rather than promoting their self-care; also the involvement of patients in their own self-care may be resisted by some patients. Lacey sees this resistance as being particularly relevant for psychiatric nursing in the UK. Two further concepts that caused a problem for Lacey were that self-care may be ideal in a health care system based on privately funded health care, but not so appropriate in a public service such as the UK system. Furthermore, that some people are unable to have any control over their environment, often as a result of social class, is not consistent with notions of promoting self-care.

Last, a paper by Kelly (1995) considers the care of a retired man with multiple cerebrovascular accidents which have resulted in mild right-sided weakness. Kelly finds Orem's model entirely appropriate and claims to have improved this man's state of health as a result of promoting his self-care following permanent residence in a hospital ward. This again shows the acceptability of Orem's model in a variety of nursing settings in the UK.

Although these last four papers are based very directly on Orem's model, all, apart from Lacey, are uncritical of the model in use. However, MacDonald does give some indication that changes are needed for the model to entirely meet the requirements of rehabilitation from long-term care in psychiatry. Although three of the papers describe patient care situations, Lacey's article is more of a critique of the concepts of the model for use in psychiatry. All of the papers show the growing exploration by and acceptability of Orem's model to nurses in the UK in a variety of settings.

CONCLUSIONS ON THE USE OF THE MODEL FROM ITS DEVELOPMENT TO 1995

From the considerable number of studies so far completed and published in the literature, Orem's model is felt to be a good framework to use in assessing people's self-care agency and deficits. The studies that have investigated this so far have been in the areas of:

- diabetes;
- well children;
- the well elderly living at home;
- people with dementia;
- levels of stress following myocardial infarction;
- patients with tiredness, nausea and vomiting during chemotherapy;
- self-care at home after discharge from hospital following lung surgery;
- chronic schizophrenic patients' social skills;
- chronically mentally ill people's morning care skills;
- elderly people's self-care abilities and deficits;
- self-care agency and deficits in self-selecting people with mitral valve prolapse.

Many of these studies have shown that Orem's assessment methods are very suitable in the situations and with the patients that have been studied. However, the validity of some of the tools used to assess the self-care agency and deficits has been queried, for example in the assessment of anxiety following myocardial infarction. Also just by the use of some of the tools developed from the model, it cannot be assumed that the social construction of some of the concepts of the model itself are necessarily adopted, for example in the translation of the Appraisal of Self-Care Agency scale.

Although assessment of self-care agency and deficits has been reasonably successful using Orem's framework, the same cannot be said for nursing intervention using her 'helping methods'. A large number of helping methods have also been developed in the published papers. These include:

- structured and unstructured teaching in book and leaflet form as well as verbally and through the use of videos with a number of different groups of people;
- social skills training using social dramatics;
- behaviour modification methods;
- nursing as support;
- the ward sister in care of the elderly wards having a self-care philosophy.

Many of the interventions were effective, for example teaching children to be involved in activities that promote self-care, teaching chronically mentally ill patients how to undertake morning care, supporting patients with mitral valve prolapse and the philosophy of the ward sister as promoting self-care on wards caring for elderly people. However, many of the nursing interventions to promote self-care have a more dubious beneficial effect; these are:

- teaching patients following myocardial infarction in order to reduce their anxiety;
- teaching self-care to patients who are experiencing nausea or vomiting during chemotherapy for cancer (although this has not been widely investigated);
- teaching patients self-care at home after lung surgery;
- teaching patients how to control their hypertension;
- teaching chronic schizophrenics social skills by the use of social dramatics;
- assessing elderly women's willingness to comply with a care plan by participating in the planning of care.

Therefore in these areas the interaction between Orem's model and the practice of nursing is less clear. In fact, it could be said that in many areas of nursing practice, particularly those that involve teaching the patient, the model currently cannot help nurses to provide effective care.

However some researchers, such as Dodd, have based their research programmes on the use of the model in practice. This can only help to develop our understanding of the relationship of the model to the practice of nursing. In this way it may help us to improve the effectiveness of interventions by a deeper understanding of the issues involved.

A further aspect of Orem's model is the extent of its use and the interest in it worldwide. Apart from clearly being widely used in North America it has also been used in Sweden and the UK. Parts of it, for example the ASA scale, have been translated into seven languages including Norwegian and Dutch. There is also evidence of interest being expressed in China: the paper by Morales-Mann and Jiang (1993) explores the use and comparability in cultural terms of the model for Chinese nurses who, we are told, are keen to develop their professional skills, including decision-making. Therefore, whether we agree with it or not, Orem's model is becoming known world-wide in many different settings.

REFERENCES

Ackerman, A.M. (1977) Patient education and its relevance to compliance, in *Hypertension, the Nurses' Role in Ambulatory Care* (ed. M.H. Alderman), Springer, New York, pp. 110–19.

American Psychiatric Association (1980) *Quick Reference to the Diagnostic Criteria from DSM-III*. American Psychiatric Association, Washington.

Bayley, J. *et al.* (1980) The effectiveness of registered nurses in breast self-examination. *Australian Nurses' Journal*, **9**, 42–4.

Blair, C. (1985) Behaviour modification in nursing practice and research: a case study. *Journal of Advanced Nursing*, **10**, 165–8.

Blazek, B. and McClellan, M.S. (1983) The effects of self-care instruction on locus of control in children. *Journal of School Health*, **53**(9), 554–6.

Braimner, L.M. (1973) *The Helping Relationship. Process and Skills*, Prentice-Hall, Englewood Cliffs, NJ.

Buros, O.K. (ed.) (1972) *The Seventh Mental Measurements Yearbook I*, Gryphon Press, Edison, NJ.

Caplan, G. (1974) *Support Systems and Community Mental Health*, Human Science Press, New York.

Chang, B.L., Uman, G.C., Linn, L.S. *et al.* (1982) The relationship of participation in care planning and patient satisfaction. Paper presented at the American Educational Research Association, New York.

Chang, B.L., Uman, G.C. Linn, L.S. *et al.* (1985) Adherence to health care regimes among elderly women. *Nursing Research*, **34**(1), 27–31.

Dodd, M.J. (1984a) Measuring informational intervention for chemotherapy knowledge and self-care behaviours. *Research in Nursing and Health*, **7**, 43–50.

Dodd, M.J. (1984b) Self-care for patients with breast cancer to prevent side-effects of chemotherapy: a concern for Public Health Nursing. *Public Health Nursing*, **1**(4), 202–9.

Dodd, M. (1984c) Patterns of self-care in patients receiving radiation therapy. *Oncology Nurses Forum*, **11**(3), 23–7.

Dodd, M. (1987) Efficacy of provative information on self-care in radiation therapy patients. *Heart and Lung*, **16**, 538–44.

Dodd, M. (1988) Efficacy of proactive information on self-care in chemotherapy patients. *Patient Education and Counselling*, **11**, 215–25.

Dodd, M.J. and Mood, D.W. (1981) Chemotherapy: helping patients to know the drugs they are receiving and their possible side-effects. *Cancer Nursing*, **4**, 311–18.

Donohue-Porter, D. (1985) Insulin-dependent diabetes mellitus. *Nursing Clinics of North America*, **20**(1), 191–8.

Dunn, L.M. (1965) *Peabody Picture Vocabulary Test Manual*, American Guidance Service, Circle Pines.

Edelson, R.I. and Seidman, E. (1975) Use of videotape feedback in altering perception of married couples: therapy analogue. *Journal of Consulting and Clinical Psychology*, **43**, 244–50.

Edgar, L., Shamian, J. and Patterson, D. (1984) Factors affecting the nurse as a teacher and practitioner of breast self-examination. *International Journal of Nursing Studies*, **21**(4), 255–65.

Evers, G.C.M. (1989) *Appraisal of Self-Care Agency (A.S.A) Scale*, Van Gorcum, Assen, Maastricht.

Evers, G.C.M., Isenberg, M.A., Philipsen, H. *et al.* (1993) Validity testing of the Dutch translation of the appraisal of the self-care agency (ASA) scale. *International Journal of Nursing Studies*, **30**(4), 331–42.

Fernsler, J. (1988) A comparison of patient and nurse perceptions of patients' self-care deficits associated with cancer chemotherapy. *Cancer Nursing*, **9**(2), 50–7.

Finestone, A.J. and Boorujy, S. (1967) Diabetes mellitus and periodontic disease. *Diabetes*, **16**, 336.

Foster, S.B. (1974) An adrenal measure for evaluating nursing effectiveness. *Nursing Research*, **23** (March–April), 118–24.

Fretwell, J.E. (1982) *Ward Teaching and Learning: Sister and the Learning Environment*, Royal College of Nursing, London.

Glaser, B.G. (1978) *Advances in the Methodology of Grounded Theory, Theoretical Sensitivity*, The Sociology Press, Mill Valley, CA.

Glaser, B. and Strauss, A. (1967) *The Discovery of Grounded Theory: Strategies for Qualitative Research*, Aldine, Chicago.

Goodwin, J.O. (1979) Programmed instruction for self-care following pulmonary surgery. *International Journal of Nursing Studies*, **16**, 29–40.

Grancio, S.D. (1979) Strategies for patient education. *Mass Nurse*, **48**, 4.

Griffiths, R.D.P. and Gillingham, P. (1978) The influence of videotape feedback on self-measurement of psychiatric patients. *British Journal of Psychiatry*, **193**, 156–61.

Hanucharurnkul, S. (1989) Predictors of self-care in cancer patients receiving radiotherapy. *Cancer Nursing*, **12**(1), 21–7.

Heine, A.G. (1981) Helping hypertensive patients help themselves: the nurses' role. *Patient Counselling and Health Education*, third quarter, 108–12.

Himmelhoch, A. (1980) Patient adherence in the treatment of hypertension. *Australian Family Physician*, **9**, 229.

Hirschfeld-Bartek, J. (1982) Health beliefs and their influence on breast self-examination in women with breast cancer. *Oncology Nurses Forum*, **9**, 77–81.

Honigfeld, G. (1974) NOSIE-30: history and current status of its use in pharmaco-psychiatric research. *Modern Problems of Pharmacopsychiatry*, **7**, 238–63.

Kelly, G. (1995) A self-care approach. *Nursing Times*, **91**(2), 40–1.

Kitson, A.L. (1986) Indicators of quality in nursing care – an alternative approach. *Journal of Advanced Nursing*, **11**, 133–44.

Kockar, M.S. and Daniels, L.M.M. (1978) *Hypertension Control for Nurses and other Health Professionals*, CV Mosby Co., St Louis.

Krug, S.E., Scheier, M. and Catell, A. (1976) *Handbook for the IPAT Anxiety Scale*, Institute for Personality and Ability Testing, Champaign, IL.

Kubricht, D. (1984) Therapeutic self-care demands expressed by outpatients receiving external radiation therapy. *Cancer Therapy*, **7**(1), 43–52.

Kyes, J. and Hofling, C. (1974) *Basic Psychiatric Concepts in Nursing*, 3rd edn, JB Lippincott, Philadelphia.

Lacey, D. (1993) Using Orem's model in psychiatric nursing. *Nursing Standard*, **7**(29), 28–30.

Larsen, D.E. (1982) Social work: independent daily living skills training for the chronically mentally ill. Unpublished PhD thesis, University of Utah, Salt Lake City, UT.

Lasky, P.A. and Eichelberger, K.A. (1985) Health-related views and self-care behaviours of young children. *Family Relations*, January, 13–18.

Li-Hua Lo (1990) Assessing breast cancer patients' self-care behaviours for nausea and vomiting. *Oncology Nurses Forum*, **17** (2 Suppl.), Abstract 15, 141.

Lorensen, M., Holter, I.M., Isenberg, M.A. and Van Achterberg, T. (1993) Cross-cultural testing of the "appraisal of self-care agency: ASA scale" in Norway. *International Journal of Nursing Studies*, **30**(1), 15–23.

MacDonald, G. (1991) Plans for a better future. *Nursing Times*, **87**(31) 42–3.

McNair, D.M., Lorr, M. and Droppleman, L.F. (1971) *Profile of Mood States*, Educational and Industrial Testing Service, San Diego.

Meleis, A.I. (1991) *Theoretical Nursing: Development and Progress*, 2nd edn, J.P. Lippincott, Philadelphia.

Miller, J.F. (1982) Categories of self-care needs of ambulatory patients with diabetes. *Journal of Advanced Nursing*, **7**, 25–31.

Morales-Mann, E.T. and Jiang, S.L. (1993) Applicability of Orem's conceptual framework: a cross-cultural point of view. *Journal of Advanced Nursing*, **18**, 737–41.

Moreno, J.L. (1946) *Psychodrama*, Beacon House, New York.

Musci, E. and Dodd, M. (1990) Predicting self-care with patients and family members' affective states and family functioning. *Oncology Nurses Forum*, **17**(3), 394–402.

Muss, H.B., White, D.R., Michielutte, R. *et al.* (1979) Written informed consent in patients with breast cancer. *Cancer*, **43**, 1549–56.

Neufeld, A. and Hobbs, H. (1985) Self-care in a high rise for seniors. *Nursing Outlook*, **33**(6), 298–301.

Orem, D. (1971) *Nursing: Concepts of Practice*, McGraw-Hill, New York.

Orem, D. (1980) *Nursing: Concepts of Practice*, 2nd edn, McGraw-Hill, New York.

Orem, D. (1985) *Nursing: Concepts of Practice*, 3rd edn, McGraw-Hill, New York.

Orton, H.D. (1981) Ward learning climate: a study of the role of the ward sister in relation to student nurse learning on the ward. Royal College of Nursing, London.

Parcel, G. and Meyer, M. (1978) Development of an instrument to measure children's health locus of control. *Health Education Monitor*, **6**(2), 149–59.

Rhodes, V., Watson, P. and Hanson, B. (1988) Patients' descriptions of the influence of tiredness and weakness of self-care abilities. *Cancer Nursing*, 11(3), 186–94.

Richardson, A. (1989) Self-care, a study of the behaviours initiated by chemotherapy patients to control nausea and vomiting. MSc Thesis, King's College, London.

Richardson, A. (1992) Studies exploring self-care for the person coping with cancer treatment: a review. *International Journal of Nursing Studies*, 29(2), 191–204.

Rivera-Alsina, M. and Willis, S. (1984) Needle and catheter colonisation in pregnant diabetic patients using continuous subcutaneous insulin infusion pump. *Diabetes Care*, 7, 75.

Ryan, C. (1980) Controversies in the treatment of hypertensives. *Comprehensive Therapeutics*, 6, 65.

Sackett, D.J. (1980) Compliance with antihypertensive therapy. *Canadian Journal of Public Health*, 71, 153.

Sackett, D.L, Haynes, R.B., Gibson, E.S. *et al.* (1975) Randomised clinical trial of strategies for improving medication compliance in primary hypertension. *Lancet*, 1, 1205.

Sandman, P.O., Norberg, A., Adolfsson, R., Axelsson, K. and Hedly, V. (1986) Morning care of patients with Alzheimer-type dementia. A theoretical model based on direct observations. *Journal of Advanced Nursing*, 11, 369–78.

Schoenbaum, S. (1982) Infection in diabetes, in *Clinical Diabetes*, ed. G. Kozak, W.B. Saunders, Philadelphia.

Schoenhofer, S.O. (1984) Support as legitimate nursing action. *Nursing Outlook*, 32(4), 218–19.

Sienkiewicz, J.I. (1984) Patient classification in Community Health Nursing. *Nursing Outlook*, November/December, 319–321.

Skyler, J. (1982) Self-monitoring of blood glucose. *Medical Clinics of North America*, 66, 1227.

Spencer, P.G., Gillespie, C.R. and Ekisa, E.G. (1983) A controlled comparison of the effects of social skills training and remedial drama on the conversation skills of chronic schizophrenic patients. *British Journal of Psychiatry*, 143, 165–72.

Spradley, J.P. (1989) *The Ethnographic Interview*, Holt, Reinhart & Wilson, New York.

Steckel, S.B. and Swain, M.A. (1977) Contracting with patients to improve compliance. *Hospitals*, 51, 81.

Stern, P.N. (1980) Grounded theory methodology: its uses and processes. *Image*, 12, 20–3.

Stillman, M.L. (1977) Women's health beliefs about breast self-examination. *Nursing Research*, 2, 121–7.

Tierney, J., Taylor, J. and Closs, S. (1989) A study to inform nursing support of patients coping with chemotherapy for breast cancer. Report, Nursing Research Unit, University of Edinburgh.

Todd, B. (1981) Twenty seven reasons people don't take their meds. *RN*, 44–54.

Toth, J.C. (1980) Effect of structured preparation for transfer on patient anxiety on leaving the Coronary Care Unit. *Nursing Research*, 29(1), 28–34.

Turnbull, E. (1977) Breast examination practices. *American Journal of Nursing*, 1450–1.

Underwood, P.R. (1978) Nursing: nursing care as a determinant in the development of self-care behaviour by hospitalised adult schizophrenics. Unpublished PhD thesis, University of California.

Utz, S.W. and Ramos, M.C. (1993) Mitral valve prolapse and its effects: a pro-gramme of enquiry within Orem's Self-Care Deficit theory of nursing. *Journal of Advanced Nursing*, **19**, 742–51.

Vicary, B. (1974) Final report on practice as Nurse Clinicians – 1. Thoracic surgery – Pulmonary. Unpublished report. The University of Michigan Hospital, Ann Arbor, MI.

Watson, D. (1979) Health education for hypertensive patients. *American Family Physician*, **8**, 315.

Weir, L. (1993) Using Orem's model. *British Journal of Theatre Nursing*, **3**(6), 19–22.

Weisman, A.D. and Worden, J.W. (1975) Psychological analysis of cancer deaths. *Omega*, **6**, 61–75.

Wheat, L. (1980) Infection in diabetes mellitus. *Diabetes Care*, **3**, 187.

Whetstone, W.R. (1986) Social dramatics: Social skills development for the chron-ically mentally ill. *Journal of Advanced Nursing*, **11**, 67–74.

FURTHER READING

Aggleton, P. and Chalmers, H. (1986) *Nursing Models and the Nursing Process*, Macmillan, London.

Chapman, C.M. (1985) *Theory of Nursing: Practical Application*, Harper and Row, London.

Chinn, P.L. (1983) *Advances in Nursing Theory Development*, Aspen.

Chinn, P.L. and Jacobs, M.K. (1987) *Theory and Nursing*, C.V. Mosby, St Louis.

Fawcett, J. (1984) *Analysis and Evaluation of Conceptual Models of Nursing*, F.A. Davis, Philadelphia.

Fitzpatrick, J.J. and Whall, A.L. (1983) *Conceptual Models of Nursing: Analysis and Application*, Prentice-Hall, Englewood Cliffs, NJ.

Griffith-Kennedy, J.W. and Christensen, P.J. (1986) *Nursing Process. Application of Theories, Frameworks and Models*, C.V. Mosby, St Louis.

George, J.B. (ed.) (1985) *Nursing Theories: A Base for Professional Nursing Practice*, 2nd edn, Prentice-Hall, Englewood Cliffs, NJ.

Kershaw, B. and Salvage, J. (1986) *Models for Nursing*, John Wiley, Chichester.

Marriner, A. (1986) *Nursing Theorists and their Work*, C.V. Mosby, St Louis.

Parse, R.R. (1987) *Nursing Science*, W.B. Saunders, New York.

Riehl, J.P. and Roy, C. (1980) *Conceptual Models for Nursing Practice*, 2nd edn, Appleton-Century-Crofts, Norwalk, OH.

Johnson's behavioural systems model

5

Table of chapter contents

Johnson's behavioural systems model

Topic researched	Model components	Results
Systems balance in chronically ill children	Assessment of achievement behaviours	Chronically ill children have behavioural systems imbalance in achievement
Systems balance in chronically ill children	Assessment of attachment behaviours	Mothers of chronically ill children show behavioural systems imbalance in attachment
Cancer patients	Behavioural systems balance	Imbalance found in all behavioural systems
Helping in nursing	The nurse as a helper	Problems with model identified
A tool to measure patient care	Second level of instruction	Physiological outcomes in infection, immobility and fluid balance identified
Evaluating Johnson's model in practice	Assessment to intervention	Assessment, diagnosis and identification of behavioural subsystems malfunctioning are impressive. Model does not prescribe nursing actions

THE AUTHOR

Dorothy Johnson was born in 1919. She obtained her Bachelor of Science in Nursing from Vanderbilt University, Tennessee in 1942, and her

Master's degree in Public Health from Harvard University, Boston in 1948.

From 1949 until her retirement she was Assistant Professor of Paediatric Nursing, Associate Professor of Nursing and Professor of Nursing at the University of California, Los Angeles.

THE MODEL

Dorothy Johnson is one of the most prolific authors on a whole variety of nursing topics and issues. Her model of nursing practice forms only a very small part of her total output; however, it has been used quite widely by nurses to analyse practice situations.

Three papers directly explain Johnson's model and can be found in the literature. These are her paper presenting the model at Vanderbilt University in 1968 (Johnson, 1968b); a chapter in Riehl and Roy (Johnson, 1980); and papers presented at the Second Annual Nurse Educator Conference in New York in 1978, available in audiotape format (Johnson, 1978). The first two of these references are the most frequently cited as providing the underpinning for nursing practice research.

Two further papers discuss other issues concerning nursing models. In *Nursing Research* Johnson (1968a) discusses the nature of theory in nursing practice; and in the same journal Johnson (1974) discusses three criteria for evaluating nursing models.

I will now give a brief outline of Johnson's behavioural systems model, followed by discussion of the work that has used her model in clinical practice along with critical analysis of the model in practice-based research.

SUMMARY OF JOHNSON'S BEHAVIOURAL SYSTEMS MODEL

According to Johnson, nursing is concerned with promoting efficient and effective behavioural functioning in order to prevent illness, during illness and following illness. Therefore the patient in this model is a behavioural system; here Johnson makes the analogy with medicine, where the patient is seen as a biological system.

The knowledge needed for this model comes from the holistic understanding of humans and their behaviour, which asks the questions: what does the individual do, why does he or she do it, and what are the consequences of that behaviour? Therefore the knowledge would need to be from the social sciences, in particular social learning theories and motivation, the biological sciences, particularly the genetic, neurological and endocrine bases of behaviour, and from the study of animal and human behaviour. This knowledge would be directed towards the outcome of interactions between different people in different situations, the processes that these interactions go through, how they are coordinated and how they respond to changes in levels of stimulation.

This model is based, at present, on a systems approach in an attempt to understand the functioning of the individual as a whole, until knowledge of behaviour of the whole person has been developed. Therefore using a systems approach it is possible to look at the functioning of subsystems in relation to the whole, where an imbalance in one subsystem will inevitably have an effect on many other systems; and where the functioning of the whole system will depend on the functioning and integration of the subsystems.

This model is based on four assumptions: first, that a person strives for a continual state of balance of the behavioural system by adjusting to outside influences; second, that the person seeks new experiences that may disturb the existing balance, and these will need behaviour modifications to re-establish the behavioural balance; third, a behavioural system which is constant is essential to the functioning of the person for the sake of him/herself and his/her social life; and fourth, that behavioural systems balance of the individual is the result of successful adaptations and adjustments, even though observed behaviour may not match cultural norms. Therefore most of the time an individual would be able to sustain a behavioural systems balance in the face of change.

Johnson (1980) sums up her model as follows:

> ... all the patterned, repetitive, and purposeful ways of behaving that characterize each man's life are considered to comprise his behavioural system. These ways of behaving form an organized and integrated functional unit that determines and limits the interaction between the person and his environment and establishes the relationship of the person to the objects, events, and situations in his environment. Such behaviour is orderly, purposeful and predictable; that is, it is functionally efficient and effective, most of the time, and it is sufficiently stable and recurrent to be amenable to description and explanation.

(p. 209)

However, where the disturbance to the systems balance is so grave as to need assistance to restore it, then the role of nursing is needed.

According to Johnson, with any system the more developed it is the more specialized, integrated and complex will be its subsystems. Each subsystem has a set of behavioural responses that share a common goal or motivation. These responses are developed by the individual and modified by physical, psychological and social factors over time, due to maturation, learning and experience. According to Johnson's model each subsystem has structure and function. There are four structural elements in each of the seven subsystems.

- The goal or motivation for the action; there will be differences between individuals in what they strive for, in the value they place on the goal, and the energy they are willing to expend to achieve the goal; also all of these may change over time.
- The individual's set, or their predisposition to act in a certain way towards a goal; this can be determined by observation.
- The choice of behaviours open to the individual for achievement of their goal; it can be assumed that the larger the repertoire of the individual, the more adaptive they are likely to be.
- The individual's behaviour; this is the only element which can be observed directly.

In this model the concern is how effective and efficient the behaviour is in achieving the individual's goals. Johnson (1980) describes this element as follows.

> Is the behaviour succeeding or failing to achieve the consequences sought? Are more skillful motor, expressive, or social skills needed? Are the choices appropriate? Is the sequence of action purposeful and orderly; does it demonstrate economy of action; is the action socially and biologically appropriate?
>
> (p. 211)

Seven subsystems have been identified that have needs which must be met by the individual or through outside assistance in order for the individual to grow and remain viable. These needs are for protection from harmful influences, nurturing by appropriate supplies from the environment, and stimulation to promote growth and prevent stagnation. The system and its subsystems tend to be self-maintaining as long as the internal and external environment is predictable and orderly, their requirements for functioning are met, and the interrelationships between the subsystems is harmonious; otherwise malfunctioning may occur.

The seven subsystems are as follows.

- **Affiliative:** during childhood the formation of attachment bonds is seen as essential to well-being; during adulthood the formation of social bonds which can include intimacy are a means of security.
- **Dependency**: this can be seen to be a developmental phenomenon, however even in adulthood a certain amount of interdependence is essential in order for social groups to survive. The consequences of dependency behaviour are approval, attention or recognition, and assistance.
- **Ingestive:** this is concerned with 'when, how, what, how much, and under what conditions we eat' (Johnson, 1980, p. 213). In affluent societies this has as much to do with social and psychological considerations as with satisfaction of purely physical needs.

- **Elimination:** this is concerned with when, how and under what conditions an individual eliminates. With this subsystem each individual must learn expected behaviours in excreting waste products, and these learned behaviours take precedence over purely physical functioning.
- **Sexual:** the beginnings of this subsystem are the learning of gender role identity. Adult behaviour will depend on cultural norms of behaviour, and has the dual function of procreation and gratification.
- **Aggressive:** this subsystem is aimed at protection rather than injury of others, and here the norms of society demand that only certain levels of aggression are allowed in order to safeguard the person and his or her property.
- **Achievement:** this has the function of mastery of the self or the environment on some standard of excellence. Areas where achievement behaviour has been recognized are intellectual, physical, creative, mechanical and social.

It is possible to view this model as a grid, as shown in Table 5.1.

Table 5.1 Representation of Johnson's (1980) model

	Goal	Set	Choice of behaviours	Behaviours
Affiliative				
Dependency				
Ingestion				
Elimination				
Sexual				
Aggression				
Achievement				

The seven subsystems function together to create harmony and stability in the system; where this does not occur disturbances in the structure and function are caused. The goal of nursing is to restore or to maintain behavioural systems balance at the highest level achievable by the individual, by acting as an external regulatory force to control behaviour to preserve the integrity and organization of the individual's behaviour.

Johnson recognizes that the knowledge base for this approach is very much in its infancy, therefore progress will be slow. She advocates research to strengthen the approach which she says is defensible and promising.

The published papers to date have mainly analysed problem identification using Johnson's model, in a variety of situations and have also helped to show the potential use of the model in some nursing settings. However, the research has all been generated in North America, which again may show resistance by British nurses to this particular theoretical perspective, or to its presentation to a British profession.

This chapter is divided into sections, following the format of other chapters. However, only three sections are necessary due to the amount of literature found, i.e. identification of problems or behavioural systems imbalance, implementation of nursing care, and the development of tools to assess standards of nursing care.

IDENTIFICATION OF PROBLEMS (BEHAVIOURAL SYSTEMS IMBALANCE)

In this section two major areas of practice were investigated, each producing two papers: the chronically ill child; and cancer patients. The methods of investigation used are questionnaire, literature search and observation.

SYSTEMS IMBALANCE IN CHRONICALLY ILL CHILDREN

Two interesting papers by the same author (Holaday, 1974, 1981) have been produced on this topic; they demonstrate how Johnson's model can help to analyse patient problems. Each of the papers investigates one of the components of Johnson's model in relation to the behaviour of chronically ill children.

The first paper examines the **achievement** behaviours exhibited by chronically ill children. It shows how these behaviours differ from the behaviours of well children.

Holaday (1974) examined the extent to which chronically ill children felt in control of their current situation. She felt that if she was able to identify the levels of internal control in chronically ill children, this could predict these children's possible levels of success, which could then be compared with well children. She also compared demographic variables with the level of internal control in chronically ill children. Where there were differences between well and ill children Holaday went on to make some suggestions about how the nurse might help to improve the sense of internal control felt by chronically ill children.

Johnson's model is able to provide a theoretical framework by examining the balance of the subsystem of achievement, through the nurse assessing:

- the goal of each achievement activity;
- the set, or the tendency to act in a certain way to achieve the goal; and
- the choice of alternative behaviours open to the individual.

The fourth of Johnson's structural elements, the efficacy of the behaviour in achieving the goals, is not considered by Holaday.

Holaday uses the concept of internal and external loci of control (Rotter *et al.*, 1972) to develop ideas of how the child may learn achievement behaviours. She says that if chronically ill children consistently view others, or events outside their control, as causing their success or failure, this will produce different levels of striving and a different perception of the difficulty of the tasks, than if such children view their own actions as causing success or failure.

She assessed the achievement behaviours of chronically ill children using the Intellectual Achievement Responsibility (IAR) questionnaire developed by Crandall *et al.* (1962) and Crandall (1965). The questionnaire contains 34 forced choice items, each asking the child to indicate which they feel is the most likely reason for achievement or failure in events they experienced. Each item indicates either achievement or failure in a particular instance. Reasons are always phrased so that the child has to indicate either an internal or an external cause. The final score for each child is the difference between the positive events for which the child takes credit, and the negative events for which she or he similarly takes credit.

The IAR scale is also able to identify the amount of ability individual children demonstrate, and the amount of effort they put into various experiences described in the items, as opposed to the level of difficulty they perceive in the tasks or the amount of luck they had in achieving them.

Crandall *et al.* (1962) and Crandall (1965) demonstrated validity for the IAR scale using these concepts, although Holaday does not appear to have estimated the validity of the questionnaire with her sample.

The subjects in the study were 24 chronically ill children, comprising 10 girls and 14 boys randomly selected from current in-patients in a university hospital in North America. The criteria for selection were that the child had been diagnosed as having a chronic illness, but with an expected survival of at least 30 years of age; that there was no diagnosis of mental retardation or a learning disorder; that children were currently between the ages of 8 and 17 years of age; and that, although they were at present in hospital, they would be discharged within the next 2 days.

The child's socio-economic group was estimated from the occupation of the father; age, sex, position in the family and age when the diagnosis was made were all obtained from the child's records.

The comparison between the chronically ill children and well children was made by selecting children from two other studies. The first of these was by Cook (1970), where 39 children were selected from 63 in the total study, according to their California Achievement Test scores; 10 were shown to be achievers and 19 underachievers. The second group of well children was chosen from Crandall's (1965) group, a sample of 923 children of various ages drawn from five schools. The IAR questionnaire was administered to both these samples of well children in their school. However, with Crandall's group the younger children had a verbal questionnaire, while the older children and all the children in Cook's sample had a written questionnaire. Holaday makes no mention of the effect of this difference of administration in her paper; it could be that verbal administration altered the responses considerably. Also the verbal presentation was used for the younger children only; therefore as well as reading ability there may be a difference in comprehension between written and verbal presentations. The lack of validity testing in the study will compound these problems.

The mothers of the chronically ill children were asked to participate in the study. Those who agreed were interviewed by Holaday to assess their goals for the child. However, as Holaday indicates, no further use was made of this data; she does not comment on the reasons for this.

The questionnaire was administered by the researcher reading it to each chronically ill child. Holaday states that the mother was not present, but no indication is given of the setting in which the questionnaire was administered. This might make a considerable difference to the confidence with which the child was able to respond to the researcher, and therefore the level of commitment she or he had to answering the questions.

The first finding is quite dramatic. It shows that the chronically ill children felt that luck, the task being too easy or too difficult, or other people preventing them from achieving or helping them to achieve were more often the reasons for failure than their own abilities or persistence. However, no tests of significance were made to show the strength of these differences; this would have increased confidence in a difference between the chronically ill and the well children. The attribution by the chronically ill children of external factors being responsible for success or failure means that these children will tend to avoid feelings of pride in their achievements, but probably more importantly will avoid feelings of shame for failure. Holaday comments that increasing maturity in children should produce an increased internal sense of control; however, with the chronically ill children, those over 12 years of age had similar scores to those under 12, showing no increase in internal control of this group compared with well children.

A further equally dramatic finding is that children diagnosed as chronically ill from birth or within the first year tended to attribute their success and failure to ability or lack of ability, rather than to persistence or the lack of it. This again shows that chronically ill children tend not to persist in the tasks they undertake, as they feel effort will not make any difference to whether they succeed or not. As Holaday suggests, the small sample size may have an effect on the findings, as the dimension of ability versus persistence was not statistically significant.

With the chronically ill children demographic variables played an important role. Boys generally had a higher sense of internal control, although this was not statistically different between the groups. The main difference within the sample of chronically ill children was the age at which diagnosis was made. Children who were diagnosed from birth as chronically ill attributed success or failure statistically more often to their ability than did children who were diagnosed at the age of 1 year (p = 0.01). Therefore those who were diagnosed from birth could be expected to have less persistence, as they would typically say that trying harder would not make any difference to their success, as they do not control what happens to them. This sense of lack of internal control means that these children would have low needs for achievement. Therefore, it could be expected that they would be less likely to approach tasks where achievement was possible than would well children or those who were diagnosed as chronically ill after the age of 1 year.

The importance of this finding is that it shows that the first year of life is crucial to the development of a sense of confidence in one's own ability to influence events affecting oneself. It would have been useful to know if up to 1 year was the most significant period, and what effects greater or lesser periods had on the sense of internal control. If, as Holaday suggests, there is a critical period for the formation of this sense of ability to achieve, then this would be crucial for health professionals and others to know. Holaday's article could have gone further to discuss this question and to suggest further research.

Analysis of socio-economic group showed only a slight difference in relation to internal control, and this was not statistically significant; similarly, findings in relation to the position of the child in the family showed the eldest child to have only a slightly greater sense of internal control than subsequent children.

When the sense of responsibility for failure only was examined a significant difference (p = 0.05) was found between the boys and the girls, with the boys having a greater sense of responsibility for negative outcomes. A greater difference (p = 0.020) was found between boys and girls when the age of diagnosis of chronic illness was also taken into account. This score showed that, particularly with the chronically ill boys, there was a tendency to avoid achievement situations. As Holaday points out, this could affect sex stereotyping of these boys where independence and assertiveness are expected qualities.

Holaday makes the link between these findings and Johnson's model of behavioural systems balance by stating that the chronically ill children in her study showed an imbalance in the achievement subsystem. She says this is so because the achievement subsystem is not developed to its fullest extent in chronically ill children when compared with well children. Chronically ill children are therefore deficient in the goal of the subsystem 'achievement'.

This raises major ethical issues for the chronically ill, which Holaday does not address, but which have to do with the North American and other cultures where achievement is a dominant value. Anyone unable to adopt these values will feel of less worth. The question here is whether nurses should be concerned with trying to make up for this imbalance, as Holaday suggests they should, and the model has as its basis; or whether an alternative lifestyle for chronically ill people would be more desirable as a nursing aim. As Johnson's model has the nurse in a dominant role, should nursing goals be to increase the frustration of the chronically ill by teaching them to be more competitive, when this involves competing against those who do not have physical disabilities? In other words, is this model appropriate for the chronically ill? Indeed, the dilemma of how to encourage chronically ill children is summed up by Krulik and Florian (1995) as 'On the one hand these children are encouraged to feel "normal" … and on the other, they may be overprotected, distressed and discouraged from fully participating in relationships and contacts due to their illness' (p. 172).

These ethical issues related to the paper and therefore to the Johnson model cause a major dilemma for the nurse in relation to chronically ill children. On the one hand the nurse would be helping the patients by increasing their internal locus of control which will help them to view effort and persistence as worthwhile attributes, and therefore, according to Johnson, promote behavioural systems balance; however, if this leads the chronically ill to experience increasing frustrations, then the model will also promote behavioural systems imbalance. Perhaps the alternative approach would be to help the chronically ill patient to be realistic in their choice of goals while encouraging persistence. However, Johnson's model does not allow for this. It is also uncertain from Holaday's study whether she has considered realistic goal choice for chronically ill children, or the attributes that encourage or inhibit this.

The second study (Holaday, 1981) assesses the imbalance in the behavioural subsystems. This paper considers the **attachment** subsystem, within the framework of Johnson's model, and in particular the mother's response to her chronically ill infant's crying behaviour.

Holaday considers crying as an infant's method of exhibiting the need for attachment. She examines attachment from the perspective of the mother's usual behaviour towards the infant when crying (the mother's behavioural set), and the mother's goal for action with her infant.

The subjects in the study were six white, middle-class mothers and their chronically ill infants who were part of a stable family. The criteria for inclusion in the study were that the infant was diagnosed as chronically ill by 3 days old, but was likely to survive for at least 10 years; that the chronic illness did not involve mental retardation or retardation of the senses; and that discharge from hospital occurred within 10 days of birth. The sample included equal numbers of male and female infants, and also equal numbers of first and subsequent born infants. However, of note here is that the available sample was 15 mother/ill infant pairs, but nine of the sample refused to participate; this is only cursorily acknowledged in the article. The very high number of refusals could well indicate that those in the study were not representative of the behaviour of the majority of mother/ill infant pairs. This problem of access throws the whole study into question.

A comparison sample of well infants was used. It is unclear from the article whether this involved secondary analysis of already collected data from the study by Bell and Ainsworth (1972), but the implications are that this was the case. This type of comparison using observational data must be suspect and is discussed further below.

Data for Holaday's study were collected through observation over a 3-month period starting when each infant was 4 months old. Mothers and infants were visited every 3 weeks for 2 months. The visits involved 4 hours of observation of the baby. This design replicated a study by Bell and Ainsworth (1972) whose sample of 26 well children was used as the comparison group for Holaday's study. Although great care was taken by Holaday to ensure that the definition of terms and the method of data collection was the same as used by Bell and Ainsworth, there is a definite possibility that many design problems may have occurred – such as the time lapse between the two studies; the possibility of differences in geographical location of the two samples; and the researchers not coordinating their efforts sufficiently. These differences would undoubtedly result in inconsistencies in data collection and subsequent analysis; such issues, however, are not considered by Holaday.

Holaday's observations involved taking notes of the infant's behaviour and the mother's reactions to the behaviour. She used a stop watch to time the period over which the infant cried, the length of time before the mother responded to the cry, and the length of time the infant was held. She also recorded where the baby was and the event immediately before the cry, the type of cry (although how this was determined is unclear), and the successful or unsuccessful maternal interventions.

To assess reliability of the observations another researcher accompanied Holaday; there was agreement of between 71% and 95% between them. These observers were trained in the data collection methods required for the study. Holaday mentions the effect which the presence of the observers may have had on the behaviours of both mother and child, and in order to minimize this the observations were centred on the child, while the mother was observed only when she attended to the child. However, this is not entirely satisfactory as no data were discarded from the initial recordings with each mother/child pair, which is more usual practice in data collection by observation.

The results showed that mothers of ill infants did not leave their infants to cry as frequently as mothers of well infants did, the mean length of the cries of all infants being 10 minutes per hour, whereas the well infants cried on average for 17 minutes per hour. The cries of the ill infants were also seen to differ in intensity, whereas the well infants' cries did not. Holaday mentions that, because the mothers pick up their ill infants very soon after they begin to cry, this may make it more difficult for the mother with an ill infant to distinguish between the reasons for her infant's crying. Analysis also showed that the mothers spent much more time in close proximity to their ill infants than the mothers of well infants. These two findings show the mothers' quick response to their chronically ill infants by a variety of actions such as picking the infant up, talking to it, patting and giving it a pacifier (dummy). This pattern of response differed from that of the mothers of well infants, where there was usually a single response, i.e. picking the infant up. Therefore the mothers' 'set' with chronically ill infants is increased, as their repertoire of actions is increased compared with the mothers of well infants.

These differences between the groups show how the mothers of ill infants attribute every cry as being a sign of urgency that needs attention. Therefore mothers are seen to exhibit a considerable amount of anxiety in relation to their ill infants. However, Johnson's model does not lend itself so easily to questioning patients, so the researchers were unable to ask the mothers this and had to rely more on observation of their behaviour. Therefore information which may have been gained from conversations between the researchers and the mothers, which in other approaches could have been used as further evidence of their levels of anxiety, cannot so easily be used with this model.

The patterns of intervention by the mothers in both groups showed that the most effective intervention to stop the infant crying was picking it up. Although the mothers of ill infants adopted other behaviours also, these were not seen to be any more effective than simply picking the infant up, and were therefore more likely to be related to the mother's general anxiety about the child. Therefore Johnson's model shows that the behaviour of mothers in relation to the goal differed between the two groups of mothers, although effectiveness of their behaviour was only achieved by a single action.

Further analysis of the data from both groups showed that the mothers' response to their infants differed significantly when the position of the infant in the family and its sex were taken into consideration. Mothers of both well and ill infants responded significantly faster to the firstborn child than to subsequent children ($p = 0.011$); also mothers responded faster to their male infants than to their female infants ($p = 0.048$). However, ill infants were seen to cry more often than well infants.

The ill and seriously ill infants cried more often than the well infants. Although the mothers responded to more of their cries than did the mothers of well infants, and their interventions were equally effective, this did not lessen the number of crying incidents. This feature of the ill infants is commented on by Holaday as being frustrating for the mothers. In relation to the number of refusals to be involved in the research from the mothers of ill infants, it could be that frustration by the mother with her ill infant is a common feature, which could lead to behaviour on the part of the mother that she finds unacceptable, but difficult to avoid.

In terms of Johnson's model the above findings indicate that the mothers of chronically ill infants have a difference in behavioural set from the mothers of well infants. This is seen in a narrower behavioural set by the mothers of ill infants in order to achieve their assumed goal of pacifying the infant, therefore responding to almost every cry. A widening of the behavioural set was seen in these mothers by their responses to pacifying, by picking up the infant as well as adopting a number of other strategies. A third area of difference in the behavioural set was the constant proximity of the mother to her ill infant.

This is an interesting use of Johnson's model, and apart from evident problems with the research design of the study, has shown some interesting results. However, the intervention of nursing strategies in such a situation must be very problematic. It is not certain whether, as Holaday suggests, the nurse would have any more success in being able to discriminate between the different cries of the ill infant than the mother would. Therefore the suggestion by her that the nurse can teach the mother how to discriminate seems very ambitious. Also, even if the nurse is able to do this, it will not be at all certain that this will change the mother's continual proximity to the child, nor her wish to respond to almost every cry. In other words the nurse's intervention may not lessen the mother's anxiety about her ill infant, nor the infant's associated behaviour.

In both papers by Holaday (1974, 1981) there is emphasis on the chronically ill person, or to use Johnson's terms, the person with a chronic behavioural systems imbalance, being returned to the status of the well person. In this the nurse is seen to decide, through research, what is 'normal' and to then create a programme for the patient or client to return him or her to this 'normal' position. What the nurse using this model will have to decide is whether this is appropriate with the chronically ill or their carers. Herein lies a moral dilemma.

Both these studies by Holaday took aspects of Johnson's model and based the study directly upon them. Therefore both studies are theory led, and the reasoning used to define the variables in the two studies is derived directly from the model. Both studies are designed as cause and effect studies, as they consider the effects of different aspects of chronically ill children's and infants' behaviour either upon their future potential or upon the behaviour of the mother. The fourth feature of these two studies is that the chronically ill children and infants were examined in their natural environments. Both these studies therefore have sound research designs, although, as mentioned above, the 1981 study has a problem in the execution of the research as many mothers eligible for inclusion declined to take part.

BEHAVIOURAL SYSTEMS IMBALANCE IN CANCER PATIENTS

Further studies that consider the identification of problems were found in two papers, which describe an instrument developed to measure cancer patients' problems, or behavioural changes. Both of these papers describe in considerable detail the way measures were developed and tested, and in this respect they offer excellent guidance for nurses aiming to produce measurement tools.

Derdiarian (1983) aimed to develop the concepts of Johnson's model by the production and testing of an instrument. This was based on Johnson's 1972 model which included a restorative subsystem (deleted in the 1980 version of the model). Derdiarian chose the situation of the nursing care of cancer patients.

Her first step was to review the literature on each of Johnson's sub-systems. She found the following.

- In the **achievement** subsystem achievement behaviour is determined by inborn factors as well as learned abilities; the main dimensions were the goal, the individual's ability, and the importance of the achievement.
- The **affiliative** subsystem has the goal of being involved in interpersonal relationships with others, and the drive is to belong; from the literature affiliation was determined by dimensions that included other people, the need to belong, and the degree of association.
- The **aggressive/protective** subsystem was viewed as a complex system of inborn factors which tended to involve biophysical mechanisms and learned factors, both of which were designed and organized to protect and preserve the individual; the dimensions which determined the goal and the drive were therefore the individual's ability and the need for protection.
- The **dependency** subsystem has the goal of obtaining support and nurture, the drive being the need for help or assistance; therefore when needs cannot be met without help from others the main dimensions of this subsystem are need, others, dependence and functionality or instrumentality.
- The **eliminative** subsystem has the consequences of constipation, diarrhoea, vomiting, distension, amenorrhoea, oedema, pain, restlessness and anxiety where there is ineffective elimination, therefore the main extrapolated dimensions of this subsystem are quality, nature and pattern and the consequences of elimination.

- The **ingestive** subsystem has the main extrapolated variables of the ability to obtain and to prepare food, and the satisfaction of eating.
- The **sexual** subsystem is viewed as the same as gender identity which includes role identities; the dimensions extrapolated were the characteristics associated with gender, and the biopsychosocial factors which lead to sexual function.
- The **restorative** subsystem has the goal of relief from fatigue, the drive being use of energy and overstimulation. The extrapolated dimensions of the restorative subsystem are the ability to sleep and to relax, and the ability to maintain physiological equilibrium.

Most of this literature is from North America, but there is no reason to believe that cultural factors play a crucial role in many of the dimensions of each subsystem. As a result of this literature search and subsequent extrapolation, Derdiarian was able to state that cancer patients have behavioural instability in each of the subsystems of Johnson's model. A further literature search was able to identify the nature of this instability in the subsystems of cancer patients as follows.

- The **achievement** subsystem shows a reduction in ability at work, as well as in the home and with the family as a result of lessened physical ability. The lower ability at work due to decreased mental abilities created anxiety. Also reported was a lessening of mental and cognitive ability; patients were less able to concentrate and had increasing absentmindedness. These reductions resulted in cancer patients altering both their short-term and their long-term goals.
- The **affiliative** subsystem showed cancer patients placing increased importance on relationships with the family, relatives and close friends. There was also a perceived increase in the importance of relationships with the church or religious organizations; these increased relationships were reported to give cancer patients a sense of sharing feelings, seeking advice and overcoming crises. A decrease was noted in relationships with work and with other social groups.
- The **aggressive/protective** subsystem showed patients reporting a decrease in physical ability due to pain, fatigue and immobility. Also reported by patients were changes in blood, hormonal, immunological, digestive and skin functions due to the cancer and its treatment. Reports were also noted of inability to concentrate and solve problems and to handle emotions. Patients expressed a wish to maintain their emotional stability.
- The **dependency** subsystem showed cancer patients' dependence on their close family and friends, and also on psychotherapy and on the health care team. They reported a decrease in reliance on themselves due to physical discomfort and pain, and also fatigue and gastrointestinal symptoms.

- The **eliminative** subsystem showed patients to have an increase in the frequency of constipation and diarrhoea, and also changes in the amount of stool passed. Increased urinary output and frequency were reported. Patients also reported increased perspiration and body odour and frustration due to changes in elimination, whether natural or as a result of surgery, and depression due to oedema, skin changes and amenorrhoea.
- The **ingestive** subsystem found patients reporting increased incidence of nausea, problems with eating due to dryness and problems of the mouth, and a decreased appetite and enjoyment of food.
- The **sexual** subsystem showed cancer patients having physical dysfunctions due to their drugs and to the site of their cancer and the surgery performed. Psychological tension between partners was also reported.
- The **restorative** subsystem showed patients with cancer reporting disturbances with the quality and quantity of sleep and with bad dreams. This was due to discomfort and resulted in daytime 'catnaps' and changes in patterns of sleep at night. Patients found an increased need to relax, and to take on less demanding physical and mental pursuits.

From this extensive literature search and extrapolation it was possible to construct an instrument to measure the frequency with which behavioural subsystems imbalance occurs in patients suffering from cancer. This instrument consisted of 121 items identifying changes as a result of cancer; 59 were physical and 62 were psychological or emotional changes in behaviour.

In the second paper (Derdiarian and Forsyth, 1983) the instrument is tested. Piloting involved three male and three female patients. Observations by the researcher of the patients' reactions to the instrument, their ability to understand the questions and the time needed to complete the instrument were noted.

Content validity of the instrument was tested using six experts, three of whom were clinical nurses in cancer nursing, two who were specialists in critical care nursing and one who was a graduate student in nursing who had cancer; all were experts in the use of the Johnson model. This group was divided in half: three members assessed the comprehensiveness of the Johnson framework, its underpinning theories, and the consistency of the instrument's operational definitions with this framework; the other three members assessed the consistency of the operational definitions with the instrument's categories and items.

Results showed 100% agreement that the framework was comprehensive and consistent with the underpinning theories; there was 97.8% agreement that the operational definitions in the instrument reflected the framework; and 95.4% agreement that the items in the instrument reflected the definitions.

Validity was additionally assessed through estimation of the theta coefficient from factor analysis. This showed a high degree of internal consistency for the items in each subsystem, but lesser values for the subsystems of elimination and restoration, which would lead to further investigation of the items in the subsystem.

Reliability of the instrument was assessed through test–retest using Pearson's product–moment correlation. Two hours were allowed between the two tests. Correlation between each test was positive showing good correlation of the measure of change and its direction, and therefore strong reliability was demonstrated. This extent of testing was an impressive feature of the design of the instrument.

The instrument was administered to 163 patients between the ages of 20 and 70 years with the diagnosis of cancer. However, patients with neurological, head and neck cancers, or cancers needing extensive disfiguring surgery were excluded due to the researcher's need to have a sample which was as homogeneous as possible. Care was also taken not to administer the instrument to patients who were starting a new course of treatment on the same day, in an attempt to minimize stress.

Patients were asked to complete the instrument in a private room in the hospital they were attending. A standard form of instructions was given to the patients verbally by a research assistant before they were asked to complete the questions on the instrument. The research assistants were trained and their performance with the patients was tape recorded. Derdiarian states that reliability of their performance was achieved; this was reviewed by two independent raters and evaluated according to the assistants' ability to instruct the patient; their style of interaction, for example, friendly/formal; and their handling of patient interruptions and questions.

As well as testing for validity and reliability, Derdiarian also used the instrument to test whether the patients noticed an increase or decrease in their ability on the item in each question; whether this had a positive or negative quality; how important this change was on a rating from 0 to 100; and what effect this change had on them. Patients were also asked to add changes which were not included in the instrument, and the effects of these changes as they had experienced them. These items added by the patients were judged, using content analysis, by a panel of three clinical nurses who were considered to be experts in nursing cancer patients. The judgement was based on whether the changes and their effects were consistent with the model and its operational definitions. This is the most serious difficulty in the paper, because it supposed that some of the problems noticed by the patients did not 'fit' either the model or its operational definitions as defined by the instrument. There were 196 'other' changes mentioned by the patients, which is more than the total number of items on the instrument. This issue is not tackled by Derdiarian, and she gives no indication as to why so many other problems should have been indicated, nor what happened to all these problems mentioned by the patients. In a study which is so well controlled in other ways, this leaves the reader wondering if the model is wholly appropriate for patients with cancer. It may also indicate the extent of the professional model of nursing being at the expense of a patient-centred model, which in a country that boasts patient satisfaction as a regular feature of assessing quality of care, leaves a lot to explain.

At the end of the section of questions relating to each subsystem, and also at the end of the instrument, patients were asked which was the most important change that had happened to them. To minimize bias the subsystems were placed in differing random order, but the sexual subsystem was always placed fourth due to the sensitive nature of the questions, which was noted by the researcher during the piloting stage.

This study is a model for designing and testing questionnaires. The extent of the 'other' items mentioned by the patients is a disturbing feature; however, it is clear that the patients related to the questions asked. Therefore the Johnson model is seen as relevant for some areas of difficulty for cancer patients.

The two studies undertaken by Derdiarian are directly based on Johnson's model, therefore they are theoretically driven. The combination of both studies leads to a very well-prepared descriptive study, but there is no suggestion that this tests for cause and effect. What makes for an interesting study is to assess the level of agreement between the literature and professional views on the one hand and the patients' experience on the other, the latter finding many new areas of problems that the former had not uncovered.

CONCLUSIONS

Four papers were found that identified behavioural systems imbalance in patients; all these papers adhere closely to the model. However, they also highlight many of the problems inherent in the model.

NURSING ACTIONS TO PROMOTE BEHAVIOURAL SYSTEMS BALANCE

There is only a single paper in this section, which perhaps reflects the limited use of this model, not only in America but also internationally. The paper does not deal with the components of the model directly, but analyses the concept of 'helping' in relation to nursing models.

HELPING IN NURSING

Cronenwett (1983) says that the concept of helping is implicit in most nursing models, and most of the authors mention helping as a function of nursing, but do not make this concept explicit in the construction of their models.

Cronenwett uses the definition of Brickman *et al.* (1982) to define the concept of helping; they use the notions of responsibility to show how helping can be seen as the responsibility of the individual or of others, and can be viewed in four different ways (Table 5.2). These ways are the result of either attributing the responsibility for the problem or for the success to oneself or to others.

Table 5.2 Helping model described by Cronenwett (1983)

Attributing responsibility for problem to self	Attributing responsibility for solution to self	
	High	Low
High	Moral	Enlightened
Self-perception	Lazy	Guilty
Actions expected of self	Striving	Submissive
Others who must act	Peers	Authorities
Actions expected of others	Urging	Discipline
View of human nature	Strong	Bad
Potential pathology	Loneliness	Fanaticism
Low	Compensatory	Medical
Self-perception	Deprived	Ill
Actions expected of self	Assertive	Acceptant
Others who must act	Subordinates	Experts
Actions expected of others	Mobilization	Treatment
View of human nature	Good	Weak
Potential pathology	Alienation	Dependent

In applying these concepts to Johnson's (1980) model of nursing, Cronenwett crystallizes helping in Johnson's model as being the responsibility of the nurse:

> Nursing is thus seen as an external regulatory force which acts to preserve the organization and integration of the patient's behaviour at an optimal level under those conditions in which the behaviour constitutes a threat to physical or social health, or in which illness is found.
>
> (p. 214)

This quotation therefore shows Johnson's view of nursing, as the nurse using this model in its intended sense has the responsibility to attain, restore and maintain the systems balance for the patient. It is the nurse who defines the problem and who acts as a regulating force in controlling the solutions for the patient. As Cronenwett says, Johnson believes that the patient should move from dependence on the nurse or others, to independence, but her model does not allow for that change to occur.

Although this is only a short paper and Johnson's model is analysed only briefly along with many others, the problems it identifies reflect the nature of some of the problems of the studies cited in the first part of this chapter.

Cronenwett's may only be one model of helping, but its implications in pointing to some of the major issues in the use of the Johnson model in nursing practice are very explicit.

THE DEVELOPMENT OF STANDARDS OF CARE USING JOHNSON'S MODEL

No papers were found which investigated the evaluation by nurses of their care using the Johnson model. Therefore this section moves on to look at a single paper that studies how nursing care may be evaluated more globally, through the use of patient indicators.

THE DEVELOPMENT OF A TOOL TO MEASURE PATIENT CARE

The study by Majesky, Brester and Nishio (1978) looks at the development of outcome measures in terms of physiological problems exhibited by the patients, and develops the idea of measuring patient outcomes as a way of measuring nursing care. They state that measurement of nursing care should be 'quick and easy to administer, and serve as a model for the identification of other indicators' (p. 365).

They selected physiological outcome measures as these are more overt than psychosocial ones. Johnson (1980) terms this the second level of instruction: '... appropriate at this level of instruction ... is the study of pathophysiology of the biologic system, of medicine's clinical science, and of the health system as a whole' (p. 214).

Majesky, Brester and Nishio argue that the development of this instrument will give the framework for measuring other dimensions of patient outcomes.

The physiological outcomes the researchers chose were the complications of infection, immobility and fluid imbalance. These were chosen because it was felt that they were directly related to nursing care; in North America this may be so, but in Britain particularly infection and fluid imbalance must be equally attributable to medical treatment, as must be the patient's recovery from such problems, particularly in the case of surgical patients. Therefore the choice of these measures cannot be totally satisfactory in Britain as indicators of nursing care alone.

A selection of criteria for measuring infection, immobility and fluid imbalance were carefully chosen from a review of the literature and tested in practice settings. The indicators finally decided upon were the following.

- Infection: urinary tract infections, respiratory infections, skin and subcutaneous infections with a purulent discharge, and raised oral temperature.
- Immobility: lightheadedness or dizziness when moving from a lying to a sitting position, or from a sitting to a standing position, a respiratory rate of less than 12 or more than 16 breaths per minute, dry stools, a red area on the skin which remains with pressure, contractures and a positive Homan's sign.
- Fluid imbalance: 5% increase or decrease in body weight, dry mucous membranes, a red and furry tongue, decreased skin turgor, and an abnormally high urine specific gravity.

The final list of patient complications due to nursing interventions consisted of 24 items, of which seven were related to infection, 12 to immobility and five to fluid imbalance. The scoring system for each item was presence/absence on admission, and presence/absence on discharge of the patient.

The researchers say that content validity was established when they judged the items for 'observability, availability, and credibility' (p. 370). However, this implies that they carried out the content validity themselves, rather than recruiting others who were not involved in constructing the items. Therefore their procedure is liable to bias the judgement of the items in favour of accepting them.

The instrument was tested using 124 patients: 28 from high dependency areas, 38 from general areas, 30 from long-stay areas and 28 from nursing homes. Each group was found to have its own mean scores, which differed from one group to another. The instrument was tested through split-half reliability and item analysis which reduced the original 27-item list to 24 items with good reliability estimates.

Inter-rater agreement was assessed by two raters on 31 patients from four health care settings. Correlation was found to be very satisfactory at 0.797 ($p < 0.01$).

The method used for assessing the effectiveness of the instrument is thorough but, as mentioned above, the content of the questions cannot be solely related to nursing care. Only using physiological measures is a further cause for concern in assessing standards of nursing care.

CONCLUSIONS ON THE USE OF THE MODEL TO 1990

Four papers investigated the nature of behavioural systems imbalance; one developed the concept of helping in nursing; and one considered monitoring standards of nursing care using the Johnson model.

Identification of behavioural systems imbalance investigated the achievement subsystem in chronically ill children, and the attachment subsystem of mothers with chronically ill infants. Both these studies showed considerable ethical difficulty for the nurse in attempting to restore behavioural systems balance. Identification of behavioural systems imbalance also investigated cancer patients.

Nursing intervention sees the nurse as the dominant partner. The model is criticized as it does not allow for the patient to regain independence. Monitoring standards of care when using only physiological measures is not seen as a true reflection of nursing care alone.

A further problem with this model would seem to be its limited use outside North America, as reflected in the research studies found. Further, the limited number of settings in which it has been used, even within North America, adds some question to its acceptance by nurses in general; although some settings are still developing the model for use in practice and research.

DEVELOPMENTS SINCE 1990

My searches through the literature since 1990 showed that no new papers had been published in the use of Johnson's model in practice. I also could find no evidence that further editions of the model had been published. However, one paper has been published which evaluates this model by collecting data on its use in the USA.

AN EVALUATION OF JOHNSON'S MODEL

Two British authors, Reynold and Cormack (1991), were involved in an evaluation of Johnson's model in action in the University of California, Los Angeles (UCLA) Neuropsychiatric Institute and Hospital and School of Nursing, USA, where the model has been widely used for about 12 years. Their paper emphasizes the application of the model to practice. They raise a number of questions about the usefulness of the model in practice.

Reynolds and Cormack apply their criteria of the relevance of the model to clinical practice, as they perceive the model working in UCLA:

1. To what extent does the model assist with the identification of the range of human responses to actual or potential health problems?
2. How does the model enable a nursing diagnosis to be made, and what is the basis of that diagnosis?
3. Does the model explain why individuals respond to health problems in the way that they do?
4. Does the model inform clinicians of the nursing interventions required to enable the client to move towards optimum health?

5. Does the model help to provide an understanding of the desired outcome of nursing intervention?

(p. 1123)

In answer to Question 1, they found that the model did form the basis of nursing assessment. As such it helped nurses to assess patients' needs, although they query whether there was an element of fitting these needs into the elements of the model. However, they do comment that the identified malfunctions were good examples of the patients' ineffectual coping, such as denial of illness or overeating.

With regard to Question 2, they show a number of stages that the nurse goes through before a nursing diagnosis is made. These stages are: the identification of one or more malfunctions of the subsystems; determination of how effectively the subsystem is working in achieving its purpose; the search for regulators in the environment that are having an effect on the subsystem (this can involve a wide-ranging search); and finally, once all the data are assembled, a complete nursing diagnosis is made which involves the interaction of all the subsystems with each other. This last stage involves a very complex conceptual analysis. It is interesting to note from Reynolds and Cormack's paper that 33% of the nursing staff are educated to Masters' level and 5% to doctoral level, while 50% hold a degree in Nursing Science.

The authors conclude that the Johnson model not only allows a nursing diagnosis to be made, but also allows nurses to describe how the diagnosis was made.

In answer to their Question 3, Reynolds and Cormack say that the nurse identifies why the behavioural subsystems are malfunctioning, for example, whether only one subsystem is malfunctioning, or if it is a combination of many of them and one is dominating the others. To do this the influencing environmental factors, identified during Stage 2 above, are used. These factors can include family dynamics, past learning or physical disabilities. The authors seem very impressed with the model in action at this stage, as they comment 'Thus the Johnson model provides nurses with the means with which to explain why individuals respond to health problems in the way that they do' (p. 1127).

Concerning Question 4, they seem less certain, as they say that the model does not prescribe nursing actions to promote behavioural systems balance, 'it does not provide a direct link between diagnosis and intervention' (p. 1127). At the intervention stage nurses were seen to select work from other areas, such as client-centred therapy or cognitive therapy, which the staff readily accepted that they did: 'we select interventions from the literature' (p. 1127).

Regarding the last question the authors' asked, Auger and Dee (1982, 1983) have developed a patient classification system to assess the amount of nursing and the level of nursing skill needed. According to Reynolds and Cormack, this tool helps to provide the answer to Question 5, although they give no details of this.

In conclusion, the authors feel that a weakness of the model is its inability to prescribe nursing actions. They also feel that the link between nursing diagnosis, nursing input and the outcomes of intervention need validation: I would entirely agree with this last statement.

This paper has provided us with a very good feel for what it must be like to use a model of nursing in an institution. Some points are good, for example definition of the patients' problems is very thorough. However, other aspects are very weak, even at their best, for example the ability to judge or measure the effectiveness of nursing interventions. This is not solely a problem for this model, however; many of the other models seem also to be weak in this area.

CONCLUSIONS ON THE USE OF THE MODEL FROM ITS DEVELOPMENT TO 1995

There are few further conclusions to add to those that I wrote in 1990. The one additional paper that I found shows that the use of and interest in the model has spread from the USA to the UK. However, this paper defines further problems for the model; while the assessment process is obviously very sophisticated in a setting that has used it for a long time and in which the majority of staff are highly educated, the link between assessment, nursing intervention and evaluation is weak. On considering this again looking at the papers by Holaday and Derdiarian, it becomes more obvious how Johnson's model gives no guidance on the way the nurses should help to restore the patients' behavioural systems imbalance. Therefore to use a decision-making process, as nursing is pledged to do, leaves a very tentative link between assessment, intervention and evaluation when this model is used.

The further problem of the nurse being in the dominant position over the patient, as indicated by Cronenwett, adds another difficulty to the use of Johnson's model in practice, where patients' and citizens' charters are now important. These charters combined with official complaints procedures make everyone's right to be heard and to decide what is right for them an important step in nursing practice.

REFERENCES

Bell, S. and Ainsworth, M. (1972) Infant crying and maternal responsiveness. *Child Development*, **43**, 1171–90.
Brickman, P., Coates, D., Rabinowitz, V.C., Karuza, J., Cohn, E. and Kidder, L. (1982) An attributional analysis of helping behaviour. in *Advances in*

Experimental Social Psychology (ed. L. Berkowitz).

Cook, R. (1970) Relation of achievement motivation and attribution to self-rein-forcement. Doctoral dissertation, University of California.

Crandall, V.C. (1965) Children's beliefs in their own control of reinforcements in intellectual–academic achievement situations. *Child Development*, **36**, 91–109.

Crandall, V.C. *et al.* (1962) Motivation and ability determinants of young children's intellectual achievement behaviours. *Child Development*, **33**, 643–61.

Cronenwett, L.R. (1983) Helping and nursing models. *Nursing Research*, **32**(6), 342–6.

Derdiarian, A.K. (1983) An instrument for theory and research development using the behavioural systems model for nursing: the cancer patient. *Nursing Research*, **32**(4), 196–201.

Derdiarian, A.K. and Forsythe, A.B. (1983) An instrument for theory and research development using the behavioural systems model for nursing: the cancer patient. *Nursing Research*, **32**(5), 260–6.

Holaday, B.J. (1974) Achievement behaviour in chronically ill children. *Nursing Research*, **23**(1), 25–30.

Holaday, B.J. (1981) Maternal response to their chronically ill infants' attachment behaviour of crying. *Nursing Research*, **30**(6), 343–8.

Johnson, D.E. (1968a) Theory in nursing: borrowed and unique. *Nursing Research*, **17**, 206–9.

Johnson, D.E. (1968b) One conceptual model of nursing. Paper presented at Vanderbilt University, Nashville, TN, April 1968.

Johnson, D.E. (1972) Lecture quotes.

Johnson, D.E. (1974) Development of theory: a requisite for nursing as a primary health profession. *Nursing Research*, **23**, 372–7.

Johnson, D.E. (1978) Application of theory in education and service. Papers presented at Second Annual Nurse Educator Conference, New York, December 1978. Audio tapes available from Teach 'em, Inc., 160 E. Illinois Street, Chicago, IL 60611, USA.

Johnson, D.E. (1980) The behavioural systems model for nursing, in *Conceptual Models for Nursing Practice* (eds J.P. Riehl and C. Roy), 2nd edn, Appleton-Century-Crofts, New York.

Krulik and Florian (1995) Social isolation of school-age children with chronic ill-nesses. *Social Sciences in Health*, **1**(3), 164–74.

Majesky, S.J, Brester, M.H. and Nishio, K.T. (1978) Development of a research tool: patient indicators of nursing care. *Nursing Research*, **27**(6), 365–71.

Reynolds, W. and Cormack, D.F.S. (1991) An evaluation of the Johnson behav-ioural systems model of nursing. *Journal of Advanced Nursing*, **16**, 1122–30.

Rotter, J.B. *et al.* (1972) *Application of Social Learning Theory of Personality*, Holt, Reinhart and Winston, New York.

FURTHER READING

Chapman, C.M. (1985) *Theory of Nursing: Practical Application*, Harper and Row, London.

Chinn, P.L. and Jacobs, M.K. (1987) *Theory and Nursing*, C.V. Mosby, St Louis.

Fawcett, J. (1984) *Analysis and Evaluation of Conceptual Models of Nursing*, F.A. Davis, Philadelphia.

Fitzpatrick, J.J. and Whall, A.L. (1983) *Conceptual Models of Nursing: Analysis and Application*, Prentice Hall, Englewood Cliffs, NJ.

Griffith-Kennedy, J.W. and Christensen, P.J. (1986) *Nursing Process: Application of Theories, Framework and Models*, C.V. Mosby, St Louis.

Kershaw, B. and Salvage, J. (1986) *Models for Nursing*, John Wiley, Chichester.

Marriner, A. (1986) *Nursing Theorists and their Work*, C.V. Mosby, St Louis.

Riehl, J.P. and Roy, C. (1980) *Conceptual Models for Nursing Practice*, 2nd edn, Appleton-Century-Crofts, Norwalk, OH.

Rogers' model of unitary human beings

6

Table of chapter contents

Roger's model of unitary human beings

Topic researched	Model components	Results
Wound healing	Reciprocy and helicy	Pig/environment interaction seen
Changes in body image during and after pregnancy	Change in pattern and organization	Both spouses body image showed change
Healthy women	Human–environment interaction as molecular structure	Inconclusive results
Screening ambulatory patients	Human–environment interaction	Creation of tool
Experience of passage of time: 1. Elderly women living at home	Life bound in space–time (4-dimensionality)	Life satisfaction; high self-esteem and inner calm
2. In different ages	4-dimensionality	Movement helps accuracy in time perception
3. During bed-rest	Human–environment interaction	Feeling rested associated with time passing quickly
Restfulness resulting from varied harmonious sounds	Integrality	A harmonious auditory environment helps to create restfulness
Support conflict of new mothers	Integrality and helicy	Creation of a theoretical model
Changes resulting from pregnancy and post-partum	Pattern and organization	Inconclusive findings
Alterations in circadian rhythms of hospitalized patients	Helicy	Both morning and evening types have changes in their sleep patterns during hospitalization

Topic researched	Model components	Results
Near-death experience	4-dimensionality	Literature review
Operationalizing Rogers' model	All components	Unclear
Effects of physical activity on growth in young children	Reciprocy and helicy	Physical stimulation promotes growth and development
Effects of therapeutic touch on tension headache	Synchrony and helicy	Therapeutic touch can relieve tension headache
Learning to use therapeutic touch	Synchrony and helicy	Personal experience of becoming a therapist
Relief of stress by social support	4-dimensionality, helicy, resonancy and integrality	Theoretical model
Closed urinary catheter instillation and irrigation	Reciprocy	Review of literature and recommendations
Movement therapy in the elderly	Helicy	Planned movement is associated with improved morale and attitudes to own ageing
Acceleration of time with age	Perception of time	No evidence for acceleration of time with age
Assessment of pattern manifestation appraisal	Human–environment interaction	Case study of assessment
Assessment of mothers' abilities to cope with a new-born baby. Assessment tool used	Assessment using a tool	Few details of use of tool or model given
The experience of undergoing therapeutic touch before, during and after treatment	Promoting harmony between human beings and environment	Linear process of unmet need, treatment, followed by prolonged and intense personal change for the better

THE AUTHOR

Martha Rogers was born in 1914. After completing nurse training she obtained a Bachelor of Science degree from George Peabody College, Nashville, Tennessee in 1937. She graduated with a Master of Arts in Public Health Nursing Supervision in 1945 from Columbia University, New York. In 1952 she obtained a Master of Public Health degree, and in 1954 a Doctor of Science degree, both from the Johns Hopkins University in Baltimore. From 1954 until 1975 she was Professor and Head of the

Division of Nursing, New York University, and since 1979 she has been Emeritus Professor.

Colleagues say she is one of the most original thinkers nursing has produced and is years ahead of her time.

THE MODEL

Rogers' model has been developed since the publication of her first book *An Introduction to the Theoretical Basis of Nursing* in 1970. This volume sets out the major tenets of her theory, and how the model should be used in practice-based research; it is the major work cited by researchers. Also available is an audiotape (Rogers, 1978) that develops and criticizes the ideas set out in the 1970 model.

Rogers has also published two chapters in edited books. The first to appear was in Riehl and Roy's *Conceptual Models for Nursing Practice* (Rogers, 1980). This work has also been frequently cited in research that uses Rogers' model as its conceptual base. The chapter 'A science of unitary man' saw modifications from her previous work. The second chapter is in Clements and Roberts *Family Health: A Theoretical Approach to Nursing Care*, entitled 'Science of unitary human beings: a paradigm for nursing' (Rogers, 1983). These two chapters are discussed briefly below before research using the model is developed.

SUMMARY OF ROGERS' MODEL OF UNITARY HUMAN BEINGS

In her 1970 publication Rogers continually states that a human being is an indivisible whole and cannot be divided into constituent parts, because the nature of a human being is to be unified. She states that there are currently two ways of misperceiving wholeness: to attempt to combine the sciences such as biology, psychology, sociology and physics, and through an interdisciplinary method to arrive at holism; or to use systems theory, where the smallest structures are examined and built up hierarchically to form the whole. This latter approach is seen where the structure of atoms leads to a higher order of the structure of cells, then tissues, then organs. Rogers says both of these methods – interdisciplinary and systems – cannot lead to the study of the human being as a whole, as the properties of the whole are not those of the parts: 'Man is a unified whole possessing his own integrity and manifesting characteristics that are more than and different from the sum of his parts' (p. 47).

According to Rogers, the human being is an open system that is constantly interacting with the environment, and vice versa; therefore each is being constantly affected by and affecting the other, through a continuous interchange of materials and energy. However, the effect one open system will have on the other cannot be predicted, as outcomes are often uncertain.

The environment also has its own unity, and both humans and the environment have the properties of continuous repatterning in their transactions with each other. The environment, says Rogers, is everything external to the human being, so, as an open system, the environment must stretch to the boundaries of the universe: 'Man and the environment are continuously exchanging matter and energy with one another' (p. 54).

The evolution of life shows a one-way trend that leads to evolutionary change, where the passage of time is integral to the everyday life of human beings. Unidirectionality means nothing will ever be the same again; time is unidirectional and irreversible. The process of life is bound up with the three dimensions of space and the dimension of time, which is characterized by increasing complexity and innovation. The development process of the human being is predictable from life to death. Evolution of human beings is simultaneous with that of the universe which exhibits continuous pattern and organization. Both human beings and the universe are subject to the laws of probability, so knowledge will rely on the estimation of probabilities of events. Change is not constant in speed, sometimes it is accelerated, at other times reduced; however, some features of human life remain relatively constant, for example its expected length: 'The life process evolves irreversibly and unidirectionally along the space–time continuum' (p. 56).

Pattern and organization are basic to the development of human life, and are observable phenomena. The energy field imposes pattern and organization on human beings and the environment, but it is recognition of this pattern that we see as wholeness. Therefore pattern and organization are unifying concepts; without them everything would be chaos, dynamic and ever-changing. The change in pattern is towards growing complexity (not towards stability) and together with organization they reflect the nature of unidirectionality. However, human beings have the ability to regulate their own changes and those of their environment by exercising choices, an expression of wholeness that reflects pattern and organization: '[these] identify man and reflect his innovative wholeness' (p. 65).

The preceding sections argue for the characteristics of all living things, not merely humans; however, humans are different from, and more complex than, other living forms. They are characterized by the capacity for abstraction and imagery, language and thought, sensation and emotion. These feelings and sensations, such as love and fear, cannot be studied as parts of the human being. Language is the means by which humans transmit their feelings and thoughts, particularly abstract thought that enables the development of understanding.

In developing a model of nursing from these assumptions, Rogers affirms that human beings are integral to the universe and that they are complementary. The conceptual boundaries of human beings touch those of the environment and are identified by an energy field which is electrical in nature and in a constant state of flux varying in intensity, density and extent. The boundaries of the human being's energy field are irregular, sometimes expanding and at other times retreating; they vary between individuals and also at different points in time. Similar properties are put forward for the environmental energy field, and interaction between human and environmental fields takes place across boundaries, the two fields extending to the universe.

Increasing complexity and organization grow out of the many interactions between human and environmental fields and continue throughout life, until they cease at death where integrity of the human field is lost. The human field is embedded in a four-dimensional space–time continuum that extends into the future as well as reaching back into the past. It has rhythmical qualities that spiral throughout life, constantly shaping and being shaped by the environment and widening or narrowing depending on the speed of change in the field. The events along the spirals are not repetitious, but similar, as the unidimensional nature of human beings does not allow for repetition of events; each is unique.

From the above developments of her model Rogers moves to develop further the ideas into testable hypotheses; these she calls principles, and they are intended to be provisional. The principles of the life process are homodynamic, and are *reciprocy*, *synchrony*, *helicy* and *resonancy*.

Reciprocy has the basic assumption of wholeness and openness. The human energy field is identified as that which is human, while the environmental energy field is everything that is external to this, and the two fields continuously and simultaneously interact with each other producing constant change. Therefore human beings are inseparable from the environment and the changes in both are probabilistic: 'Reciprocy is a function of the mutual interaction between the human and the environmental field' (p. 97).

The principle of **synchrony** has the basic assumptions of reciprocy plus the life process evolving unidirectionally in a four-dimensional space–time matrix. This has properties of increasing complexity and patterning and organization, but there is no returning to previous states. The past is non-repeatable, but it is important in the development of the future:

> Synchrony is a function of the state of the human field at a specified point in space–time interacting with the environmental field at the same specified point in space–time.

> (p. 99)

The principle of **helicy** contains the basic assumptions of synchrony and reciprocy, but also that life develops rhythmically, with greater organization as human beings constantly interact towards achieving greater complexity, not homeostasis. The interactions are also probabilistic, where similarities occur, but change in one field cannot predict with absolute certainty the change that will occur in the other fields, although rhythmical similarities can be identified and probabilities determined: 'Helicy is a function of continuous innovative change growing out of the mutual interaction of man and environment along a spiralling longitudinal axis bound in space–time' (p. 101).

The principle of **resonancy** has as its basic assumption that the pattern and organization changes in both the human and the environmental fields are transmitted by waves. These have different frequencies, and there is a continuous rhythmical flow of waves between human beings and the environment. The way a human being experiences the environment is through these waves. Rogers has supervised a series of doctoral students who have completed theses testing this principle, but none has been able to show that human and environmental interactions are transmitted by electrical waves, therefore this concept remains uncertain. Unfortunately these theses have not been published.

The principle of **homodynamics** assumes that changes in human beings are inseparable from those in the environment, and are both irreversible and unrepeatable. They result in continuous pattern and organization transmitted by waves.

Despite the disappointing findings of the research students investigating the nature of waves, Rogers has supervised many other students to doctoral level who have developed her model. Two of these studies have been published and are available for scrutiny and evaluation (Porter, 1972; Strumpf, 1978). They are discussed later in this chapter.

Rogers sees her model being used in practice in a number of ways. She defends her broad principles, as a wide variety of unpredictable circumstances require such a broad approach. She also defends practice being based on knowledge and intellectual judgement; therefore there are no rules of thumb, no room for memorizing rules, and all nursing intervention strategies should be questioned. Nursing intervention is therefore selected according to intellectual skill, and the techniques for intervention will be wide and varied. Nursing practice has its basis in the holistic nature of human beings and their integrity with the environment, therefore nursing must promote harmony between the interactions of humans with the environment; this may mean teaching people how to live in harmony with their environment while helping to direct changes. Probabilistic goal-setting which allows for the changing nature of definition and promotion of health, but also recognizes the developmental nature of people, is the domain of nursing. Human beings must recognize in daily activities the rhythmical nature of human life and the openness of human and environmental fields that will aid repatterning of both; an example of this is overstimulation or understimulation that has serious consequences for humans, as shown in studies of patients in intensive care units. Nursing must also be directed to correcting health problems that arise from social inequalities, technological advances and other public events; so, there is an acute need for large-scale community health services that recognize the wholeness of human beings.

Rogers sees that the human being is an integral participant in nursing intervention. The latter is not directed to disease categories, although these may form supplementary and relevant data in deciding on nursing intervention, but based on the wholeness of human beings and on determining the state of the human being in relation to the environment and the preceding states that have led up to the present state. Nursing must be concerned with evaluation that will help to estimate probabilities in achieving a predetermined goal.

Rogers' (1970) work concludes by saying that human beings have major resources within themselves to determine the direction taken by development. Nursing intervention should be directed towards helping people to mobilize their resources in order to strengthen the human–environment relationship and heighten the integrity of the individual. It must also take into account the human being as a thinking, feeling being who relies on humanitarian goals.

In her 1980 work Rogers reasserts that the assumptions on which her model is based are four-fold.

- That human beings and the environment are energy fields extending to infinity; however, she no longer asserts that these fields are electrical in nature – each field is an entirety that cannot be broken down into parts, such as biological, psychological and social.
- Openness of the energy fields is continuous, so there is no room for concepts such as equilibrium or adaptation.
- Pattern and organization are how the energy fields are identified; these are continuously changing in an innovative and creative way, the human and environmental fields being characterized by wave patterns that show increasing diversity.
- The human and environmental fields are four-dimensional – the three dimensions of space and the dimension of time, which is evidently different from a three-dimensional world and requires substantial abstract thinking. It may be that the four-dimensional human being is embedded in a four-dimensional environment, where the former has continuous fluctuating boundaries. Therefore the present becomes irrelevant in this model, it is only the 'relative present' that is important; this makes paranormal events possible in this model.

In 1980, Rogers' four principles were reduced to three: **helicy** and **resonancy**, which remained unchanged from her 1970 work, and **complementarity**, combining the previous principles of synchrony and reciprocy: 'The interaction between human and environmental fields is continuous, mutual and simultaneous' (p. 333). Within this system change is still unidirectional, probabilistic and moving towards increasing diversity of field pattern and organization.

In her 1983 work Rogers further amends the principle of complementarity, now calling it **integrality**, although its contents remain substantially the same as those of complementarity.

The research following these publications has been devoted to developing many of the assumptions and principles of the model, involving the nature of human–environment interaction, the identification of the individual's and the environment's current state, and the evaluation of certain nursing actions to promote improved human–environment interaction.

This model is possibly one of the most developed in terms of practice research; one of the reasons for this may be the large number of doctoral students supervised by Rogers. One of the studies (Gill and Atwood, 1981) received critical appraisal in the nursing press, which gave considerable insight into the nature of the differences in interpretation of the model. These papers are discussed in this chapter.

The first section in this chapter is devoted to studies that identify the unitary state and health; the second section examines studies devoted to nursing intervention in promoting health or recovery from illness. No studies were found that dealt predominantly with planning or evaluating nursing care using Rogers' model. However, two papers showed how identification of the unitary state led through intervention to evaluation; these are included in a supplementary section following identification.

IDENTIFICATION OF THE UNITARY STATE

This section contains a number of quite novel studies developed around Rogers' model. They take a variety of areas of nursing practice and examine particular aspects of them: reciprocy and helicy in wound healing; unidirectionality and pattern and organization in changes during and after pregnancy; the nature of wave patterns investigated through perceived body size in relation to space and conversational distance; three studies on the experience of the passage of time (in the elderly, in relation to movement, and to resting in bed); human–environment interaction seen in support as experienced by new mothers; and change in pattern and organization in sleep–wake rhythms of patients in psychiatric hospitals.

The number of studies found, and the rigour of many of them is an unexpected and commendable feature in the acceptance of the challenge that this model has created. Unfortunately none of these studies was conducted outside North America.

A STUDY OF RECIPROCY AND HELICY IN WOUND HEALING

The first study (Gill and Atwood, 1981) uses the area of wound healing to examine the relationship between the environment and the individual. It examines the extent that manipulation of the environment will influence the change in the individual's state over time, or, more precisely, one part of the individual – the skin. To this extent one could argue that the study is not really based on holism, as the skin is only one part of the total individual. However, the authors set out to test Rogers' principles of reciprocy and helicy directly, and state this at the outset of their paper.

Gill and Atwood (1981) examined the effects of epidermal growth factor (EGF) on wound healing. Using Rogers' model they operationalized the human–environment interaction as being represented by the keratinocyte of the skin at the wound edge which is the boundary of the human field; anything external to the cell membrane of the keratinocyte comprises the environmental field. This represented operationalizing the principles of **resonancy**, 'a function of the mutual interaction between the human field and the environmental field' (Rogers, 1980, p. 97). The authors' use of the principle of **helicy** was through the rate of healing of the wound, incorporating the idea of the space–time continuum that Rogers saw as having rhythmic qualities and that she visualized as the 'Slinky': 'Helicy is a function of continuous innovative change growing out of the mutual interaction of man and environment along a spiralling longitudinal axis bound in space–time' (Rogers, 1970, p. 101). This rhythmic quality was seen as each turn of the spiral containing all the four stages in the cycle of the keratinocyte. According to Howard and Pelc (1953) these are: the pre-DNA synthesis period; the DNA synthesis period; the post-DNA synthesis period; and mitosis. The rate of each cycle is usually steady in order to maintain the relationship of cell production to cell loss.

The study investigated the rate of wound healing seen to occur when EGF is added in different strengths to wounds. Because the dose–response curve needed to be defined, an initial study on humans was felt unethical, so the study was conducted on a young Yorkshire-mix pig. The choice of this animal was due to the documented similarities in skin structure between humans and pigs. Apart from defining the dose–response curve, three hypotheses were also tested (p. 71).

- Topical application of EGF will increase the migration of keratinocytes over the wound.
- Topical application of EGF will increase the mitotic index.
- Topical application of EGF will increase the rate of differentiation of keratinocytes over the wound.

A number of small epidermal incisions were made on the back of the pig, and into these was applied concentrations of 10 ng/ml, 20 ng/ml and

40 ng/ml of EGF every 2 hours for 6 hours, then every 6 hours for 24 hours. Sodium chloride (NaCl) was applied to control wounds according to the same schedule. Biopsies of wounds taken in random order were performed at 12, 24 and 27 hours.

The results of healing were reported at the end of 27 hours only. Results showed that there was poor epithelialization with the 10 ng/ml solution; there were some areas of epithelialization with the 20 ng/ml solution; and there was a triple layer of keratinocytes over much of each wound with the 40 ng/ml solution; the control wounds showed only a single cell layer. The researchers report that this did not show a definite dose–response curve as a function of the different strengths of EGF. However, there is support for the principle of reciprocy, as the environmental field (the EGF) is seen to interact positively with the porcine field (the wounds) during the period of the study. The principle of helicy is also supported, as changes in the porcine field are seen at the time of changes in the environmental field – when the concentrations of EGF are increased and result in better wound healing. The researchers also claim that the 'Slinky' with the varying size of its spirals is an ideal representation of the differences in wound healing according to the varying times of cell generation and growth. However, the evidence in their paper is insufficient to support this claim.

Although this is a well-controlled study, it presents two main problems. First, it questions the validity in the application of a model of human beings to an experiment that uses an animal as its subject. There is still much debate about the extent to which human behaviour can be discussed or predicted as a result of animal studies. For ethical reasons it is now also becoming less justifiable in some quarters to use animal experimentation before subjecting humans to treatments, but for the researchers to make such a direct link between the process seen in an animal and a model intended for the study of humans is taking things a little too far. The second problem is that using a holistic model to examine one system – the skin – is directly opposed to Rogers' assumptions about holism.

However, the study is based directly on Rogers' model and is a cause and effect study which is well controlled. Therefore the results can be seen as reliable. The results are however difficult to interpret in relation to Rogers' model due to the problems discussed in the previous paragraph.

Following the publication of this study a critique was published (Kim, 1983) that addressed some of the major problems of any study related to practice issues using a model of nursing. This paper used Gill and Atwood's study to demonstrate three specific questions (p. 89).

- Is the logic used to derive the research hypotheses adequate, and rigorous?
- Is the research methodology used in the study appropriate for testing Rogers' model?

- If problems exist with respect to the above questions, how might they be resolved?

Kim first argues that the nature of the human and environmental fields is different; that is, they are governed by different patterns of interaction so the changes that occur in either field are not necessarily similar. However, taking Rogers' principle of reciprocy as a function of the interaction between the human and environmental fields, Gill and Atwood alter the environmental field in order to measure the human, or in this case the porcine, reaction. This is clearly a different interpretation of Rogers' principle of reciprocy than the theorist intended. Second, Kim argues that Rogers did not intend the human and environmental fields to be seen as governed by causal laws; contrary to this she says that Gill and Atwood have used 'positive association' as the basis of the relationship between changes they have observed in their experiment.

Kim's argument with operationalizing the principles as used by Gill and Atwood is the same as I have mentioned above – that is, that Rogers says the human being is a unitary energy field; therefore to say that the 'human field is the keratinocyte adjacent to the wound edge' (Gill and Atwood, 1981, p. 70) is not consistent with Rogers' holistic concept. Second, Rogers does not see changes in terms of positive or negative, but in terms of greater organization and complexity. Therefore, again Gill and Atwood's use of the model is not consistent with the intention of the theorist.

Kim also criticizes Gill and Atwood by quoting Rogers: 'the characteristics and behaviour of unitary man are specific to unitary man' (Rogers, 1980, p. 330). This shows quite clearly that Rogers would have considered experiments on animals to be unsuitable as a testing ground for her model of the human–environment interaction, as she says unequivocally that knowledge of human phenomena can only be derived from humans.

Kim accepts that the principles of holism and reciprocy are difficult to operationalize, but advocates repeated testing to produce refinements of the concepts.

Gill and Atwood defend their study, and in a subsequent article (Atwood and Gill-Rogers, 1984) show a wider interpretation of Rogers' principles than those used by Kim in her critical analysis. They view reciprocy in a number of ways, which will take different forms as the model and its principles are refined. In the Kuhnian sense (Kuhn, 1970) this is quite acceptable as the development of metatheory. They also claim that Gibbs' (1972) paradigm helped them to move between levels of abstraction to arrive at their operational level, and they have used this paradigm not only in their 1981 study but also on other occasions and found it useful. Atwood and Gill-Rogers also say that Gibbs' paradigm is consistent with Rogers' model where causality is specifically precluded:

however, for probability to be able to explain or describe a set of circumstances, several conditions must occur, as they say: '(1) temporal priority; (2) covariation in dependent and independent variables; (3) specified nature (positive or negative) and preferably the form of the association' (p. 88).

In their experiment Attwood and Gill-Rogers say that temporal priority operated through the time lapse between the wound being made and the different applications of EGF. They also say that the language used to describe the subsequent healing process was consistent with covariation between the strength of EGF and the rate of healing. The form of the association, they state, is not specified in causal terms as a value judgement, but in terms of covariation.

Atwood and Gill-Rogers also refute the accusations of Kim in relation to testing partial theories. They say that Hardy (1978) set a precedent for testing partial theories and that they concentrated on one side of the relationship between human beings and the environment while holding the other side constant. Therefore they refute the accusations made by Kim in her arguments of logical adequacy in their study.

Atwood and Gill-Rogers defend their operationalization of Rogers' model as being part of the process of building up an understanding of the workings of a systems model. They say that in order to test the latter a number of substeps would need to be completed first, otherwise to test all the variables at once in such a complex situation would lead to 'non-significant findings for unknown reasons' (p. 89). It is only through carefully validated research that the nature of relationships will be known.

With regard to their methodology, Atwood and Gill-Rogers say that while Rogers recognizes that humans are different from other forms of life, she also says that there are some attributes in common. At this early stage of the development of the model, in order to test rigorously many variables, the only ethical option is to use animal experimentation. They recognize the results will need to be critically examined in relation to humans but feel at present 'we ... must measure holism the best way possible' (p. 90).

This debate is the most challenging work found in the literature on the use of any of the models in practice research. It shows the enormous gulf in thinking between various researchers on how to interpret and use this model; it also shows the amount of debate needed before even the basic premise of the model becomes accepted. It is interesting that the debate should have centred around the use of Rogers' model, as the abstract principles involved are arguably more challenging than those in many of the other nursing models.

Many nurses in Great Britain find the principle of holism attractive, and therefore would wish to develop their thinking around this central premise, but to date no studies have been found in this country using Rogers' model as a framework for practice. This begs the question whether Rogers' principles are acceptable or usable in Great Britain.

PATTERNS OF CHANGE IN BODY IMAGE DURING AND AFTER PREGNANCY

This section outlines one of the best known and frequently cited papers on the use of Rogers' model in practice research (Fawcett, 1977). It develops the assumptions in Rogers' model as: 'Man and environment are complementary energy fields characterized by wholeness, openness, uni-directionality, pattern and organization, sentience and thought' (p. 199). The researcher develops these ideas around the family as an open system, as she says that any change in one family member is reflected in changes in other members. Therefore the natural occurrence of pregnancy should show these changes taking place. The research evidently began before 1975, as a paper in 1975 makes the case for Rogers' model to be developed around the family as a system (Fawcett, 1975). It makes a strong case for systems theory being similar to the way a family operates, as an open system interacting with the environment. It therefore makes the case for Rogers' model as conceptualizing all the features of the family in oper-ation.

Fawcett (1977) takes Rogers' principles of change in pattern and organization and studies the changes that occur during pregnancy. These changes, as women perceive them, can be measured as perceptions of the amount of space their bodies occupy, and the changes between their body boundaries and the environment during pregnancy.

There is evidence, says Fawcett, to show that women are not alone in experiencing pregnancy; it affects the whole family, particularly the husband or partner. Her literature review shows that husbands in many cultures experience various symptoms of pregnancy during their wife's pregnancy. On this evidence Fawcett hypothesizes that the husband's body image will change during the wife's pregnancy, and the closer their relationship the more they will influence each other. Therefore the hus-band's response to his wife's pregnancy would further demonstrate changes in his pattern and organization with his wife's changes as the pregnancy progresses.

The evidence quoted in the literature review by Fawcett is not sufficiently convincing to suggest that the type of changes experienced by the husband are similar enough to the wife's experiences to be taken as completely synonymous; therefore testing with the same tools may well lead to non-significant findings.

On the basis of her literature review, Fawcett formulated four hypo-theses (p. 203).

- Spouses' patterns of change in perceived body space during and after pregnancy will be similar.
- The stronger the identification between spouses, the greater the similarity in their patterns of change in perceived body space during and after pregnancy.
- Spouses' patterns of change in articulation of body concept during and after pregnancy will be similar.
- The stronger the identification between spouses, the greater the similarity in their patterns of change in articulation of body concept during and after pregnancy.

The tools used to test these hypotheses – administered to both parties equally – were the following.

- A semantic differential, designed to measure the strength of identification between the spouses, which used concepts that had previously been validated. Adjectives which represented the opposite ends of poles were chosen to represent these scales – evaluation, power and activity. The difference of the scores between spouses was the difference between their meanings of events.
- A device to measure the perceived body space of each subject, which was composed of concentric circles 2.5 cm apart, from 27.5 to 135 cm in diameter, on a piece of clear vinyl. Each circle was numbered randomly so that distance was not indicated by increasing numbers. The testing of this device was through piloting on a sample of 32 subjects, and test–retest reliability was obtained using both non-pregnant and pregnant women and their husbands; reliability scores ranged from 0.56 to 0.89. Despite the lower reliability scores, no further comment or amendments were made to the device. Clear and precise instructions were given to the subjects that they were to estimate their body space using the device.
- A figure drawing test to measure the way the body was seen, which required each subject to draw a male and a female figure. The drawings were rated according to a predetermined scale that considered the shape, personal identity, sex differentiation, and amount of detail in the drawings. Witkin *et al.* (1974) had previously determined the reliability of this rating scale to be from 0.65 to 0.92, i.e. an acceptable level of reliability. Following the figure drawing test further reliability was obtained by a professional artist, who rated independently of the rating scale. This gave a correlation of 0.92, which is a very high level of reliability and gives confidence in the scale.

The subjects were 50 married couples who were living together during the study. They were both free from illness or disability, including uncorrected vision. They had all attended childbirth preparation classes. The couples were recruited from numerous sources including childbirth classes, obstetric groups and referrals from other members of the group.

All subjects were Caucasian and each social group was represented, although the top three groups predominated. The mean age of the women was 26.5 years, and of the husbands was 28.7 years.

The couples were interviewed in their homes on two occasions, the first between the eighth and ninth months of pregnancy, and the second during the first and second months post-partum. All the instruments were administered to each partner with the figure drawing test and the semantic differential given before the topographic device. Fawcett gives no reasons for this choice, which was clearly stated, although she evidently felt that this sequence would have an effect on the results.

Data were analysed using multiple regression techniques which showed that although each spouse's body image did change, the pattern of change was different. This was seen by the women as the perception of an increase in their body size during the eighth and ninth months of pregnancy, a decrease in the first month post-partum, but an increase again in the second month post-partum. However, the perception by the men of their body size showed an increase in the eighth and ninth months of their wife's pregnancy, but a decrease in both the first and second months post-partum. Moreover, the women showed a more dramatic decrease in body size after the birth of the baby than did the men. Therefore, neither hypothesis could be supported by the data collected. In addition, the strength of the identification between the spouses did not make a difference to the similarity of their perceived body shape.

One of the most convincing arguments put forward by Fawcett for the lack of support for her hypotheses is that husbands may merely imitate the body image of their wife, which may account for the perception by the husband of change in his own body shape during his wife's pregnancy, rather than identification with her body shape as Fawcett had hypothesized. Lazowick (1955), she says, maintained that imitation indicates similar behaviour, while identification indicates similar frames of reference; the difference therefore, according to Lazowick, is between observing and mimicking (imitation), or internalizing the entire being of another (identification). These two concepts would both need a different form of investigation to access them. However, according to Rogers, imitation could be seen as a less well-developed stage of identification, therefore as patterning and organization achieve greater diversity and complexity imitation may be one of the stages leading to identification. As Rogers (1970) says: 'Developmental events along life's axis express the growing complexity of pattern and organization evolving out of multiple previous man–environment interactions' (p. 98).

Following from the rejection of the first and second hypotheses, it is no great surprise that the third and fourth hypotheses were also rejected.

Therefore, Fawcett was unable to show that changes in body shape, as indicated through similar identification, figure drawings and estimated body size, were similar between spouses.

Fawcett comments that the concept of identification changes and increases as pregnancy progresses and remains strong following the birth. She says that this supports the notion that as a task becomes more crucial, identification between the parties increases. However, she feels that the evidence in her study supports the notion that identification is generally a labile measure. This would tend to support the quotation above which refers to development of field pattern and organization over time. We might therefore tentatively say that the development of field pattern and organization is not a constant or one-way process; it varies, but its general direction over time is towards increasing, growing complexity and increasing organization.

This is a useful study, and although the hypotheses were not supported it has a number of interesting features.

- The way in which the individual interacts with the environment is unclear, but that she or he does so is made very plain in this study. This interaction is shown predominantly in Fawcett's sample of husbands who were unaware of perceiving changes in their own body shape; this only becomes apparent through psychological testing.
- The principles of pattern and organization along the space–time matrix become clearer when interpreting the data showing changes in the perception of body shape.
- The very abstract nature of Rogers' model is given form with a study such as Fawcett's, as it shows how the principles of energy fields and simultaneous interactions with the environment can be used and developed by nurses in practice with patients.

As Fawcett's study is based directly on Rogers' model, we can see from the above features of the study how Rogers' concepts have been developed. The study shows cause and effect, between pregnancy and its effects on both partners. The study was conducted in the couples' own home, and we can assume that this enhanced the study, as the couples' natural family environment was chosen.

INDICATORS OF THE RELATIONSHIP BETWEEN THE HUMAN FIELD AND SELF-ACTUALIZATION IN HEALTHY WOMEN

This study by Clarke (1986) set out to test directly the nature of the energy fields proposed by Rogers as the method of human–environment interaction. In this respect it is an ambitious study. It requires development of the holistic nature of the model, which has humans and the environment as discrete yet interacting fields. Since Rogers' (1980) work these energy fields have not been viewed as electrical or magnetic. This demands a considerable amount of resourcefulness on the part of a researcher to develop a rigorous, researchable study.

There are certain similarities between this study and Fawcett's; both examine the effects between individuals on each other, and both use a topographic device to do so; however, this is where the similarities end.

Clarke says that Rogers' model is frequently referred to as being untestable; however, she gives no references to back up this statement. Undeterred by this she sets out to test Rogers' model directly using concepts from field theory of living systems.

According to Clarke, energy fields and pattern and organization are basic features of the universe; although the nature of the energy fields is very unclear, analogies with electromagnetic fields must remain as analogies only. She feels that one of the basic elements of energy fields is an open system which could be measured through energy exchange using the framework of molecular structure by body weight, as this is one indicator of the exchange that occurs daily between humans and the environment.

In terms of wave patterns in the environment, Clarke again uses the principles of molecular structure. She says that less weight should be an indication of a faster field motion of waves exchanged between the individual and the environment. Therefore if fat is viewed as one of the behavioural manifestations of waves, then more fat will suggest longer waves and therefore slower exchanges between the individual and the environment. This will mean that obese individuals will be slower to change their weight than thinner people, and slower activity levels in the obese would be consistent with this principle of slower field motion.

These logical extensions put forward by Clarke are not based on any evidence of adequacy other than an attempt to operationalize Rogers' model. Therefore the suppositions she makes must be inventive speculation.

Clarke operationalizes these extensions of Rogers' model by using various devices.

- The topographic device as used by Fawcett in the study described above. Clarke uses this to demonstrate the exchange of energy between the individual and the environment. She follows her argument that as obese subjects perceive themselves as smaller than in reality, their human field is dense and contracted; this is similar to electrons being close together, moving more slowly and having lower energy levels, the opposite of that in thinner people. Therefore the topographic device will measure perceived body space (PBS), which will reflect the speed of the energy exchange between the individual and the environment.

- A measure of personal space to define further the density of the field. Again using concepts from molecular structure she extrapolated that a field with more energy would be less dense as the molecules would be moving faster and be further apart; this would mean a greater inter-action with the environment. Therefore measurement of preferred conversational distance (CD) between two people was the method chosen to demonstrate these ideas.
- The individual's actual weight. Clarke suggested that if the obese indi-vidual had slower interaction with the environment, then using the principles of molecular structure a greater preferred CD would be seen in obese people compared with thinner people.
- The personal orientation inventory (POI). Clarke used this measure to demonstrate levels of self-actualization. She says:

The inherent assumption is that those with self-actualizing values and behaviour will be at a higher developmental level than their less actualizing counterparts. It was hypothesized that those with an expanded field of decreased density would demonstrate a higher level of self-actualization.

(p. 32).

The hypotheses generated as a result of this use of concepts were (Clarke, 1986, p. 33):

- an inverse relationship between body weight and PBS;
- a direct relationship between body weight and CD;
- an inverse relationship between PBS and CD;
- an inverse relationship between self-actualization and body weight;
- a direct relationship between self-actualization and PBS;
- an inverse relationship between self-actualization and CD.

The use of Rogers' model as developed by Clarke shows hypothesized properties that have similar features in both the individual and the environment, namely the molecular structure. Using these features Clarke has hypothesized that similar reactions will occur in the individual, between the individual and the environment, and within the environ-ment. Therefore the hypotheses she proposes would only be examples of the whole variety of interactions occurring continuously.

Subjects recruited for the study were 130 female college student volun-teers who were screened for perceptual, hearing and visual problems. Their ages ranged from 18 to 51 years (mean 25.7).

All subjects were measured first using the measure of CD. Subjects were asked to begin 3.6 m away from the researcher and to gradually walk towards her until the most comfortable conversational distance had been reached. This method had previously been tested elsewhere (Pedersen, 1973) for reliability using a test–retest method; reliability was found to be high, at 0.93.

Second, subjects were tested using the topographic device as described by Fawcett (1977). However, Chodil (1979) reported that subjects found the instructions given to them confusing; therefore these were modified and subjects were asked to 'identify the circle that best reflects the place where you stop and the environment begins' (Clarke, 1986, p. 34). However, according to Clarke, subjects still found difficulty with the device, and frequently referred to particular parts of their bodies. This would suggest that the device or the instructions need further modification if the device is to reflect body boundaries adequately, as in its present state the device does not appear to be a totally valid indicator.

In the Personal Orientation Inventory (POI) (Knapp, 1976) there were 150 two-choice items, and the scale was developed around the type of behaviours self-actualizing people reported themselves. Reliability for the test had previously been achieved (Shostrom, 1973) at between 0.91 and 0.93; Shostrum was also able to show significant discrimination between those who had been identified as self-actualizing and those who were not. Construct validity had also previously been ascertained for this scale.

Data collection also included subjects' reported weight, demographic data, and data on the subjects' diet and exercise behaviour. Lastly subjects were weighed to ascertain their true body weight.

Analysis of the data collected was by Pearson's product moment correlation. Results showed that only the sixth hypothesis was statistically significant ($p = 0.02$), i.e. those subjects with a high level of self-actualizing as measured by the POI had a statistically smaller conversational distance than subjects with a lower level of self-actualizing. However, the factors associated with this interaction are very unclear, and it is uncertain from this study whether molecular structure is the contributing factor. Of all the proposed hypotheses, the sixth makes the greatest assumptions, based on very flimsy evidence that molecular structure could have a bearing on the expected interaction.

Clarke makes considerable criticism of her study, and of its relationship to Rogers' model. The topographic device was evidently not a valid measure of body boundaries; furthermore the position of the researcher in relation to the subjects was not systematically evaluated during use. As conversational distance was taken as the first measure, subjects became confused when asked to estimate their body boundaries using the topographic device as the second measure; they frequently asked what was the relationship between the two measures, and therefore may have seen the topographic device as a further indication of their conversational distance.

Perceived body size and weight are also suspect measures due to society's current expectation of the female figure. Perceptions of body size and weight are bound to be influenced by these prevailing expectations, therefore the pattern of interaction between the individual and the environment is bound to be unstable. However, Clarke suggests that the molecular structure she advocates is a stable feature of the individual's interaction with the environment, which is why obese individuals lose weight more slowly. Moreover, Rogers (1970) frequently states that the energy fields are continually in a state of flux:

> An energy field identifies the conceptual boundaries of man. This field is electrical in nature, is in a continual state of flux, and varies continuously in its intensity, density and extent.
>
> (p. 90)

Despite these findings, Clarke's study is useful in pointing out the difficulty of operationalizing and measuring aspects of Rogers' model. It shows that some indicators, namely conversational distance, can demonstrate human–environment boundaries but the other measures used in this study to define boundaries should be carefully considered before further use.

There is also a need to develop more valid measures of openness and human–environment interaction if Rogers' model is to be successfully used in practice settings, as it is questionable whether energy is transmitted by molecular structure.

Clarke's study was also based directly on Rogers' model, so Clarke is attempting to operationalize and to measure Rogers' concepts by a descriptive study. The fact that she is unsuccessful does not deny the validity of Rogers' model, however, it does limit the options by which energy fields can be measured. To this extent it adds to the knowledge of the model.

A TOOL FOR SCREENING AMBULATORY CLIENTS

The main aim of this study (Anderson, 1980) was to develop a tool for assessing the psychosocial health status of patients visiting an ambulatory clinic in Detroit, Michigan, USA. It was hoped to develop a brief, comprehensive assessment tool that could be used to guide initial assessment of clients in this centre, as a method of demonstrating efficiency. It was hoped that this instrument would compare favourably with other longer measures already known to be valid and reliable.

Anderson uses Rogers' (1970) concepts in her initial opening statement: 'The patient's total environmental field (internal and external) should be assessed during the initial visit in order to plan comprehensive health care' (p. 347). However, Rogers asserts that we should not use a single area, such as psychosocial:

Human behaviour is synergistic. Behavioural manifestations of the life process are symphonic expressions of unity and cannot be dichotomized as objective or subjective, as internal or external, as mental or physical.

However, this paper does not develop the assumptions or principles of Rogers' model. The study then discusses and evaluates tools to assess patients' psychological health. But as this paper claims to use Rogers' model it is important to use it here, if only to show the problems it causes for the rigorous use of models in practice.

Anderson uses two measures, the Social Readjustment Rating Scale (SRRS) of Holmes and Rahe (1968) and the Heimler Scale of Social Functioning (HSSF) (Heimler, 1975). Both scales had previously been tested by various researchers for reliability and validity and were found to be acceptable measures; they were both tested against the Assessment of Life Conditions Scale (ALC) (Harrington, 1978). The ALC scale consisted of 23 items, and subjects had to tick which of the items referred to themselves. The items contained 17 negative phrases, for example being 'uptight a lot of the time'; and six positive items, for example 'satisfied with way of life'. The score on the ALC measure was obtained by summing positive and negative items indicated by the subjects. This scale was developed by the physician-in-charge of the Kaiser Permanent Health Maintenance Organization, San José, California, whose beliefs in designing the questionnaire are clearly stated in the paper:

[he] believes that a significant proportion of health care providers' practices consist of caring for patients with psychosocial problems. His research supports the notion that, if psychosocial needs could be assessed and addressed directly, health care would be more cost effective.

(p. 347)

An unfortunate feature of this paper is the impression of nurses carrying out doctors' instructions, and making an initial assessment of patients for doctors to confirm or deny.

Both the SRRS and the HSSF were assessed against the ALC scale using 40 patients with physical problems from four clinics in Michigan, each of whom was administered the three scales. The sample included 32 females and eight males; 25 were black and 15 white. Although the study mentions that the age range and social class of clients was a cross-section, no details of this are given in the article.

Differences in demographic details were found; blacks scored significantly more positive events than whites on the ALC scale ($p < 0.03$); and women had significantly higher negative scores ($p < 0.04$) and also perceived themselves to be significantly less healthy (p < 0.04) than men on the ALC scale.

When the ALC scale was examined alongside the SRRS, the negative scores on the former scale predicted the units on the latter scale when taken over the last 6 months. The regression equation showed the probability to be < 0.02. However, the high standard error of 126, and the low squared correlation (r^2 = 0.13) showed that the ALC scale is not at present useful in a clinical setting without further refining.

The negative scores on the ALC were highly significantly correlated with all the HSSF scores (significance ranged from p = 0.02 to p = 0.0001).

The study therefore showed that negative scores on the ALC were related to scores on two longer scales, the SRRS and the HSSF. However, the sample is relatively small, and is biased towards women; also, as mentioned above, the sample was not shown to be truly representative in other respects. From the point of view of this book, the most disappointing part of the study is that it did not show how Rogers' principles were used in a rigorous way to create further knowledge and understanding of her model, and one wonders why the model was quoted at the beginning of the study. Therefore there can be no conclusions drawn about Rogers' model from this paper.

THE EXPERIENCE OF THE PASSAGE OF TIME

The three studies in this section develop Rogers' principle of the perception of time. Rogers (1970, p. 55) sees time as an 'integral part of man's everyday life' but she links the life process to time and to the dimensions of space which create a four-dimensional state. She says that 'Life evolves unidirectionally along the space–time continuum' (p. 57). In her 1980 work Rogers develops this idea further, describing a human being as a 'four-dimensional energy field embedded in a four-dimensional environmental field' (p. 331). The studies in this section deal more directly with the aspect of time, although the third study, by Smith, does not involve the use of a control for environmental factors.

The first two studies (Strumpf, 1987; Newman, 1982) deal with the perception of time in the elderly and use different methods to achieve their results. The third study (Smith, 1984) investigates the experience of a limited period of enforced bedrest, examining the perceptions of time by the subjects according to differences in environmental stimulation.

All these studies raise interesting issues about the difficulty of measuring the time perception of individuals, and the importance that is attached to the perception of time by the individual and its relationship to health.

The experience of the passage of time in the elderly

The first study (Strumpf, 1987) aimed to investigate the subjective experience of time in elderly women, and to offer some speculation on the meaning of findings to the life and health of the elderly, for nurses to understand better the experiences of the elderly and relate these to the provision of nursing care.

This study was part of a larger study to explore the quality of life of the elderly living at home. Strumpf reviewed the literature on subjective time experience in relation to the elderly; he outlined the problems associated with measurement of such a concept, described his study to investigate time experience in elderly women, commented on the meaning of the findings for these women, and considered the nursing implications for care of the elderly.

The literature revealed that one of the methods of experiencing time is the subjective impression that it is moving either quickly or slowly or not moving at all. This is usually referred to in the literature as time aware-ness, and has a dimension that includes perception of events both in the past and the present. Piaget (1966, 1970) suggested that those with a per-ception of fast internal time rates found external time to be slow in the present, compared to internal events, but the passage of time in the past had been very fast.

During working life time is of the essence, but during retirement Markson (1973) suggests that adjustment and therefore health will depend on the individual's successful changing relationship to time. There were also felt to be several influencing factors in the relationship between age and the experience of the passage of time: age, imminent death, activity levels, emotional state, outlook, environment and the value of time. However, other studies have shown no relationship between age and the perception of time passing quickly (Kuhlen and Monge, 1968).

There also seemed to be considerable agreement that older people who are more oriented towards the future were also more likely to be satisfied with life, to experience a greater sense of well-being, and to be better adjusted to life in general. Considerable evidence showed that indi-viduals who were in an institution or were unwell perceived time to pass more slowly than healthier people. Generally there seemed to be a rela-tionship between increasing age, psychological well-being and the expe-rience of time passing. One of the questions asked by Rogers (1970) was 'Is the speed with which time is perceived to be passing an index of the speed with which the ageing process is occurring?' (p. 115).

Strumpf notes how difficult it is to measure the subjective experience of the passage of time, and examines the ways in which this has been achieved by others in this field. He comments that although each of the instruments used provides some useful information about the perception of time by the elderly, they do not deal adequately with the complexity of the experience of the passage of time. He is also pessimistic about such a measure being capable of being produced.

Three tools were used in this study.

- The Time Metaphor Test (Knapp and Garbutt, 1958) consists of 25 phrases that indicate poetic descriptions of the passing of time. Subjects are asked to choose the five that they feel most closely resemble how time appears to be passing for them. The test was devised through factor analysis, with the 25 phrases arranged into three groups, ranging from fastest to slowest. However, this scale was developed over 30 years ago using male undergraduate students only, so its validity must be suspect.
- The Time Opinion Survey (Kuhlen and Monge, 1968) asks subjects for their opinions on the passage of time; responses are on a 5-point scale.
- The Time Reference Inventory (Roos, 1964), measuring whether the individual has a past, present or future orientation to time, has 30 statements divided into 10 positive, 10 negative and 10 neutral. To each of the statements the subject must assign a past, present or future response.

Although Strumpf notes that validity is suspect in each of these instruments, and also with each combination, he does not mention reliability testing and whether this has been previously achieved. He also makes no mention of whether validity was a problem in administering the Time Metaphor Test, as he had previously suspected.

A sample of 86 women was tested using the measures described above. They were recruited from a large urban senior citizens' centre in North America and met the following criteria: they were over the age of 65; all reported an adequate income to provide for food, shelter and health care; they were caring for themselves at home; they were able to be actively involved in daily activities outside the home; they rated their health as fair to good; where they had been widowed, this had been for more than 6 months; and they had completed a level of education of sixth grade or above. Although criteria for inclusion in any study are important, in this study these criteria would suggest a narrow range of middle and upper class women used to above-average income and lifestyle.

The participants were asked to complete the three scales, as well as a life satisfaction and self-concept scale, and were given the opportunity to comment on the way they experienced time. However, apart from a brief mention by the researcher that these women were satisfied with life and had a strong self-concept, this area was not developed further in the article.

Results from the Time Metaphor Test showed that the women chose some of the phrases more frequently than others, these tending to be from the naturalistic–passive cluster. This cluster represents symbolic feelings of a mystical sense of time, and a feeling of time being encompassing and oceanic; the metaphors in this cluster containing phrases such as a 'vast expanse of sky', 'a quiet motionless ocean', 'a road leading over the hill'. The least chosen phrases were those in the dynamic–hasty cluster, which represented achievement, motivation, and had a more impersonal and constant sense with a feeling of forward movement of change; phrases in this cluster included 'a dashing waterfall', 'a speeding train', 'a fast moving shuttle'. The choices would imply that in addition to being satisfied with their lives and having a high self-esteem, these women also had a sense of inner tranquillity that was not associated with a sense of clock time or haste to achieve targets.

The results from both the Time Opinion Survey and the Time Reference Inventory showed that the majority of the women (75.6%) felt time was passing fairly to extremely rapidly, but most of them (83.7%) did not feel that time was 'running out'. In relation to orientation, slightly more than one-third (36%) of the women had a present orientation – the present being more important than the past – although the majority (57%) recognized the importance of the past to their current lives. Also, 46% reported having most pleasure when thinking about the past – a striking feature of the study – but this did not mean that these women lived in the past. As Strumpf says:

> Much is written about the predilection of older people for the past, without fully appreciating the fact that one need not be past-oriented or fixed in the past, to recognize its significance or to enjoy its old memories.
>
> (p. 210)

In relation to the use of the three tools together, Strumpf comments that the items on the Time Metaphor Test did not correlate well with either the Time Reference Inventory or the Time Opinion Survey, because the two measures were concerned with more factual information about time. Also the two latter scales did not correlate well with statements made by the women, which would lead one to suspect a problem of validity for these two tests.

Therefore, with this group there would appear to be a sense of satisfaction with life, and a high self-esteem. As a measure of health for these women it could be said that this is linked to a sense of inner calm where the women do not show features of being hurried by a sense of clock time, or time being shortened. Despite the limitations of the instruments used, the group was shown to have a predominant sense of living in the present, although remembering that the past has meaning and associated pleasure for them. Therefore, nurses should not assume that reminiscence as therapy for the elderly is the same as living in the past, but possibly it provides a sense of continuity with the present for the well elderly, and can therefore be linked to positive adaptation and maintenance of self-esteem.

This research helps to support Rogers' claim that ageing is a developmental process, where the present is seen as a continuation of the past, and recalling the past with feelings of pleasure is a sign of health in the well elderly. This tends to support Rogers' (1980) work: 'ageing is a continuous creative process directed towards growing diversity and field pattern and organization. It is *not* a running down' (p. 336).

Strumpf's work shows no support for the concept of perceived time passing quicker for the well elderly than for younger people. Being based directly on Rogers' model and using a cause and effect design, this study shows the relationship between this group of elderly women's perception of time and health. By doing so it adds to our knowledge of Rogers' model.

The second study (Newman, 1982) takes a very different approach and explores more directly the difference in time perception between the elderly and a younger age group in order to explore the hypothesis of expanded consciousness. This is more closely related to Rogers' (1970) statement 'Age differences, thermal and biochemical factors, occupational involvement, and sleep–wake states are some of the areas that have been implicated in efforts to explain time perception variations' (p. 115).

Although the study is not directly based on Rogers' model, the principles in her model are broad enough to encompass work such as that undertaken here. The researcher also refers to Rogers' model having similar features to those in the study.

Newman (1982) follows Bentov's (1977) principles of ageing as evolving towards increased complexity and organization with the development of higher levels of consciousness. Bentov proposes that the difference between an individual's subjective measure of time and the measure of clock time would be an index of the individual's level of consciousness. Rogers does not go quite this far, but her 1980 model moves in a similar direction: 'Perception of time as passing is clearly different from time estimation. Evolution from the pragmatic to the visionary bespeaks the fulfilment of new potentials and growing diversity' (p. 335). Newman therefore suggests that as time perception in the elderly shows an increase compared with younger people, the former have higher consciousness levels.

In a previous study Newman (1982) developed a model of subjective time, which specified that:

$$\text{perceived duration} = \frac{\text{level of awareness}}{\text{content of activity at that time}}$$

This shows that if an activity is absorbing to the person involved, then perceived time will be expanded. This is a state of altered consciousness where the individual experiences more time being available to undertake the activity than actual clock time; so the more expanded consciousness is held during the activity, the more there will be an increase in subjective time.

The hypotheses put forward by Newman (1982, p. 291) are:

- perceived duration is positively related to age;
- older adults manifest a higher index of consciousness than younger adults;
- preferred walking rate is positively related to perceived duration.

To test these hypotheses Newman chose a sample of 85 adults between the ages of 60 and 89 years (mean age 71.5 years), 80% of whom were women. They were recruited from senior citizens' organizations, were all American-born and living in Pennsylvania.

Subjects were asked to estimate the passing of time under two conditions. The first asked them to estimate 40 seconds by imagining the sweep of the second hand on a watch while sitting quietly. The second asked them to estimate 40 seconds while walking round an oval track at their preferred pace. Preparation for the second condition was by a practice walk which was recorded by the experimenter; subjects were told to signal when they were ready to start the 40 second walking. Subjects were also asked to imagine the time by imagining the sweep of the second hand on a watch.

Results showed that perceived duration of time was not related to age; therefore the first hypothesis was rejected. However, this could be due to problems of experimental design rather than real differences. The actual interval produced by the subjects – the index of consciousness – showed a trend in the direction of an increase with age, but this was not statistically significant. These data were then compared with those obtained by Newman on previous studies with younger groups of subjects; again no significant difference was found between age and index of consciousness, therefore the second hypothesis was not supported. However, the fact that data from the previous studies by Newman may not have been a good match due to the lapse of time, change of setting and other features, is not mentioned in her 1982 article.

The third hypothesis was supported, showing that people are able to make a more accurate estimation of time while moving than while sitting still. Rogers does not hypothesize about the direction or nature of differences in the perception of time, she merely raises the question 'Is time perception a reflection of the real world or is it a derivation from the real world? Can it be that time perception is a relative reality?' (p. 115).

Newman says the more accurate time estimation in her subjects may be due to them gauging clock time by their walking pattern. Therefore in relation to Rogers' questions, a rhythmic activity such as walking was seen to help the individuals to estimate clock time more accurately than when sitting still. A further significant finding was a difference between the sexes, showing that women overestimate, or have a significantly greater perceived duration of time, than men. Therefore nurses needing evidence of perceived differences in time duration in the elderly should be encouraged to carry out experimentation in this field, provided that they bear in mind the level of difficulty of such an exercise.

Despite the generally disappointing findings of this study, the fact that men and women do differ in their perception of time is worthy of further investigation. Implications that women are less governed by clock time and more by a sense of perceived time may be a result of prior socialization. With the emphasis on work outside the home, this may permanently change the perception of time and therefore the importance of clock time for women.

This paper further develops Rogers' concepts of time while also giving some helpful indicators for the way in which time perception can be measured.

The experience of the passage of time during bed rest

A single study (Smith, 1984) continues the examination of the experience of time, but relates this more to Rogers' principle of continuous and mutual interaction between human beings and the environment which has the properties of continuous pattern and organization. Smith examines how the perception of time alters with differences in the auditory environment, and how this affects feelings of tiredness or restedness when the individual is confined to bed.

Previous studies conducted by the same researcher (Smith, 1975, 1979) had failed to establish that changes in the perceived duration of time occurred with changes in an auditory environment. When the environment was quiet subjects did not perceive time as passing more slowly than when continuous audiotapes were played. A significant finding in these studies was the relationship between the experience of time dragging and a feeling of tiredness.

Although Smith uses Rogers' (1980) model in its broadest sense in this study, the findings can be related to the model in a number of different areas, for example Rogers' questions:

> Age differences, thermal and biochemical factors, occupational involvement, and sleep–wake states are some of the areas that have been implicated in efforts to explain time perception variations. Is time perception a reflection of the real world or is it a deviation from the real world? What kind of relationship exists between time perception and sensory phenomena?
>
> (Rogers, 1980, pp. 115–16)

In her summary of the literature Smith shows that the judgement of duration is affected by the movement of the individual, the level of movement resulting in the speed of information processing which gives the experience of the passage of time. Two of the indicators used by Smith to show movement or change are the auditory environment and the experience of restedness/tiredness. She says that where only indistinguishable sounds and a feeling of tiredness exist, this is an indication of increased information processing and therefore increased human–environment exchange. This would lead to an overestimation of clock time and produce a sense of time dragging.

The hypotheses Smith put forward to test these assertions were:

- judgement of duration will be shorter for organized environmental information than for ambient environmental information for subjects confined to bed for 150 minutes;
- judgement of duration will be shortened for subjects perceiving themselves as rested than for subjects perceiving themselves as tired at the end of 150 minutes of bed confinement.

The sample chosen was 60 men and 60 women from 18 to 35 years of age, all students at an American university, who were paid $10 for their participation. All were minimally screened as being healthy by being asked the same single question about their health. Male and female subjects were randomly assigned to one of the two experimental groups. However, before the experiment began 36 subjects were eliminated either due to non-attendance on the prescribed day, due to health problems or due to being on medication that might have influenced the results.

Subjects rested on a bed in a laboratory setting with controlled dim lighting, controlled temperature and two beds divided by a wooden screen. The experimenter measured time duration by a timer with a second hand; subjects were asked to rate their level of tiredness/ restedness on a rating scale from 6 to 20 at the end of the experimental period and before they got off the bed.

Subjects were divided randomly into two groups. The groups differed in their controlled auditory environment: one group merely received sounds from the environment, predominantly quiet; the second group received auditory information consisting of messages arranged in sequence and with a coherent pattern.

Subjects were given specific instructions, their watches were removed and they were told to remain in bed without talking or smoking. During the period of bed rest subjects saw a lighted sign display for 2 minutes which indicated that they should produce a signal of 40 seconds on a switch beside their beds. In their estimation of a 40 second interval subjects were asked to visualize a clock with a rotating second hand. Samples of the subjects' ability to estimate time were taken at 27, 75, 120 and 150 minutes; also one 40 second sample was obtained before the start of the study to give subjects practice with the equipment.

The data collected from the two groups showed that there was no difference in the perception of time according to the type of auditory information given to the subjects. However, it could be that neither type of information was sufficiently stimulating to the subjects to create the difference in time perception.

Data analysed using a *t*-test on the feelings of restedness/tiredness showed there was a significant difference ($p = 0.04$) between the numbers of subjects who felt rested and who perceived time as passing quickly, and those who reported feeling tired and experiencing time as passing slowly. A further finding was that subjects who felt rested and who experienced time passing quickly also had more unusual sensory experiences – such as dreams, trance-like states, unusual sounds, smells and tactile feelings – than the tired subjects.

It would appear from this study that the experience of feeling rested after a period of enforced bed rest is related to the experience of time passing quickly in healthy subjects. Individuals experiencing a feeling of rest in these circumstances also reported more unusual sensory experiences. However, what other contributing factors are associated with these feelings are unclear from this study. Smith has been unable to isolate the role of environmental factors in contributing to this effect, as the sound given to the subjects made little difference to their feelings of restedness. It could possibly be that varied sounds or a combination of sounds might have made a difference. The factors that affect Rogers' principle of human–environment patterning and organization could not therefore be isolated here in relation to the passage of time; only the factors involving the human field were isolated.

It is important for nurses to know the environmental factors that lead to differences in the perception of the passage of time, particularly with patients confined to bed, and the relation of these factors to health. This would be significant research which could use Rogers' model as its framework.

TESTING ROGERS' PRINCIPLE OF INTEGRALITY

In a 1985 conference address, Rogers defined the principle of integrality. The conference paper (Rogers, 1985) has not been published in Britain, but the principle of integrality is defined by Smith (1986, p. 21) as 'the continuous mutual human–field and environmental–field process'. The study in this section sets out to test integrality through exploring the experience of the environment during enforced bed rest.

Smith (1986) conducted this further study which she claimed was derived directly from Rogers' model. She also based the work on her previous studies in a similar area (Smith, 1984), and claimed that the auditory input from the environmental field meets with the individual's perception which goes to make up the individual's state of restfulness in the human field; this operationalizes the principle of integrality. The question she asked was: 'How do changes in environmental resonance change a person's perception of rest?' (p. 22).

In this study the environmental field is patterned at different frequencies structured by the experimenter: (a) relative quiet; (b) music; and (c) the human voice. The human field was tested by the level of restfulness experienced by the individual at the end of the period of rest.

The hypothesis was: 'perception of restfulness will be lower (subjects more rested) for confined subjects who experience varied harmonious auditory input than for those who experience quiet ambience' (p. 23).

The study comprised 120 healthy subjects, 60 men and 60 women between the ages of 18 and 25, who were randomly assigned to one of two groups of auditory input on the day they arrived in the laboratory; each was paid $10 for participation.

The method used to assess the level of restfulness/tiredness at the beginning and end of the study was Borg's (1971) tool of perceived exertion. However, the tool was substantially changed by Smith, as were the terms used to describe the state of the individual; this change was from 'light to heavy' (Borg), to 'rested to tired' (Smith). The rating scale was left as from 6 (very, very rested) to 20 (very, very tired), but in Borg's scale these figures represented heart rate, whereas in Smith's study they described the degrees of feeling either tired or rested. This amount of change would not justify the tool being used in such different circum-stances without further validity testing. Smith carried out further testing using a test–retest reliability measure on a sample of 20 healthy women, which gave acceptable results.

One group received a varied auditory input, the second a quiet auditory input. The varied auditory input had controlled time periods for specific inputs and for silence, in sequence – specific pieces of music, followed by silence, followed by a story, followed by silence. This sequence was repeated using different pieces of music and different stories until the end of the 150 minutes of the experimental period. The music was chosen by four musicians, who rated different pieces accord-ing to a scale of musical selection associated with mood; similarly the stories were chosen by a panel who rated the ones which were clearest and most interesting from a series of stories. In the quiet auditory environment only muffled sounds could be heard throughout the 150 minutes.

The experiments took place in a non-soundproofed room in a quiet location, with the experimenter sitting behind a wooden screen and viewing subjects through a one-way mirror. Each subject was confined to a single bed; the room was lit by controlled dim lighting and had controlled heating.

Subjects were told they were to stay in bed and could not talk or smoke. They rested in bed for 15 minutes before the start of the auditory input after which they were asked to complete the initial tool of perceived restfulness; following this the auditory input was begun. At the end of 150 minutes of bed rest the perceived restfulness tool was again given to subjects.

The mean restfulness/tiredness score for subjects in the quiet environment was 12.35, and for subjects in the mixed auditory environment was 10.85. Testing the differences in responding according to the two environments showed a statistically significant difference ($p < 0.05$) between the two groups of subjects; subjects in the mixed auditory environment felt significantly more rested than those in the quiet environment.

The results showed that both the human and the environmental fields do interact to the extent that the controlled environmental field produced an effect on the subjects in a controlled setting by creating a feeling of a greater or lesser degree of restfulness. However, this should not be viewed as a causal relationship, as Rogers rejects causality, but rather be thought of as probabilistic: 'continuous, mutual simultaneous interaction, evolving towards increased differentiation and diversity of field pattern and organization' (Rogers, 1980, p. 333).

These findings are of considerable importance to nursing, as patients in bed can be helped to feel more rested, and therefore perhaps recover from illness quicker, if their environment has a structured auditory input. This is seen by Smith as preferable to merely a quiet environment, which she says may produce tension and irritation, and may therefore interfere with rest. The mixed auditory sounds structured the environment for the subjects, whereas the quiet environment meant subjects had to impose for themselves a structure on the environment in the presence of very little information; this creates work for the subject.

This study, based directly on Rogers' principles, helps to support the principle of integrality by showing the mutual interaction between human and environmental fields. Further work in this area is undoubtedly essential, especially with ill people and those of varying ages, to assess the kind of environmental sounds that are most conducive to a feeling of restfulness, and the relationship of this feeling to the promotion of health.

THE SUPPORT CONFLICT EXPERIENCED BY NEW MOTHERS

The single paper in this section (Crawford, 1985) loosely examines Rogers' principles of integrality and helicy from a theoretical perspective. The study is not based entirely on Rogers' model, but examines the continuous and mutual interaction between the human and environmental fields. It takes the human field as the new mother and the environmental field as the nature and type of support she receives from others after the birth of the baby.

Crawford says that the birth of a first baby can be seen as a crisis for the couple, both in adjustment to the birth and also in the incompatibility between the new role of parents and other existing roles.

Hobbs (1965, 1968) found that where close relatives gave extra help, this resulted in increased difficulty in the parents adjusting to their new roles. But provided help was given by close relatives in a way that did not intrude on the couple's privacy, or judge their abilities as parents, the relatives were viewed as helpful. However, as Crawford points out, there is undoubtedly room for seeing this support as a source of conflict.

On this evidence Crawford decided to build a theoretical model of the properties of support network relationships, particularly to examine the factors that influence conflict in these relationships. Rogers' model was used to provide a nursing perspective 'because it is concerned with the interaction between the person and the environment' (p. 101). Crawford selected Rogers' principle of helicy as she wanted to examine the diversity of the environmental field pattern, or the different ways in which support could be given; and she used integrality to conceptualize the properties of support that might create conflict. However, this is not the strict use of the model as Rogers intended; Rogers' intentions were that both the environmental and human fields had different properties but were continuously repatterning and reorganizing in relation to each other, changes in both occurring through their mutual interaction. Further, it seems unclear whether examining helicy in the environmental field alone will lead to results that can be compared with data collected from the human field using the integrality principle.

Taking Rogers' principle of helicy, Crawford concentrates on diversity in the environmental field by selecting the number of different ways in which support can be given by a relative; she also chose a concept of 'partiality' which indicated 'more than one person providing a particular type of support' (p. 101). However, this again shows that Rogers' model is being examined from one perspective only, namely the environmental field, not from mutual interaction of the environmental and human fields as is intended by the principle of helicy.

Crawford links the concepts she has proposed to show that the environmental field has forms in which support can be given and a variety of people who can give it, while the human field shows conflict as a result of the support given and received by the new parents. Also included in Crawford's model were features such as age and socio-economic group of the new mother, which Crawford saw as influencing conflict (Figure 6.1).

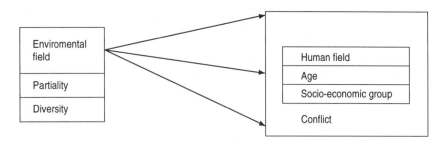

Figure 6.1 Model of support conflict as in Crawford (1985)

From the model in Figure 6.1 Crawford suggests that the lower the age and socio-economic group of the new mother, the smaller number of support relationships she is likely to have, and the greater the potential conflict in these relationships.

Research is needed to demonstrate the adequacy of the model to explain and predict the relationships proposed. However, even if empirical support is given to the model through research in practice, it can at best give support to a limited aspect of Rogers' model, and one that is unlikely to reflect the nature of continuous mutual interaction between the human and environmental fields. In order to show this interaction further, modifications to Crawford's model would be needed to show the types of changes that occur in both fields.

CHANGES IN ROLE IDENTITY AND SELF-CONCEPT FROM PREGNANCY TO THE POST-PARTUM

Brouse (1985) elaborated Rogers' model by studying certain aspects of the human field. It is argued that one of the times when the most dramatic changes occur to a woman is during pregnancy and immediately after the birth of the baby, particularly if it is her first child. These changes were examined using Rogers' model to show the developmental changes in the human field pattern and organization and the increasing complexity, differentiation and diversity that occur. The effect of the environment on socializing the individual that creates further pattern and organization changes in the human field is also examined.

Brouse (1985) felt that the changes happening to a woman during pregnancy and the early post-partum could be viewed as possibly the most dramatic life changes to happen to her. These changes could clearly show the development that occurs in the way the woman views herself and identifies with her role. The feedback that others give her on the way she is performing the role adds to her feelings of self-worth. Brouse suggests that there may be a relationship between female role identity, self-concept and successful mothering.

Brouse uses Rogers' (1980) principle of helicy:

> The nature and direction of human and environmental change is continuously innovative, probabilistic, and characterized by increasing diversity of human field and environmental field pattern and organization emerging out of the continuous, mutual, simultaneous interaction between the human and environmental fields and manifesting non-repeating rhythmicities.
>
> (Rogers, 1980, p. 333)

The Nurse Theorist Group (Kim and Moritz, 1982) identified nine patterns of a unitary person. These patterns vary in intensity, duration and rhythm and were categorized into three factors:

- interaction (exchanging, communicating and relating);
- action (valuing, choosing and moving); and
- awareness (waking, feeling and knowing).

Brouse uses these categories to develop role identity and self-concept scores in a woman throughout pregnancy and immediately after the birth of the baby. She sees socialization of the individual as patterning behaviour in appropriate ways, and gender identity as the result of this pattern and organization, which becomes the self-concept. She sees the gender identity becoming more complex as the individual develops, and that in some individuals gender identity will be stronger, or more intense, than in others.

Brouse extrapolates that femininity will intensify in a woman particularly at the end of pregnancy, where she sees the need for an intensified human–environment interaction when the mothering role is begun, especially in relation to the first child. With successful mothering the woman's self-concept is increased. Therefore Brouse operationalized Rogers' principle of helicy by examining the relationships between gender role identity, femininity, self-concept and comfort with the mothering role from the last month of pregnancy until 5–6 weeks post-partum.

Brouse proposed four hypotheses.

- A greater increase in self-concept and femininity scores will occur in primiparous as opposed to multiparous women during the last stage of pregnancy and up to 6 weeks post-partum.
- Women with high levels of both masculine and feminine behaviours, and those with high levels of feminine behaviours will have a greater increase in feminine and self-concept scores than women with masculine and undifferentiated behaviours during the last stages of pregnancy and up to 6 weeks post-partum.

- Self-concept scores will be significantly related to feminine scores.
- The woman's self-concept score will be significantly related to the comfort she feels in meeting the infant's needs 5–6 weeks after the birth.

The sample was 73 women who were selected at childbirth classes; 52 were primiparous and 21 multiparous. They were all tested on three occasions. Demographic data were: a mean age of 27.4 years; education for an average of 14.2 years; 80.6% employed outside the home; above average mean socio-economic group; and predominantly Catholic (52.1%).

The women completed the questionnaire on three occasions – during the last month of pregnancy when questionnaires were given to them to complete at home and collected during the following childbirth class; during the second and third weeks post-partum; and during the fifth and sixth weeks post-partum. These two later sets of questionnaires were posted to the women during the first and second weeks post-partum, respectively. The sample size of 73 subjects represented 52.5% of all subjects approached to take part in the study (initial sample 139). This is an average level of response rate, particularly with a postal questionnaire; however, Brouse does not suggest reasons for non-response, nor the more important question of whether the non-responders may have been different in some way from those who completed the questionnaire. If non-responders were different from responders this would be a source of bias.

The following scales were used to test the subjects.

- The Bem Sex Role Inventory (Bem, 1981), which is designed to measure masculine and feminine attributes. This categorized each woman into one of four gender role identities: androgynous; feminine; masculine; or undifferentiated. The scale comprises 60 adjectives: 20 socially desirable feminine, 20 socially desirable masculine and 20 neutral. Subjects marked each on a 7-point scale according to how they felt each adjective described them-selves.
- The Tennessee Self-Concept Scale (Fitts, 1965), which consists of 100 items. Subjects rate themselves on each item from five responses ranging from 'completely false' to 'completely true'.
- The Maternal Attitude Scale (Cohler, Weiss and Grunebaum, 1970). Only one of the five factors in the scale was administered to this group of women which consisted of 33 statements; the women selected from 'strongly agree' to 'strongly disagree' on a 6-point scale. These items reflected the extent that the women felt they understood their infant's needs and were able to meet them.

The results showed that the first hypothesis, when analysed using an analysis of variance, was not supported: primiparous women did not have higher feminine and self-concept scores than multiparous women over the period of time studied. Therefore the principle of development through time was not demonstrated in this work; so the women having their first child did not show a greater increase in self-concept and feminine characteristics compared to their scores before the birth of the baby, than increases in the same measures in women having their second or subsequent child. Primiparous women did however show higher self-concept scores than multiparous women at all the times measured. However, Brouse says there is evidence from Rubin (1975) that an increase in self-concept in primiparous women occurs earlier in pregnancy and has slowed down by the last trimester.

The second hypothesis was also not supported using an analysis of variance, but it was shown that women who possessed more masculine or undifferentiated behaviours had the greatest increase in feminine and self-concept scores during the period studied; however, this increase was not significantly different between gender identity groups. Despite this, the self-concept of the feminine group of women did not show the expected increase; Brouse says this would have indicated that the value society places on feminine behaviours during pregnancy and mothering was not felt by these women, but by those with masculine behaviours. Brouse wonders whether women in the latter group are therefore more aware of society's expectations and more able to make an appropriate response, thus showing greater flexibility in behaviour. These findings, although not in the ways hypothesized by Brouse, show inconclusive support for Rogers' principle of helicy by not clearly showing the nature of the inter-action between the human and environmental fields. What may be concluded is that some fields may have greater density and intensity than others, so there may be a greater ability for change in some fields than others.

The third hypothesis was supported; feminine scores were significantly related to self-concept scores on each of the occasions studied. However, when each of the role identity groups was examined individually, the androgynous and also the undifferentiated group had statistically significant correlations between feminine and self-concept scores only during the last month of pregnancy and at the sixth week post-partum. The masculine group had statistically significant correlations between femininity and self-concept scores at each of the periods studied; whereas the feminine group had no significant correlations at any of the periods studied. This shows that the model proposed by Brouse as derived from Rogers' model does not stand up, as the influence of the environmental field on the female behaviours of the feminine group after childbirth is not correlated with an increase in this group's self-concept. Alternatively it could be that Rogers' model itself has weaknesses in human–environmental field relationships that this study has identified. However, a great deal of further work must be conducted before it can be demonstrated which of these alternatives is the most likely.

The fourth hypothesis was not supported: there was no relationship between self-concept and the mothers' feelings of comfort with their mothering role at between 5 and 6 weeks post-partum. However, as Brouse points out, she did not use any measure to show the value of the mothering role in these women. This may have shown some interesting findings, particularly as 80% of the women were employed outside the home before the birth of their baby, and at 6 weeks post-partum 10% had already returned to work and 39% intended to do so within the next few months. Therefore the instrument to measure comfort with the mothering role needs to be developed with a greater emphasis on reliability.

The findings from this study show that gender role identity is variable and changes with different patterns of feminine behaviour and with self-concept during a stage of maximum development in a woman. Therefore from this study it can be concluded that the human field does achieve pattern and organization which is faster at some times than at others, and will have different speeds or density for some people than for others. To this extent it supports Rogers' model. However, the study does not conclusively show the influence of the environmental field, a weakness due mainly to its design. Brouse says that the implications of the findings for nursing should be towards helping women with low femininity to develop mothering skills; however, this seems to demand a very prescriptive approach which does not allow for individual variation according to the needs of the mother.

ALTERATIONS IN CIRCADIAN RHYTHMS OF SLEEP–WAKE PATTERNS IN HOSPITALIZED PSYCHIATRIC PATIENTS

Floyd's (1984) paper studied Rogers' principle of helicy:

> Life evolves along a spiralling longitudinal axis bound in the curvature of space–time. With each turn of the spiral along the axis, similarities appear. Spirals along the axis are further embedded within the spiralling of the axis itself. Rhythmic phenomena are expressions of the reciprocal relationship between man and environment.
>
> (Rogers, 1970, p. 100)

In exploring the sleep–wake rhythms of psychiatric patients the study shows how patients who are predominantly morning, predominantly evening or intermediate types will exhibit shifts in their sleep–wake patterns, depending on whether they are in hospital or being treated as out-patients and living at home. The study shows clearly how the hospital environment alters the sleep patterns of each type.

Floyd used Horne and Ostberg's (1977) findings which showed how people differ in their circadian rhythms: morning types feel best early in the day, and evening types feel best later in the day. These two types also differ in their preferred time of going to bed and rising in the morning, with the morning types preferring to go to bed and rise early, while the evening types prefer to stay up late and rise later in the morning. Floyd also found evidence that morning types had more difficulty changing their sleep–wake cycles than did evening types (Foulkard, Monk and Lobban, 1979).

The bases for Floyd's hypotheses were that:

Rhythms of living systems tend to become shorter and faster with the development of the system; and changes that occur naturally with the development of the system are speeded up during periods of disruption or change.

(Floyd, 1984, p. 225)

Her hypotheses were:

- psychiatric patients in hospital would have shorter and faster sleep–wake rhythms than those treated from home;
- evening-type hospitalized psychiatric patients would have shorter and faster rhythms than morning-type hospitalized psychiatric patients.

These shorter and faster sleep rhythms were defined as shorter and more frequent periods of sleep during the 24 hour period.

The research design used 35 pairs of hospitalized and out-patients, matched for psychiatric diagnosis and gender. All patients met the criteria of being over 18 years of age, mentally able to participate in the study, free from other chronic illnesses, having had at least one admission for a psychiatric illness, and had been in their present environment for at least 2 weeks. This last criterion was particularly important in order to allow subjects to stabilize the biochemical rhythms that affect sleep–wake patterns (Sollberger, 1965; Reinberg, 1970). The study took place in a small urban psychiatric hospital in a midwestern American state. All the patients in hospital were encouraged to rise by 7 a.m., although there was flexibility in the time they went to bed.

Patients were asked to self-administer the Self-Assessment Questionnaire to Determine Morningness–Eveningness (SAQDME) (Horne and Ostberg, 1976) and a Modified Sleep Chart (MSC) (Lewis and Masterson, 1957), and asked to complete them over 24 hours starting at noon of the chosen day. So that patterns of sleeping–waking were not altered by weekend activities, the schedules were only completed on Tuesdays, Wednesdays and Thursdays.

Additionally patients were asked to complete a Chemical Substance Record devised by Floyd to record prescribed and other drugs taken, including caffeine, nicotine and alcohol. This record was subsequently compared with medical prescriptions to minimize distortions. Two of the out-patients' records were considered questionable, and these patients were removed from the study.

The validity of the SAQDME had been previously established by the developers, using food intake and measures of oral temperature to establish the difference between morning and evening types. Subsequent use by the developers further showed its discriminating ability; however, reliability measures had not been carried out prior to Floyd's study.

The MSC used boxes on a graph, each box represented 20 minutes within a 24 hour period. Subjects were instructed to place an S in each box where they judged themselves to have been asleep for more than 10 minutes, otherwise they were to place an A in the box. The reliability and validity of the MSC had not been established by the developers, but Floyd says she did this by comparing the patients' self-reports with records from nursing staff who were also asked to complete the MSC for 20 of the 35 in-patients in the study; this correlated to 97% of the estimations by patients. The validity of the Chemical Substance Record was checked so that estimations of sleeping time could be controlled according to hypnotics taken. A panel of four pharmacologists rated 138 substances as having an effect on sleeping time; there was broad agreement on the substances and their effects between the four raters (0.86), and these effects were added as a covariate analysis.

The results, using analysis of covariance (ANOVA), showed that hospitalized subjects were asleep statistically less than out-patients ($p < 0.05$), amounting to 0.6 hours less sleep in a 24 hour period. When adjustment for drug effects was taken into account the amount increased to a 1 hour difference. However, the average age of out-patients was greater by 6.6 years than the average age of in-patients, which may have had an effect on the amount of sleep needed; when this age difference was added as a possible covariate the effect of age on sleep was found to be insignificantly small in this sample.

Results of the SAQDME showed both groups of subjects fell into categories:

- eight moderate evening types;
- 37 neither morning nor evening types;
- 23 moderate morning types;
- two definite morning types.

Because of the small number of definite morning types Floyd combined the 23 moderate morning types with the two definite morning types. The combined categories were: eight (11%) evening, 37 (53%) intermediate, and 25 (36%) morning types. The small number of evening types may lead to the suspicion that this group is not representative of the wider population. Also of concern is that Floyd did not mention whether there was a predominance of any of the categories in the hospitalized or out-patient groups.

The hospitalized patients showed no significant difference from the out-patients in their times of falling asleep at night; however, a significant difference was found ($p < 0.05$) between hospitalized patients and out-patients in the time of waking up, the former waking more than 1 hour earlier than the out-patients. When differences between patients were analysed using the SAQDME the three types of hospitalized patients did not show any significant difference between time of falling asleep at night and waking up in the morning. However, with the out-patients the different circadian types showed significant differences in the time of falling asleep ($p < 0.05$), a difference of 3½ hours between evening and morning types. In spite of the small number of subjects in the evening group, it can be seen that both morning and evening types have to change their sleep–wake pattern during hospitalization. In this study the change during hospitalization for morning types was a delay of ¾ hour in falling asleep and 3 hours in waking up; whereas the change in evening types was to advance their falling asleep time by 1½ hours and their waking time by 3 hours. Intermediate types had no change in their falling asleep, but they woke up approximately 1½ hours earlier than normal.

The second hypothesis was not supported, i.e. hospitalized evening types were not shown to have significant differences in sleep patterns compared with morning types. However, there is evidence (Hildenbrandt and Stratmann, 1979) that morning types have more difficulty than evening types in adjusting to different sleep–wake patterns.

This study was based directly on Rogers' model. As such it helps to support her principle of helicy by showing that the rhythms of sleep–wake patterns differ with the environmental field in which the individual is situated, as it is shown clearly that adjustments have to be made by hospitalized psychiatric patients to their usual sleep–wake patterns. What is not addressed in this study is the effect these changes had on the patients, whether they experienced discomfort, or whether these changes adversely affected their health.

What is also not fully answered in this study is the difference in length of rhythms between psychiatric hospitalized patients and out-patients. Although Floyd obtained measures on the Modified Sleep Chart from all patients in the study in 20 minute periods, she does not comment on the lengths of periods of sleep seen in the different groups, or in the different locations of patients, apart from one brief mention that hospitalized morning types have more episodes of waking at night than other patients. It can be assumed from this that both hospitalized intermediate and evening types have a loss of sleep of 1½ hours in 24 hours, but this was not compensated for by 'napping' during the day. Therefore, although Rogers' principle of a change in the length of the rhythm has not been seen here, it does not deny the principle of helicy.

THE NEAR-DEATH EXPERIENCE

This short paper (Papowitz, 1986) does not set out to collect data scientifically nor to analyse it, however it does make a contribution to Rogers' model in terms of four-dimensionality (Rogers, 1980, pp. 331–5), where Rogers sees paranormal events as being possible:

> Consider the point made ... that 'human field' and 'relative present' are identical. Examine the implications for explaining pre-cognition, déjà vu, clairvoyance and the like. [This] is rational in a four-dimensional human field in continuous mutual, simultaneous interaction with a four-dimensional environment.
>
> (p. 335)

The contribution of this paper to Rogers' principle of four-dimensionality is in the description of the near-death experience. The paper describes two types of five stages of a near-death experience, and how it affects those subject to it.

Papowitz described two types of near-death experience. The first of these is defined by Grosso (1981) as a deathbed vision where someone close to death suddenly becomes alert, coherent and speaks in an elevated mood. In this state, a person may speak of seeing or talking to dead members of the family or dead friends. Shortly after this the person returns to his or her previous morbid state and dies soon afterwards. This experience can be very disturbing for the relatives, and counselling by someone who has knowledge of these events can help to relieve anxiety.

The second type of near-death experience is that described by Ring (1980) and has five stages. Papowitz says patients must have experienced passing through at least one of these stages for researchers to identify this as a near-death experience. The five stages are as follows.

- Euphoria: here the person has a peaceful feeling with the overwhelming experience of happiness and joy, and no pain or other bodily sensations.
- Out-of-body state: in this stage people experience a humming or buzzing sound and find themselves above their body looking down on it in a detached manner. They are aware of what is happening to their body but are unable to intervene and can act as a spectator only. At this stage they may encounter dead relatives or friends who lead them to the next stage.
- Entering darkness or a tunnel: the person experiences a loud buzzing or ringing sound at the same time as moving quickly through darkness or a tunnel. Those encountered during the previous stage are still present and act as a guide to the next stage.
- Unearthly world of light: the experience during this stage is one of floating and being peaceful and serene, at one with the universe and being very loving and forgiving. There is no awareness of time or space, and the person feels all-knowing. Awareness of a 'presence' in an unearthly light is encountered, but this is a brief experience.
- Entering into the light and making a decision: during this stage the 'presence' asks non-verbal 'questions' about the person's life, with an instant non-judgemental playback of the life events. Family and friends met in previous stages are warm and welcoming, but a barrier is reached where the person knows they must make a decision, either to remain in this place or to return to an earthly life. This is not always a pleasant decision, as the desire is often to remain, but the persuasion is to return, and when the decision is made individuals find themselves returned to their own body.

According to Sabom (1982) 40% of survivors of an incident such as cardiac resuscitation have a near-death experience.

When Papowitz asked patients she nursed if they had told anyone of their near-death experience they frequently said they thought they would not be believed and were also fearful of being thought mentally unbalanced. Also people said they were unsure what was happening to them, and thought that they may have been dreaming. This led Papowitz to believe that patients have unresolved concerns about their near-death experiences, which can be relieved by counselling from someone who is aware of the phenomenon.

This evidently well-documented phenomenon strengthens Rogers' assertion of the 'relative present' (Rogers, 1980) being related to a four-dimensional model of the human field of life events; so, the near-death experience is conceptualized as one of the experiences of the relative present.

CONCLUSIONS

In this section a number of Rogers' assumptions and principles have been developed which have led to a clearer understanding of the implications of the model for clinical practice in nursing. They have also led to knowledge of the model and its authenticity. In a controversial paper Gill and Atwood (1981) have shown reciprocy and helicy in wound healing on the skin of a pig; the perception of time is shown by time perception having a deep significance for the elderly (Strumpf, 1987); Smith (1986) added to our knowledge of integrality by showing that differences in feeling rested after lying in bed depended on the auditory environment; Brouse (1985) also showed that the speed of pattern and organization changes in time and between people. Further support for Rogers' principles came from Floyd (1984) who showed that helicy is able to be adjusted by some people when their sleep rhythm has to be adjusted; and the near-death experience adds to our understanding of four-dimensionality and the relative present.

However, none of the studies examined in this chapter so far was conducted outside North America. This indicates a current lack of acceptance in other cultures of Rogers' model of unitary human beings and of the principles of reciprocy, synchrony, helicy and resonancy in nursing.

Before moving to the next section on intervention using Rogers' model I will discuss two remaining papers that take a broader perspective than identification: they deal with this and also other stages of problem-solving – identification through to evaluation. The first paper is an attempt to operationalize Rogers' model for use with the nursing process; the second paper is an investigation of how increased activity affects infants' growth and development.

AN OPERATIONALIZATION OF ROGERS' MODEL

This paper by Whelton (1979) attempts to show how Rogers' model can be used by practising nurses in each stage of the nursing process. It is not based on research, but as it claims to show how the model can be used in practice, it warrants inclusion. It sets out to show how assessment can be carried out using various methods and criteria which are well known in nursing assessment, and then works through the following stages of problem-solving (based on Yura and Walsh, 1973).

Whelton outlines the five main assumptions of Rogers' (1970) model as being: wholeness; human–environmental continual interaction; a unidirectional life process; the human being's unique pattern and organization; and the human being's capacity for abstract thought, imagery and emotion. From these she derives five concepts: wholeness of the human being; openness between human beings and the environment;

pattern and organization derived from previous human–environment interactions; unidirectionality – no events can ever be repeated; and sentience and thought, understanding and experience that increase with age.

Whelton sees that from these five assumptions are derived four principles of homodynamics: reciprocy – human–environment continuous interaction; synchrony – the patient's state depending on the human–environment state in space–time; helicy – life evolving unidirectionality; and resonancy – change in pattern and organization in both human beings and the environment occurring in waves whose speed can change.

From this she moves on to look at specific medically diagnosed diseases such as decreased cardiac output and impaired neurological functioning, discussing the physiological impairment in these two diseases and the decreased perceptual ability in neurological malfunctioning. Whelton then discusses compensations which these patients will have to make in order to live with their limitations; these are based on fluid intake and output, activity and rest, dependence and independence:

> When a balance is not maintained between fluid intake and output and/or activity and rest and/or dependence and independence, disharmony within the pattern and organization of the body system occurs and decompensation ensues.
>
> (p. 9)

Although at this point she quotes Rogers as saying that when pattern and organization are absent the human field ceases to exist, she relates this to the physical needs of the patient, their emotional state and their social interactions. Therefore from the end of the description of Rogers' model this paper runs into severe difficulties, mainly due to the way operationalization views a human being as a series of biological, psychological and social systems and not, as Rogers' intended, holistically. Rogers (1970) is very clear about this approach of holism:

> The properties of man cannot be derived from the study of biology, physics, psychology, and sociology any more than psychological properties can be deduced from the study of atoms and molecules.
>
> (p. 45)

Whelton develops an assessment strategy that she bases on wholeness, openness, pattern and organization, unidirectionality, and sentience and thought; but within these she breaks assessment down into physical systems, for example:

Areas of assessment for the patient with decreased cardiac output as organized by the nursing concepts cited by Martha Rogers

Wholeness
Physical integrity
   Respiratory systems
      Respirations, rate and character
      Breath sounds
      X-ray reports
      Laboratory findings, i.e. arterial blood gases
      Orthopnea
      Paroxysmal nocturnal dyspnea
      Cough
      Sputum, quantity and character

(p. 10)

Each of the systems is dealt with similarly. However, Whelton does recognize that the use of a very structured assessment tool could be restrictive and prevent open interaction between the nurse and the patient. She also assumes from the assessment criteria that although the tool is only intended as a guide, assessment by the nurse takes place by interview; this again is a restrictive approach which does not look at the wider implications of synchrony as Rogers intended.

This use of medical/nursing systems is further evidenced by Whelton discussing how a nursing diagnosis is made following assessment. In the patient with decreased cardiac output she states the nursing diagnosis as 'body fluid excess as evidence by continued weight gain, jugular venous distension, peripheral oedema, decreased urinary output, hypertension and tachycardia' (p. 14). She then makes out a nursing care plan to deal with these problems which relies on measurement of vital signs and monitoring patients' weight and fluid intake and output. The plan is based on the scientific principles of biology, behaviour and nursing sciences; thus again a deductive approach derived from the academic and nursing disciplines is used, in opposition to Rogers' intentions of holism.

The implementation phase is discussed by Whelton as 'setting the environmental changes into effect that will result in or compensate for changes in the patient' (p. 18). However, this implies a cause and effect relationship between the environment and the patient, in that the environment (the nurses' actions) will cause the changes in the patient's condition. This again is directly opposed to Rogers' intentions of changes in the human being and the environment being probabilistic – not occurring by causal relationships.

In summary, this is a rather confused and confusing paper. In attempting to combine Rogers' model with the nursing process Whelton has taken parts from each, but as far as Rogers' model is concerned, she has missed the essential features of the model. Much work will have to be undertaken into the nature of the human–environment simultaneous interaction that truly shows holism before a problem-solving approach can be used as intended by Rogers. To this extent the paper by Whelton is premature.

THE EFFECTS OF PHYSICAL ACTIVITY ON INFANTS' GROWTH AND DEVELOPMENT

This study (Porter, 1972) shows one of the most dramatic effects on the human field of any discussed in this chapter so far. It takes Rogers' principle of reciprocy, human and environmental fields being open and in constant interaction with each other, and resonancy, growth and development occurring as a result of the mutual human-environment interaction, as central.

The question that the study sets out to answer is whether an increased environmental input would improve the existing changes in the growth and development of infants. This environmental input was in the form of a planned programme of motion for infants.

The study shows the development level of the infants before the programme of intervention started, describes it in detail, and measures the level of development at the end of the programme; to this extent it follows the identification, intervention and evaluation stages of this chapter.

Porter (1972) found evidence to suggest that stimulation of a neuromotor or sensory nature influenced the behaviour of infants (Hasselmeyer, 1963; Neal, 1968; Earle, 1969). She developed the idea that there is an interrelationship between the factors that influence growth and development where the human field is seen as an energy field in continuous motion. The particular factors that she chose to measure growth and development in infants were weight, length, motor behaviour, adaptive behaviour, language behaviour and personal–social behaviour.

The study was conducted in the Philippines using two groups of infants. The subjects were 94 full-term infants, ranging from 4 to 40 weeks old, living in Dumaguete City. Infants for inclusion in the study had no history of premature birth, birth injury, congenital or other developmental abnormality; infants were also only chosen if their mothers had attended prenatal care. Before the study started home visits to the families were conducted to cultivate cooperation and inform the families concerned.

The infants were divided equally into control and experimental groups. The control group consisted of 24 males and 23 females with a mean age of 18.31 weeks, and the experimental group matched this exactly; there was random assignment to groups. Other factors such as socio-economic group, place in the family and nutrition were not controlled, but were assumed to be normally distributed among the infants' families.

The control group received the conventional care given by families to their infants. In the Philippines the mothers and other carers 'meet' the needs of the infants and there is a large extended family. The mother has a predominantly care-taking, affectionate and training role. However, all carers are extremely cautious of allowing infants to move about freely: they are usually carried or, when sitting, are placed on the carer's lap but receive little attention, although others freely express affection towards them by cuddling and kissing them.

The experimental group also received this conventional care within their families, but in addition received a planned regime of passive cycling exercises and rest for two 20 minute periods each day. The exercises consisted of two 5 minute cycling periods alternating with 5 minute rest periods when the infant was left to engage freely in any activity, although she or he was picked up if crying. The exercises were conducted by the mother or the major carer for 6 days a week over a period of 2 months. To ensure that the regime was being carried out properly the researcher visited each family unannounced once a week. After 1 and 2 months changes in growth and development of the infants were assessed.

The tools used to assess the infants before the study began, at 1 month into the study and at the end of the 2 month period were the following.

- A Detecto beam scale used to weigh the infants, reported as 99% accurate.
- Gesell Development Schedules used to assess the developmental status of the infants (Gesell and Amatrude, 1947). Porter provides evidence of work which shows that these tools are reliable to between 0.88 and 0.99 on 40-week-old infants; concurrent validity was also shown (-0.64) with normal infants of between 4 and 93 days.

Using the above scales, differences between the control and experimental groups were looked for in weight, height, motor development, adaptive development, language development and personal–social development. Measurements taken of all the infants before planned exercises showed no significant differences between either group in any of these measures. Also analysis of the two groups showed no significant differences between the ages of infants in the two groups.

After 1 month, the midpoint of the period in which the experimental group was given planned exercises, results using a t-test showed a significant difference between the control and experimental group ($p=$ 0.0001). In motor development the difference between the two groups was significant at $p = 0.004$; in adaptive development $p = 0.0001$; in language development $p = 0.00004$; and in personal–social development $p = 0.0005$. This shows a high level of significant difference between the two groups which cannot be attributed to chance, and is therefore likely to be attributed to the results of the planned exercises given to the experimental group.

At the end of the 2 month period, the end of the experiment, the same measures were performed on the two groups. Statistically significant differences were found in all the measures: weight showed a significant difference between the two groups at $p = 0.0001$; height $p = 0.0011$; motor development $p = 0.0001$; adaptive development $p = 0.00004$; language development $p = 0.0001$; and personal–social development $p = 0.00004$. Again these differences between the two groups are highly unlikely to be produced by chance, and are therefore much more likely to be produced by the effects of the planned exercise regime given to the infants in the experimental group. The differences between the two groups are shown in Table 6.1 at the 1 and 2 month periods.

Table 6.1 Changes in infants following the exercise programme in Porter's study

	Pretest	Gain after 1 month	Gain after 2 months
Weight (pounds)			
Control group	213.9	19.69	36.05
Experimental group	213.97	21.9	51.17
Height (inches)			
Control group	25.2	0.63	1.1
Experimental group	25.3	1.16	2.24
Motor development[a]			
Control group	92.89	1.4	12
Experimental group	94.4	15.5	29
Adaptive development[a]			
Control group	89.07	2.37	11.3
Experimental group	85.87	16.9	30.07
Language development[a]			
Control group	91.07	5.23	17.4
Experimental group	94.4	18.33	33.74
Personal–social development[a]			
Control group	93.06	4.9	17.69
Experimental group	87.98	24.07	41.4

Mean scores per group in Porter's (1972) study.
[a]Measured using the Gesell Development Schedules (Gesell and Amatrude, 1947).

Table 6.1 shows that some of the measures, namely height and language development, show an initial dramatic change in infants in the experimental group, and this difference diminishes slightly between the groups as time progresses; however, with weight, motor development, adaptive development and personal–social development, exercising the infants continues to widen the differences between the two groups until at least the end of the experimental period.

As this study is based directly on Rogers' principles of mutual interaction of human and environmental fields it therefore adds considerable weight to Rogers' principle of reciprocy, which is shown by the change in the child's environmental field through the major carer providing a planned schedule of exercise. The exercise programme coincides with changes in the child's field as shown by the measures taken at 1 and 2 months into the planned exercise regime. The study also gives support for Rogers' principle of resonancy, as the changes that occur are developmental, and show that development occurs faster in a child who is undergoing a scheme of regular planned activity, and slower in a child who does not receive this type of activity.

Although Porter does not frequently fall into the trap of suggesting causal links between activity and development of the child, on one occasion she does so: '…it is quite clear that there was sufficient evidence to infer that the difference in weight gain between the two groups was caused by the exercising' (p. 216). The notion of causality is not one that Rogers supports, preferring the principle of probability that allows both human beings and the environment to repattern and organize themselves while interacting with each other. This implies levels of probability that changes in one will affect the other.

However, the changes that are undoubtedly shown in this study demonstrate the crucial nature of infancy as being a time when there is greater potential for development at different speeds. What is unclear from this study is whether the changes shown will be maintained by the infants in the experimental group after the exercise schedule is stopped; and whether all the indicators would show such a marked difference between the two groups if the schedule of exercises was to continue for a longer period – height and language development, for example, may not show continued increase. A further feature not shown is the effect of activity schedules on infants in a wider age range, and children of different ages; similar experiments could be conducted with a wider age range to further examine Rogers' principle of resonancy.

Porter's study has also shown how physical and psychological development can be assessed in infants, how a programme to speed development can be implemented, and how evaluation of the programme of intervention can be carried out. However, this study is in danger of not adhering to holism by taking physiological measures as the basis of development.

Porter's study concludes the section on identification of needs and problems, and also studies using identification through to evaluation using Rogers' model.

No studies were found in the literature which were based on planning nursing care using Rogers' model. The next section therefore examines the studies that deal with implementation or intervention, using Rogers' model.

IMPLEMENTING NURSING CARE USING ROGERS' MODEL

To Rogers, intervention in nursing is through the principle of homo-dynamics based on holism. Therefore intervention, using Rogers' 1970 model, must include reciprocy, synchrony, helicy and resonancy. As Rogers (1970) says:

Intervention should be directed towards assisting individuals to mobilize their resources, consciously and unconsciously, so that the man–environment relationship may be strengthened and the integrity of the individual heightened. Therapeutic modalities must incorporate within them cognizance of man as a thinking, feeling being.

(p. 134)

So intervention implies that the patient's environment includes the nurse as a major feature.

Five studies were found in the literature. Two use an approach not seen in the other models, namely therapeutic touch. This is particularly appropriate to Rogers' model as it very directly demonstrates the human–environment interaction; also Rogers includes the use of therapeutic touch in the 1980 version of her model:

Clairvoyance, for example, is rational in a four-dimensional human field in continuous mutual, simultaneous interaction with a four-dimensional environmental field. So too are such events as psychometry, therapeutic touch, telepathy, and a wide range of other phenomena.

(p. 335)

The other three studies in this section use different methods of implementation: the first uses social support as a method of nursing action; the second reviews the literature on bladder irrigation techniques; the third shows the effect on the elderly of a movement therapy programme.

THE EFFECTS OF THERAPEUTIC TOUCH ON HEADACHE

The first of two studies on therapeutic touch (Keller and Bzdek, 1986) shows the effectiveness of therapeutic touch in a controlled trial of two groups of people suffering from tension headaches. This method of nursing care is strongly advocated by the researchers as an intervention method of choice. There is also evidence that it is gaining acceptance in Britain as a method of nursing care in a variety of settings.

According to Rogers' principles therapeutic touch uses the human—environment interaction, synchrony and helicy, as its method of producing change and effecting healing. The energy fields of the patient are said to be directly influenced by the therapist, as she or he directs energy into the patient for healing to occur. The therapist is also thought to redirect areas of tension away from the human field (Krieger, 1979, 1981).

In reviewing the literature Keller and Bzdek found that therapeutic touch need not necessarily involve physical contact, but contact must always be made with the patient's energy field (Krieger, 1975). The effects of therapeutic touch are said to be threefold: reducing anxiety, relieving pain and promoting healing. It is also said to be based on the principles of holism (Krieger, 1981), where the therapist acts as a channel to direct energy in the environment to the recipient, who uses energy to restore balance and promote healing.

To Keller and Bzdek it appeared that tension headaches were a good medium to demonstrate the effects of therapeutic touch, because anxiety was a known contributing cause and there had been no previous studies showing the technique in use with such problems.

They proposed three hypotheses.

- Tension headache pain will be reduced following therapeutic touch, and the initial reduction will be maintained for a 4 hour period.
- Subjects who receive therapeutic touch will experience greater tension headache pain reduction than subjects receiving a placebo simulation of therapeutic touch.
- Subjects who receive therapeutic touch will maintain greater tension headache pain reduction than subjects receiving a placebo simulation of therapeutic touch 4 hours following the intervention.

These hypotheses were tested on 60 volunteer subjects ranging from 18 to 59 years of age (mean age 30 years). Subjects were recruited from three sources, a student health clinic at an American university, the general student and staff population of the same university, and the general public via radio and newspaper advertisements. The 60 subjects comprised 75% females; 70% were college students and 30% white collar workers; subjects had a mean educational level of 16 years; 97% were white. The criteria for inclusion in the study were that subjects had a tension headache which had been diagnosed using a standardized protocol and a physical examination, and that no medication had been taken for the headache for at least 4 hours prior to the study. A feature which does not appear to have been considered by the researchers is how much any of the subjects knew of therapeutic touch, either its use or its effects, although they do mention that none of the subjects had experienced its use.

Keller and Bzdek used three scales to rate subjects' experience of pain from the McGill–Melzack Pain Questionnaire (Melzack, 1975): the Pain Rating Index (PRI), the Number of Words Chosen (NWC) and the Present Pain Intensity (PPI). The McGill–Melzack Pain Questionnaire has been shown to be reliable in its ability to distinguish between the different types of headaches (Allen and Weinemann, 1982). The scales were given to the subjects on three occasions: immediately before the intervention, 5 minutes afterwards, and subjects were also given a copy to take home to fill out 4 hours later, after which the researcher telephoned each subject to obtain the scores and to ask if any treatment had been taken for the headache.

Subjects were randomly assigned to one of two groups; they were unaware of their group assignment, but knew there was a 50–50 chance of being assigned to either a placebo or an experimental group. Analysis of demographic variables of level of education, age, sex, medication practice, religion and level of scepticism of therapeutic touch did not differ significantly between the groups.

In the therapeutic touch group the therapist made a conscious effort to help the subject, passing her hands from 15 to 30 cm away from him or her to assess the energy field and redirect any accumulated tension out of the field. The next phase involved the therapist resting her hands around the subject's head but not touching it; where areas of energy imbalance were found, she then directed energy to the subject.

In the placebo group the therapist simulated the movements carried out with the therapeutic touch group. The researchers say the motion is indistinguishable from therapeutic touch; however, instead of the therapist making a conscious effort to help the subject, the focus of attention was on mentally subtracting from 100 by 7. The intervention with each subject in each group took 5 minutes.

During the experimental period subjects in both groups were asked to sit quietly and to breathe slowly and deeply.

The scores on all three scales were not statistically different between the two groups of subjects before intervention began, showing that for this occasion an acceptable level of reliability was found. Also at the end of data collection internal consistency was found between the scales at each point at which measures were taken. However, the researchers do not mention validity measures in their study.

Data were analysed using a Wilcoxon signed rank test, which gave a significant difference in the number of subjects who felt a reduction of pain in the therapeutic touch group. This difference was seen on all scales of the McGill–Melzack Pain Questionnaire and was found 5 minutes after the intervention ($p < 0.0001$); 4 hours after the intervention subjects in the therapeutic touch group still had significantly less pain than subjects in the control group ($p < 0.0001$). Therefore the first hypothesis was supported.

Analysing the data using a Wilcoxon test showed that there was a significant difference in the amount of pain reduction in subjects in the therapeutic touch group compared to those in the control group. This difference was shown in each of the scales: the PRI showed a difference with $p < 0.005$ between the groups; the NWC a difference with $p < 0.002$; and the PPI a difference with $p < 0.0001$ between the groups. This supported the second hypothesis.

Analysis of the data using a Wilcoxon test 4 hours after the intervention showed that the therapeutic touch group had less pain by 77% compared with the pre-intervention period, and the placebo group had reduced pain by 56% over the same period. This difference between the groups was not statistically significant. Therefore the third hypothesis was not supported. However, 50% of subjects in the control group were found to have taken analgesics in the 4 hour period following the placebo intervention, whereas only 16% (five subjects) of the therapeutic touch group were found to have taken any medication during this period. In the subjects who did not use any analgesics following the interventions statistical differences were found between the groups on all three scales at 4 hours after the interventions: $p < 0.01$ for the PRI and the NWC, and $p < 0.005$ for the PPI index. Therefore for those subjects for whom therapeutic touch made a significant difference to their level of pain the third hypothesis was supported. Despite this it is evident that not all subjects benefitted equally from pain reduction by the use of therapeutic touch, and the influences involved in those not receiving pain relief are far from clear.

As this study is based directly on Rogers' concepts of synchrony and helicy it adds support to these principles by showing that interaction between human beings and the environment does occur and can be enhanced through planned intervention. In the case of therapeutic touch the therapist is seen to be able to influence the healing process of someone suffering from tension headaches more often than purely by chance. However, it is unclear why and how some subjects suffering from tension headache escape from this healing process; whatever prevents this human–environment interaction needs to be investigated further. It would appear from this study that scepticism of the effects of therapeutic touch alone is insufficient to prevent the intervention occurring; so, is a mechanism possible that can consciously or unconsciously block an intervention on the part of the recipient?

LEARNING TO USE THERAPEUTIC TOUCH

The second paper on therapeutic touch (Quinn, 1979) shows the therapist being able to use therapeutic touch in an effective manner. It is not a research study in the sense of using controlled trials, but deals with one nurse's subjective path to using therapeutic touch and her current feelings about its use and effectiveness. The paper gives little critical appraisal of Rogers' work.

Quinn tells of her initial enthusiasm for nursing in different settings after she graduated. However, this enthusiasm waned until she resigned from the profession and, in a sense of desperation, enrolled in a graduate nursing programme at New York University.

During her period as a graduate student she encountered therapeutic touch, and learned the principles of its operation using the self as an energy transmitter, which forced her to examine herself in depth. She was '...for a time, paralysed by self-doubts in terms of therapeutic touch' (p. 663) and was therefore unable to feel the cues that were discussed in relation to its use. This aroused her anxiety, which she eventually overcame, and she then intuitively became aware of what needed to be done for the patient in using therapeutic touch. She is now able to see patients relax and become pain free, those who were restless become calm, and withdrawn patients respond. She uses this as her evidence of the changes taking place in the patient.

She says that the use of this intervention requires a new way of viewing illness. The sick person is now seen as needing to be sick at that particular moment, and the therapist is encouraged to explore the events in the patient's life that lead to this need.

Quinn believes that in order for her to be most effective using therapeutic touch she must be completely open to the energy fields surrounding her, and thus the patient also has the most benefit from her healing. At those times when she is able to be completely open, at the end of healing she feels tired and ineffectual. It seems that when she is completely open she acts as a transmitter of energy, and the more closed she becomes the more she generates energy. Even after two years of practising therapeutic touch she is still perfecting her art, and is unaware of how open she is being until the end of the session when she feels the after effects. She believes that the changes in the energy patterns occurring in herself during therapeutic touch simultaneously effect changes in the patient's energy patterns.

Although, as mentioned above, this is not intended to be a scientifically rigorous study, its inclusion in a chapter on the use of Rogers' model in practice is warranted on at least two counts: to give insight into the lengthy process of learning the techniques of therapeutic touch (which Rogers says are legitimate nursing activities), which also seems to demand self-awareness; and to give a feel for the effects of the procedure on the healer as a personal experience.

SOCIAL SUPPORT AS A METHOD OF RELIEVING STRESS IN NURSING

This paper by Allanach (1988) is not a research report but an extrapolation of Rogers' model in relation to occupational stress felt and experienced by nurses. It is useful in its proposals for research to verify the model, particularly in the area of occupational stress. The paper uses four of the principles of Rogers' model, four-dimensionality, integrality, helicy and resonancy, and relates these to the work of Sarter (1987) who further develops Rogers' principles. The paper outlines each of Rogers' principles.

The paper begins with theories and models of stress from researchers outside the field of nursing, but as these are not of direct relevance to Rogers' model they have not been included here. Allanach wrote the article from the perspective of a nurse manager wanting 'to influence the phenomenon of stress in nursing' (p. 73), believing that a study of the nature of social support and its relationship to occupational stress was important to nursing knowledge.

Examining Rogers' (1970) model, Allanach took the principle of four-dimensionality, describing the human and environmental fields as constantly interacting. She then took Sarter's development of four-dimensionality which describes the energy field as a manifestation of consciousness, Sarter suggesting that evolutionary idealism explains consciousness.

Allanach describes integrality as the 'continuous, mutual exchange of energy between human and environmental fields in space–time four-dimensionality' (p. 78). In Rogers' (1970) words:

> The human field possesses its own identifiable wholeness. Despite its dynamic nature and continuous interaction with the environment, it maintains identity in its ever-changing but omnipresent patterning. Pattern and organization of the field express themselves in a wide range of ways all of which have relevance for the integrity of the field. Envision the human field in the curvature of space–time. The life process is the expression of the rhythmical evolution of the field along a spiralling longitudinal axis, bound in the four-dimensional space–time matrix and ever shaping and being shaped by the environment.
>
> (pp. 90–1)

Taking Sarter's developments we see that as energy is conscious, integrality can be seen as the consciousness of human beings and the environment interacting continuously, and therefore experienced by the individual as their reality.

On helicy Allanach says that this is the process of continual change which has properties of diverse patterning and organization of both the human and the environmental fields, which occur in non-repeating rhythms. Sarter's developments describe how the human field patterning and organization can be seen as manifestations of consciousness, and that helicy is the final development of evolutionary idealism. Helicy can therefore be viewed as the evolution of the individual's consciousness, or the refinement of understanding, motivation and emotion with the passage of time; so that one would expect individuals continually to develop a clearer understanding of themselves as thinking, feeling and doing.

Resonancy is described by Allanach as the waves that pattern and organize the human and environmental fields. These wave patterns are evolving continuously from lower to higher frequencies due to life experiences where wave patterns interrelate continuously. Sarter describes resonancy as the process of continual development of clarity and awareness of oneself, based on interactions with the environment, the most complex being with other humans in one's environment which will assist in the evolution of consciousness. One might therefore expect that, as a result of continual interaction with one or more people, an individual would achieve a greater self-understanding. Having thoughts, actions and feelings leads to an evolving sense of self through social support in stressful situations, where the individual would perceive supportive behaviours as those which promoted the ability to understand oneself. This would move the nurse from lower to higher frequencies of consciousness.

Allanach's model proposes the nurse resolving her problems of stress through discussion, which promotes her ability to determine her own reality and is non-causal. In relation to occupational stress, this prevents a narrow view that provides simplistic answers to problems likely to be very complex.

Allanach goes on to discuss how this model might be tested in practice. The main question is whether there is a relation between perceived supportive behaviour and an increasing sense of self-awareness. She proposes a qualitative methodology which would allow for description of supportive interactions, then develops a number of ideas for which of these methods would be suitable and the general problems of qualitative methodology.

The first problem of qualitative methodology she tackles is that of rigour, quoting Sandelowski's (1986) work which shows that credibility (by those involved recognizing the experiences described), fittingness (the results being able to fit into similar situations) and consistency (through an accurate description of the methods used which would allow for replication to occur) confirm that qualitative methodology can be rigorous. She mentions multiple triangulation, which compares a number of different methods, as a method which would increase the confirmation or credibility of the results.

A method she feels would be suitable for a study of this nature is a questionnaire with open-ended questions asking subjects to reflect on stressful work situations where support was obtained. The responses would be content-analysed by several analysts to reveal the conceptual system used by the nurse in linking perceived support to consciousness of self.

A further method advocated by Allanach involves Kennedy and Garvin's (1986) method of confirmation–disconfirmation. Here subjects are engaged in activities that confirm the experiences and disconfirm the worth of others. This method uses interviews to discover which situation out of a number presented is perceived as the most supportive, and further probing attempts to discover the subject's cognitive appraisal of the workings of the supportive relationship. Transcripts of the interviews are also content-analysed to determine the nature of the relationship between perceived support and the development of the self.

These methods are only two of many available to help to determine the nature of the relationship between perceived support and the development of the self, but it is clear that these important ideas put forward by Allanach need to be tested. Testing would also provide a very useful source of knowledge of aspects of Rogers' model in this situation.

One of the major functions of the nurse manager is to give support to nurses being managed. What makes support acceptable or unacceptable to those receiving it is vital for the nurse manager to know in order to be effective. Alternatively, can colleagues be equally effective in providing support for each other, in the absence of nurse managers, and is this relationship not equally as essential to determine? Would similar features be seen in the way the environmental field of the nurse manager or a colleague interact with the nurse's human field? These are important questions for nursing, but are also very relevant areas for further development of Rogers' model.

CLOSED URINARY CATHETER INSTILLATION AND IRRIGATION

This study by Burgener (1987) is only loosely based on Rogers' model, and so has a problem in showing useful developments of some of Rogers' principles. However, the problems it causes for the model give room for further thinking on the nature of human–environment interaction in a very practical area, i.e. assisting urinary drainage.

Burgener makes a reference to Rogers' model by stating that nurses need to consider the impact of the environment on the health of the individual. She says that Rogers stresses the environment cannot be separated from the individual and that the continuous human–environment interaction is important to nursing care. Burgener's assertions are found in Rogers' (1970) principle of reciprocy:

[which] postulates the inseparability of man and environment and predicts that sequential changes in the life processes are continuous, probabilistic revisions occurring out of the interactions between man and the environment.

(p.97)

Rogers (1970) also asserts that human beings have an identifiable whole-ness which is surrounded by the boundary of the human field:

[which] possesses its own identifiable wholeness. Despite its dynamic nature and its continuous interaction with the environ-ment, it maintains identity in its ever-changing but omnipresent patterning. Pattern and organization of the field express themselves in a wide variety of ways, all of which have relevance for the integrity of the field.

(p. 91)

Burgener reviews the literature on catheter irrigation/instillation and says that nursing practice has been unable to develop an irrigation/ instillation system that meets with an acceptably low level of infection where urinary catheters are in use. She uses the guidelines of Horsley (1981) as the basis of her assertions of acceptability.

If catheter irrigations are necessary, the needle syringe, 21-gauge needle, and sterile irrigant are used and then discarded. If frequent irrigations are necessary, a triple-lumen catheter permitting con-tinuous irrigation within a closed system is preferable.

(p. 5)

Burgener says that, although avoiding the use of indwelling catheters is the best answer to problems of infection, they are sometimes indicated, for example in bladder, prostate or vaginal surgery. However, whatever the indication, the process of catheter-ization has inherent risks of infection due to trauma of the mucosa which increases susceptibility, or to contamination which introduces infection.

In these two instances alone it is possible to see the human–environment interaction as the nurse inserting the catheter and the catheter itself both constitute the environment; however, it is difficult to see the exact nature of the human field. Where the catheter is contaminated and bacteria (environment) are introduced into the human field, at what point do they become part of it; and does the catheter, once inserted, also become part of the human field or does it remain part of the environmental field? These are important arguments in Rogers' (1970) model, as she frequently states the differences that occur in the human energy field:

Multiple irregularities characterize the boundaries of man's energy field. At times the field may extend further into the environment and at other times retreat in the direction of man's visible core.

(p. 90)

It is also possible that the emphasis on the urinary system creates problems of loss of holism. All these questions are ignored by Burgener's paper; however, they recur in almost every statement she makes.

Other features of the environment which predispose to infection are the level of the nurse's education, handwashing practices, and the use of larger than necessary catheters causing pressure and urethral ischaemia; also the natural cleansing of the urethra by the passage of urine is prevented which encourages pathogens to migrate to the bladder. With these factors Burgener advocates a strong suggestion of causality rather than probability, which is again inconsistent with Rogers' model. A further source of promotion of environmental pathogens is other patients in the same room (Hargiss, 1980, 1981). Reducing the environmental risk of infection is achieved by: maintaining a good level of nutrition; lack of trauma to the urethral mucosa; urine flow which is not impeded and has no backflow into the bladder; effective cleaning of the catheter–urethral junction; the maintenance of the patient's normal flora; and maintaining a closed urine drainage system.

Causality is also referred to directly by Burgener when describing types of microorganisms involved in urinary tract infection; however, she reverts to probability when discussing the influence of infection on mortality, by describing other influencing factors such as age, non-surgical disease or progressive, fatal, underlying illnesses. Also the structure of the female urethral tract is known to be more susceptible to infection than that of the male.

Burgener says that irrigation of catheters is associated with a higher or equal level of urinary tract infection than in patients without irrigation. Closed systems of irrigation have also shown this pattern, where the disconnection of bags of fluid, and contamination of irrigation fluid and equipment were thought to be probable influencing factors.

From the human field one can see the various changes that are thought to necessitate irrigation, or in Rogers' terms, intervention from the environmental field. These indications are: thick and foul-smelling urine that may or may not create a blockage (Kennedy and Brocklehurst (1982) found that 60% of nursing units carried out a weekly routine of irrigating all indwelling catheters); leakage of urine and severe infection (it was shown by Lapides (1979) that obstruction of urinary flow has a major influence on urinary infection); intervention from the environmental field in the form of irrigation should use solutions such as polymixin, neomycin or acetic acid (Andrioli *et al.*, 1968; Desautels, 1975; Schneckloth, 1975).

Recommendations involving the environmental field show that a closed drainage system is preferable to an open one (discussed previously), but only the latter can be used. As Warren *et al.* (1978) concluded, despite changes in catheter design and the use of microbial agents, continual opening of the system for irrigation means that there is no effective method of combatting infection. A further environmental hazard is the use of catheter plugs; Birum and Zimmerman (1971) showed that using these more than once gave an 80% change that they would contribute to urine contamination, and single use only was advisable.

A further problem related to the probabilistic nature of urinary tract infection is that records of the use of catheters, irrigations with catheters and the incidence of infections are not routinely kept. Therefore for adequate use of Rogers' model these probabilities need to be ascertained.

Although this article may be very useful for nurses working in areas where patients are catheterized, or for infection control nurses, using Rogers' model will lead to difficulties. These difficulties have been discussed in more detail above; they also have to do with the lack of holism in Rogers' sense, as the topic only deals with one of the parts of a human being – the urinary system. Another problem is not being able to identify what constitutes the human field. If these problems are overcome, which is not a minor undertaking, then the question of probabilities needs to be addressed in relation to human–environmental field interaction.

THE EFFECTS OF MOVEMENT THERAPY IN THE AGED

This study (Goldberg and Fitzpatrick, 1980) deals with the effects of a planned programme of movement for the elderly in an institution. The authors claim that the intervention is based directly on the principles proposed by Rogers. A controlled trial established the differences between residents who had undergone movement therapy and those who had not, and looked for specific outcomes in terms of morale and self-esteem. As outcomes are also involved in this study, it could be said to include measures of evaluation using Rogers' model.

Goldberg and Fitzpatrick do not specify which of Rogers' (1970) principles in particular they are setting out to develop and test through research, although their aim is to test a holistic nursing intervention. However, as they make it plain they are looking for change in the individual as a result of a programme of planned intervention, it is assumed that the principle of helicy is being used as a framework for this study. The authors claim that their planned intervention of movement therapy is derived from Rogers' (1970) model, and although Rogers does not specifically mention movement therapy, it is clear that this form of intervention falls well within the domain of her model.

> Intervention should be directed towards assisting individuals to mobilize their resources, consciously and unconsciously, so that the man–environmental relationship may be strengthened and the integrity of the individual heightened. Therapeutic modalities must incorporate within them cognizance of man as a thinking, feeling being.
>
> (Rogers, 1970, p. 134)

Five hypotheses were tested in this study; these were that elderly institutionalized people who participate in a programme of movement therapy will show improvement in:

- morale scores as measured by the Philadelphia Geriatric Centre Morale Scale (PGCMS) (Lawton, 1975);
- agitation scores as measured by the PGCMS;
- attitudes towards their ageing as measured by the PGCMS;
- lonely dissatisfaction scores as measured by the PGCMS;
- self-esteem scores as measured by the Rosenberg (1965) Self-esteem Scale.

All these measures were then compared with similar people who had not undergone a programme of movement therapy.

The PGCMS has the advantage of being relatively short and easy to understand. It is a 17-item forced choice questionnaire where the choices are dichotomized into high or low morale responses. The scale has three components: (1) the agitation index (which consists of six items); (2) the attitude towards one's own ageing index (five items); (3) the lonely dissatisfaction index (six items). The scale has been tested for correlation with other measures of life satisfaction by Lohman (1977) and was found to have a high value, although Goldberg and Fitzpatrick do not give a value.

Rosenberg's Self-esteem Scale (10 items) is designed to measure attitudes towards the self on a favourable–unfavourable scale. Self-esteem on this scale includes the subject's self-respect, their feelings of worthiness, their feelings of equality with others, recognition of their limitations, and that they will grow and improve. Reliability of 92% has been found by Robinson and Shaver (1972). A criticism of this scale is that it was developed for adolescents and validity across all age groups has not been tested. However, Goldberg and Fitzpatrick conducted a pilot study which found that the only change needed was reducing the four response levels of the scale to two – 'agree' and 'disagree'. These two scales (the PGCMS and the Rosenberg Self-esteem Scale) were used before the planned therapy was begun and again at the end of the experimental period.

The subjects in the study were 30 people aged 65 or older. They were selected from residents of a 100-bed nursing home in a metropolitan area in the United States. The criteria for inclusion in the study were that the subject was oriented in time and place, was able to speak English, could make the judgements required by the scales, and was able to participate in the movement therapy classes. Further details were taken of age, sex, physical disabilities and length of time subjects had been in the institution. The sample was divided into two groups by random assignment – four men and 11 women in the control group, and three men and 12 women in the experimental group. When differences were analysed between the groups using a t-test a significant difference was found between the groups in length of time in the institution, the control group being in the institution significantly longer than the experimental group. All other differences between the groups were statistically insignificant.

The control group participated in their usual wide range of daily activities in the nursing home, and the experimental group took movement therapy sessions instead of one of their daily activities. These were held two mornings a week for 6 weeks, each session lasting approximately 60 minutes, out of which 30 minutes was devoted to activity. The sessions were led by a graduate nurse who 'uses body motion and language in a dynamic process to meet therapeutic goals' (p. 342). This, the only information about the contents of the sessions given, is insufficient to allow for replication of the study.

Both the PGCMS and the Self-esteem Scale were given to subjects before and after the movement sessions. Both scales were read to subjects by the experimenter, but no mention is made in the article of what method the subjects used to rate themselves.

The results took into account the differences between the groups by analysing the length of time residents had been in the institution and the differences in responses to the scales completed after the movement therapy sessions ended, adjusting the responses to the before-session scales accordingly. The differences between the control group and the experimental group were that after the movement therapy sessions the experimental group had significantly higher total morale scores ($p < 0.05$) and attitudes towards their own ageing scores ($p < 0.01$) than the control group. There was also a trend towards greater self-esteem ($p = 0.06$) in the subjects in the experimental group, but this did not reach an acceptable level of statistical significance; however, levels of self-esteem were moderate to high in all subjects before the experiment began, therefore maybe only minimal room for improvement was possible. This level of self-esteem shows the quality of care the residents received in the institution. No significant differences were found on the agitation scores or the lonely dissatisfaction scores between the two groups after the movement therapy sessions.

Some of the factors which are unclear from this study are to do with the effect of more attention being given to the experimental group than the control group (the Hawthorn effect) as well as the way of assessing disability. During the experimental period the control group were given no attention by the experimenter, although they carried out other activities, so the results could be due to the attention of the experimenter. An attempt should have been made to minimize this effect and Goldberg and Fitzpatrick have recognized this. The second problem with the research design is the way the disability score was achieved:

> A disability score was obtained by compiling a list of current acute or chronic problems as identified by physicians or nurses in the medical record. Each independent problem was given a scoring value of one point, and a disability score was obtained by summing the total number of problems for any one individual.
>
> (p. 343)

This method is naive in that the number of disabilities found is unlikely to indicate the extent of disability of the individual; this fact is ignored, therefore this reductionist approach may well lead to inaccurate results.

Despite the problems noted with the experiment, this work adds support to Rogers' principle of helicy as it shows that change can be brought about in the institutionalized elderly by a participatory programme of environmental intervention. Although the programme lasted for a period of only 12 hours spread over 6 weeks, a significant change in at least two aspects of the experimental group was seen. However, what is not clear is the length of time over which the effects will last once the programme is withdrawn, and also the period of time which significant change in the other factors – agitation and loneliness dissatisfaction – would take to achieve. Using Rogers' principles it may be that these two factors have longer spirals than morale, attitude towards their own ageing and self-esteem scores. However, as Goldberg and Fitzpatrick point out, it may be that agitation reflects a level of caring about oneself and the environment which is a developmental trend in the elderly and shows some responsiveness; therefore it may be a feature of what Rogers (1980) calls 'continuously creative process directed toward growing diversity of field pattern and organization' (p. 336).

CONCLUSIONS

Implementing nursing care is a definite stage in Rogers' model, where she specifies particular methods of intervention. According to Rogers (1970) nursing intervention should enhance the person–environment interaction in order to strengthen the integrity of the individual through the principles of reciprocy, synchrony, helicy and resonancy.

The papers that develop nursing intervention using Rogers' model have helped to give credence to her principles. These papers show that therapeutic touch can be an effective method of relieving tension headaches, which develops our knowledge of synchrony and helicy; and that planned movement therapy with the elderly can improve morale and attitudes towards ageing amongst this group and may also have an effect on their self-esteem. One of these methods – therapeutic touch – is not found in research using other models of nursing in this book.

CONCLUSIONS ON THE USE OF THE MODEL TO 1990

In summing up the use of Rogers' model in practice settings I have found that this model has generated the largest number of studies of all the models considered in this book. This may be partly due to the programme of research instigated by Martha Rogers with her doctoral students.

Despite this amount of research, which has been generated in a relatively short time, there is no indication that this model has been used in practice outside North America. This is a shame, as many nurses in Great Britain recognize the concept of holism as entirely relevant to their work with patients and clients. It could be that the language of the model limits its use in practice settings.

The knowledge that has been gained from systematic investigation of particular settings has been shown by Fawcett (1975, 1977) in that the human field does change and develop its pattern and organization in relation to certain events. However, the nature of the environmental influence is unclear from her study. Floyd was able to demonstrate the principle of helicy by showing the effect on hospitalized psychiatric patients of changes in their sleep–wake rhythms. Browse was unable to clearly isolate features of the human and environmental fields interacting in women both immediately before and after childbirth.

The principle of reciprocy and resonancy is shown convincingly by Porter when she demonstrates human–environment interaction between children and their mothers which affects their growth. However, Clarke (1986) was unable to define the nature of waves in her study which was based on theories of molecular structure. Therefore the nature of waves in Rogers' model remains unclear.

The passage of time was found by Strumpf (1987) to be related in elderly women to a feeling of inner calm, associated with life satisfaction and a high self-esteem. Newman (1970, 1982) found a difference between men and women in their ability to estimate clock time; this may be due to socialization patterns.

Investigating the effects of intervention in nursing Goldberg and Fitzpatrick (1980) took the principle of helicy and showed that planned changes due to movement therapy made a difference to morale and self-esteem in the elderly. Helicy is also convincingly demonstrated by Keller and Bzdek (1986) who showed that a trained therapist could give sustained relief for tension headaches using therapeutic touch.

DEVELOPMENTS SINCE 1990

The development of Rogers' model has progressed apace since 1990. Not only have there been papers published outside North America which advocate the use of the model, but there have also been tributes to the author, who is seen as a controversial but brilliant leader. I will discuss the papers that have appeared to support the use of the model in practice and to show how it can be used, before concluding with an assessment of the impact of Rogers and her model.

IDENTIFICATION OF THE UNITARY STATE

Two papers published in Britain show the growing acceptability of this model here. The first is a literature review; the second, by the same author, is an account of the way in which assessment can be carried out using Rogers' model.

THE PERCEPTION OF TIME

Biley (1992) advocates Rogers' model and concepts as having 'considerable relevance for nursing practice' (p. 1141) although he acknowledges the difficulty that first-time readers may have in understanding it. He concentrates, in a literature search, particularly on the notion of accelerating evolution, and discusses its implications, i.e. that as people get older they perceive time as passing quicker than when they were younger. However, as yet there seems to be no conclusive evidence that as people age they perceive time passing more quickly; here he uses the study by Strumpf which is discussed above.

Evidence from a number of studies has shown that, as yet, research has been unable to provide any conclusion to the theory of acceleration of time with age. If the passage of time is an individual experience, then maybe nurses need to help those who are experiencing time as passing slowly, which may not necessarily, according to Rogers, be only the elderly. However, a study of Rogers' Theory of Accelerated Evolution has led to an interest in the experiences of elderly people and their perceptions of time. This could lead to the need for some sort of therapy for those who are experiencing time passing slowly.

ASSESSMENT OF ENERGY FIELDS

Biley (1993) acknowledges that Rogers' model was not intended as a framework to guide nursing action and therefore should not be used as such. He describes it as 'an abstract but scientific knowledge base from which theories and guidelines for clinical practice can and have been developed' (pp. 519–20). What Biley hopes to do in this paper is to show how guidelines developed from one aspect of the conceptual framework, namely energy fields, can direct nursing practice.

Explicit in Rogers' model is that the environment can have a positive or negative effect on the human field and vice versa. So the aim of the nurse who is incorporating the concept would be to promote a positive and continuous interaction between the human and the environmental field.

Biley gives an example of how a pattern manifestation appraisal can be carried out. However, due to Rogers' insistence on the person being holistic, a list of categories on which to question and observe the patient is not appropriate; the nurse needs to consider the whole person. The second stage, according to Biley, is to promote harmony between the person and the environment, which promotes health. The example given by Biley demonstrates well how assessment and promotion of harmony, or integrality, can occur, and can be far from complicated.

Although this is not a research paper, it is useful in helping those less familiar or less confident with the model to consider it and its implications for nursing. As Biley says, this model is now being used worldwide in guiding research, practice and curricula. He sees the model as having a lasting impact on nursing.

DEVELOPMENT OF AN ASSESSMENT TOOL FOR POST-PARTUM MOTHERS

At this point it is appropriate to include a paper from North America which discusses the development of an assessment tool to be used with post-partum mothers.

Tettero, Jackson and Wilson (1993) developed an assessment instrument to assess a new and first-time mother's ability to cope with her newborn baby. The instrument has two main sections – influencing data and energy field pattern data. However, it becomes plain at this point in the paper that the authors did not develop the tool themselves, but the paper is really about their use of Rogers' model and how the tool has helped them to collect data from post-partum mothers. The Appendix to the paper shows the tool to have been developed by Madrid and Winstead-Fry in 1986.

The influencing data section in the assessment tool is further divided into sections requiring demographic details such as name, age, marital status, occupation and medical diagnosis. The energy field pattern data section requires details such as: being comfortable with oneself (in the relative present); communication that promotes integrality; the sense of rhythm that sets the pace of the life process; a sense of feeling part of the environment outside oneself; one's personal identity held by oneself and others; and one's integrality which shows ability to accept challenges and survive crises. Each of the subheadings also has a series of substatements which, we are told, are interdependent and affect each other. The authors claim that this assessment 'represents the client's state of consciousness and reflects the integrity of one's own human–environmental energy field' (p. 779).

The last section of the paper applies the tool in a case study to show how it should work. The authors describe their 'arduous task' in understanding the model before they could consider the use of a holistic approach to nursing.

However, the paper is rather uncritical and also does not develop a systematic appraisal of the use of the assessment tool in practice. Of further note is that the paper sees the model as being applied to the clinical area. This occurs in several statements, for example:

> The purpose of this paper is to apply one particular conceptual model – that of Rogers' (1970) Science of Unitary Human Beings – to assess a new mother coping with her first newborn.
>
> (p. 776)

It seems, then, from this paper that the authors are assessing the appropriateness of the model and the tool for use with these mothers; it is therefore a shame that they did not give full details of the effects of this assessment.

EVALUATION OF NURSING ACTIONS TO PROMOTE HUMAN–ENVIRONMENT INTERACTION

One paper was found which developed the notion of evaluating the effect of nursing care on the ability to promote increased harmony between human beings and the environment. This was done by asking people receiving therapeutic touch to explain their previous situation and to compare it with their present feelings about their situation. Therapeutic touch is one of the therapies that is very appropriate in the use of Rogers' model.

Samarel (1992) investigated the experience of those undergoing therapeutic touch, as she failed to find studies in the literature which addressed this. The study was informed by phenomenology, so data were collected about the lived experience of people undergoing therapeutic touch. Twenty people who were undergoing therapy participated (12 female and eight male). They were all given written explanations of the research which was discussed with the investigator. Each participant was interviewed twice for between 15 and 45 minutes. However, we are not told the method of recording the data, although a detailed description of how the data were analysed is given.

Samarel found that the data fell into three categories: experiences before treatment, experiences during treatment and experiences following treatment. As in all good reporting of qualitative research, samples of the conversations of the participants are used in the paper. The experiences of the participants prior to treatment contained three elements of unmet needs which were physiological, mental/emotional and spiritual. However, all these descriptions were in the past tense so they were 'remembered perceptions'.

Experiences during treatment contained statements about self-awareness, which was related to physiological and mental/emotional factors, and other awareness which was related to roles and relationships. Therefore according to Samarel's study the lived experience of therapeutic touch was ' ...one of developing physiological and mental/emotional self-awareness as well as developing awareness of others' roles and relationships with the participants' (p. 654).

After treatment the experience of the changes described by the participants again fell into all three categories: physiological, mental/emotional and spiritual. The resolution of these previously unmet needs led participants to feel a prolonged and intense personal change for the better which was comprehensive and evidently involved a sense of intense fulfilment. This was described as peace, serenity and a sense of well-being.

Participants described the experience of therapeutic touch as a linear process where they began with an unmet need, sought treatment and proceeded through a number of treatments which continued to have an impact on their lives. Participants also talked about therapeutic touch being dynamic, as the nature of their experience changed as therapy progressed.

This study shows some excellent results of therapeutic touch. However, as the authors readily say, the sample is evidently biased, as participants are taken from those undergoing therapy. Therefore those for whom therapy was not successful are unlikely to be included in the sample. So the findings need to be treated with caution. Having said this, on the basis of this study the effect that therapeutic touch can obviously have is most impressive. Therefore as far as Rogers' model is concerned, this adds considerable weight to one of her nursing actions to promote human–environment integrality.

CONCLUSIONS ON THE USE OF THE MODEL FROM ITS DEVELOPMENT TO 1995

Undoubtedly Martha Rogers is a controversial figure. This is emphasized nowhere more than in a paper by Garon (1992). In terms of her model the reactions have been both very positive: 'Her greatest contribution to nursing, however, is her development of an evolutionary conceptual system that has inspired tremendous creativity, research activity, and intellectual growth in the profession' (Garon, 1992, p. 71); but also very negative: 'One of the major criticisms of the Rogers' model is that it is not applicable to clinical practice' (p. 70).

Despite the negative comments, Rogers' model is still being developed and used in practice, as we can see by the papers produced since 1990. The possible effectiveness of therapeutic touch as a nursing action is a distinct boost to the model.

Rogers' model is also continuing to gain recognition internationally. This is evident not only in the two papers from the UK by Biley, but also in the paper by Garon (1992) published in the USA where she says 'there is evidence that its use in practice is increasing' (p. 70). She cites three examples of the model being used: one in geriatric assessment, another in caring for the terminally ill and a third in nursing administration.

The abstract nature of some of the concepts, such as the nature of waves, makes it difficult to develop knowledge in nursing practice. But, as Garon says, this undoubtedly adds to the creativity of researchers and is a challenge to us all.

REFERENCES

Allanach, E.J. (1988) Perceived supportive behaviours and nursing occupational stress: an evolution of consciousness. *Advances in Nursing Science*, **10**(2), 73–82.

Allen, R. and Weinmann, R. (1982) The McGill–Melzack Pain Questionnaire in the diagnosis of headache. *Headache*, **23**, 20–8.

Anderson, M. (1980) A psychosocial screening tool for ambulatory health care clients: a pilot study of validity. *Nursing Research*, **29**(6), 347–51.

Andrioli, V.T., Kunin, C.M., Stamey, T.A. and Martin, C.M. (1968) Preventing catheter-induced urinary tract infections. *Hospital Practice*, **3**, 61–8.

Attwood, J.R. and Gill-Rogers, J.P. (1984) Metatheory, methodology, and practicality: issues in research uses of Roger's science of unitary man. *Nursing Research*, **33**(2), 88–90.

Bem, S.L. (1981) *Bem Sex Role Inventory Professional Manual*, Consulting Psychologists Press, Paolo Alto, CA.

Bentov, I. (1977) *Stalking the Wild Pendulum*, E.P. Dutton Co., New York.

Biley, F.C. (1992) The perception of time as a factor in Rogers' Science of Unitary Human Beings: a literature review. *Journal of Advanced Nursing*, **17**, 1141–5.

Biley, F.C. (1993) Energy fields nursing: a brief encounter of a unitary kind. *International Journal of Nursing Studies*, **30**(6), 519–25.

Birum, L.H. and Zimmerman, D.S. (1971) Catheter plugs as a source of infection. *American Journal of Nursing*, **71**, 2150–2.

Borg, G. (1971) The perception of physical performance, in *Fitness* (ed. R.J.

Shepherd), Thomas, Springfield, IL, pp. 280–94.

Brouse, S.H. (1985) Effect of gender role identify on patterns of feminine and self-concept scores from late pregnancy to early postpartum. *Advances in Nursing Science*, **7**, 32–48.

Burgener, S. (1987) Justification of closed intermittent urinary catheter irrigation/instillation: a review of current research and practice. *Journal of Advanced Nursing*, **12**, 229–34.

Chodil, J. (1979) *The Topographic Device: Analytical Tool or Source of Artifacts?* Read before Sigma Theta Tau, Upsilon Chapter, Research Day, New York University, New York.

Clarke, P.N. (1986) Theoretical measurement issues in the study of field phenomena. *Advances in Nursing Science*, **9**(1), 29–39.

Cohler, B., Weiss, J. and Grunebaum, H. (1970) Child-care attitudes and emotional disturbances among mothers of young children. *Genetic Counselling Monographs*, **82**, 3–47.

Crawford, G. (1985) A theoretical model of support network conflict experienced by new mothers. *Nursing Research*, **34**(2), 100–2.

Desautels, R.E. (1975) Managing the urinary catheter. *Nursing Digest*, **3**, 30–1.

Earle, A. (1969) Effect of supplementary post-natal kinesthetic stimulation on the developmental behaviour of the normal female newborn. PhD thesis, New York University.

Fawcett, J. (1975) The family as a living open system: an emerging conceptual framework for nursing. *International Nursing Review*, **22**, 113–16.

Fawcett, J. (1977) The relationship between identification and patterns of change in spouses' body image during and after pregnancy. *International Journal of Nursing Studies*, **14**, 199–213.

Fitts, W. (1965) *Manual: Tennessee Self Concept Scale*, Counselor Recording and Tests, Nashville, TN.

Floyd, J.A. (1984) Interaction between personal sleep–wake rhythms in psychiatric hospital rest–activity schedule. *Nursing Research*, **33**, 255–9.

Foulkard, S., Monk, T.H. and Lobban, M.C. (1979) Towards a predictive test of adjustment to shift work. *Ergonomics*, **22**, 79–91.

Garon, M. (1992) Contributions of Martha Rogers to the development of nursing knowledge. *Nursing Outlook*, March/April, 67–72.

Gesell, A.L. and Amatrude, C.S. (1947) *Developmental Diagnosis*, 2nd edn, Paul B. Hoeber, New York.

Gibbs, J. (1972) *Sociological Theory Construction*, Dryden Press, Hinsdale, IL.

Gill, B.P. and Atwood, J.R. (1981) Reciprocy and helicy used to relate mEGF and wound healing. *Nursing Research*, **30**(2), 68–72.

Goldberg, W.G. and Fitzpatrick, J.J. (1980) Movement therapy with the aged. *Nursing Research*, **29**(6), 339–46.

Grosso, M. (1981) Toward an explanation of near-death phenomena. *Anabiosis*, **1**, 3–23.

Hardy, M. (1978) Perspectives on nursing theory. *Advances in Nursing Science*, **1**, 37–48.

Hargiss, C.O. (1980) The patient's environment: haven or hazard. *Nursing Clinics of North America*, **15**, 671–88.

Hargiss, C.O. (1981) Infection control: putting principles into practice. *American Journal of Nursing*, **81**, 2165–86.

Harrington, R. (1978) Balm for the worried well. *Innovation*, **5**, 3–10.

Hasselmeyer, E. (1963) Handling and premature infant behaviour. PhD thesis, New York University.

Heimler, E. (1975) *Survival in Society*, John Wiley, New York.

Hildenbrandt, G. and Stratmann, I. (1979) Circadian system response to night work in relation to the individual circadian phase position. *International Archives of Occupational and Environmental Health*, **43**, 73–83.

Hobbs, D. (1965) Parenthood as crisis: a third study. *Journal of Marriage and the Family*, **27**, 367–72.

Hobbs, D. (1968) Transition to parenthood: a replication and extension. *Journal of Marriage and the Family*, **30**, 413–17.

Holmes, T.H. and Rahe, R.H. (1967) The social readjustment rating scale. *Journal of Psychosomatic Research*, **11**, 213–18.

Horne, J.A. and Ostberg, O. (1976) A self-assessment questionnaire to determine morningness–eveningness in human circadian rhythms. *International Journal of Chronobiology*, **4**, 97–110.

Horne, J.A. and Ostberg, O. (1977) Individual differences in human circadian rhythms. *Biological Psychology*, **5**, 179–90.

Horsley, J.A. (1981) *Closed Urinary Drainage Systems*, Grune and Stratton, New York.

Howard, A. and Pelc, S.R. (1953) Synthesis of deoxyribonucleic acid in normal and irradiated cells and its relation to chromosomes. *Heredity*, **6**, 261–73.

Keller, E. and Bzdek, V.M. (1986) Effects of therapeutic touch on tension headache pain. *Nursing Research*, **35**(2), 101–6.

Kennedy, A.P. and Brocklehurst, J.C. (1982) The nursing management of patients with long-term indwelling catheters. *Journal of Advanced Nursing*, **7**, 411–17.

Kennedy, C.W. and Garvin, B.S. (1986) Confirmation–disconfirmation: a framework for the study of interpersonal relationships, in *Nursing Research Methodology*, (ed. P.L. Chin), Aspen, Rockville, MD, pp. 221–35.

Kim, H.S. (1983) Use of Roger's conceptual system in research: comments. *Nursing Research*, **32**(2), 89–91.

Kim, M.J. and Moritz, D.A. (1982) *Classification of Nursing Diagnosis: Proceedings of the Third and Fourth National Conferences*, McGraw-Hill, New York.

Knapp, R. (1976) *Handbook for the Personal Orientation Inventory*, San Diego Editions, San Diego.

Knapp, R. and Garbutt, J. (1958) Time imagery and the achievement motive. *Journal of Personality*, **26**, 426–34.

Krieger, D. (1975) Therapeutic touch: the imprimatur of nursing. *American Journal of Nursing*, **75**, 784–7.

Krieger, D. (1979) *The Therapeutic Touch: How to Use your Hands to Help or Heal*, Prentice-Hall, Englewood Cliffs, NJ.

Krieger ,D. (1981) *Foundation for Holistic Health Nursing Practices: the Renaissance Nurse*, J.B. Lippincott, Philadelphia.

Kuhlen, R. and Monge, R. (1968) Correlates of estimated rate of time passage in the adult years. *Journal of Gerontology*, **23**, 427–33.

Kuhn, T.S. (1970) *The Structure of Scientific Revolutions*, 2nd edn, The University of Chicago Press, Chicago.

Lapides, J. (1979) Mechanisms of urinary tract infection. *Urology*, **14**, 217–25.

Lawton, M. (1975) The dimensions of morale, in *Research Planning and Action for the Elderly: The Power and Potential of Social Science*, (eds D. Kent *et al.*), Human Sciences Press, New York.

Lazowick, L.M. (1955) On the nature of identification. *Journal of Abnormal Social Psychology*, **51**, 175–83.

Lewis, H.E. and Masterson, J.P. (1957) Sleep and wakefulness in the Arctic. *Lancet*, **1**, 1262–6.

Lohman, N. (1977) Correlations of life satisfaction, morale and adjustment measures. *Journal of Gerontology*, **32**, 73–5.

Madrid, M. and Winstead-Fry, P. (1986) Rogers conceptual model, in *Case Studies in Nursing Theory* (ed. P. Winstead-Fry), National League for Nursing, New York, pp. 73–102.

Markson, E. (1973) Readjustment to time in old age. *Psychiatry*, **36**, 37–48.

Melzack, R. (1975) The McGill Pain Questionnaire: major properties and scoring methods. *Pain*, **1**, 277–99.

Neal, M. (1968) Vestibular stimulation and developmental behaviour of the small premature infant. PhD Thesis, New York University.

Newman, M.A. (1982) Time as an index of expanding conscientiousness with age. *Nursing Research*, **31**(5), 290–3.

Papowitz, L. (1986) During resuscitation, some patients face a life-or-death choice that no one else will know about – unless they ask. *American Journal of Nursing*, April, 419–20.

Pedersen, D. (1973) Development of a person space measure. *Psychological Reports*, **32**, 527–35.

Piaget, J. (1966) Time perception in children (trans. B. Montgomery), in *The Voices of Time* (ed. J. Fraser), George Braziller, New York.

Piaget, J. (1970) *The Child's Conception of Time* (trans. A. Pomerans), Basic Books, New York.

Porter, L.S. (1972) The impact of physical–physiological activity on infants' growth and development. *Nursing Research*, **21**(3), 210–19.

Quinn, J.F. (1979) One nurse's evolution as a healer. *American Journal of Nursing*, April, 662–4.

Reinberg, A. (1970) Evaluation of circadian desynchronism during transmeridian flight. *Stadium Generale*, **23**, 1159–68.

Ring, K. (1980) *Life at Death: A Scientific Investigation of the Near-Death Experience*, Coward, McCann and Geoghegan, New York.

Robinson, J. and Shaver, P. (1972) *Measures of Social Psychological Attitudes*, Survey Research Centre, University of Michigan, Ann Arbor.

Rogers, M.E. (1970) *An Introduction to the Theoretical Basis of Nursing*, F.A. Davis, Philadelphia.

Rogers, M.E. (1978) *Nursing Theory: Study of the Nature and Direction of Unitary Development* (audiotape), Teach 'Em, Inc., Chicago.

Rogers, M.E. (1980) A science of unitary man, *in Conceptual Models for Nursing Practice* (eds J.P. Riehl and C. Roy), 2nd edn, Appleton-Century-Crofts, New York.

Rogers, M.E. (1983) Science of unitary human beings: a paradigm for nursing, in *Family Health: A Theoretical Approach to Nursing Care* (eds I.W. Clements and F.B. Roberts), John Wiley, New York.

Rogers, M.E. (1985) Science of unitary human beings: a paradigm for nursing. Paper presented at the Nurse Theorist Conference, Pittsburgh, PA, 16 May 1985.

Roos, P. (1964) Time referenced inventor. Unpublished manuscript.

Rosenberg, M. (1965) *Society and the Adolescent Self-Image*, Princeton University

Press, Princeton, NJ.

Rubin, R. (1975) Maternal tasks in pregnancy. *Maternal and Child Nursing Journal*, **4**, 143–53.

Sabom, M.B. (1982) *Recollections of Death: A Medical Investigation*, Harper and Row, New York.

Samarel, N. (1992) The experience of receiving therapeutic touch. *Journal of Advanced Nursing*, **17**, 651–7.

Sandelowski, M. (1986) The problem of rigour in qualitative research. *Advances in Nursing Science*, **8**(3), 27–37.

Sarter, B. (1987) Evolutionary idealism: a philosophical foundation for holistic nursing theory. *Advances in Nursing Science*, **9**(2), 1–9.

Schneckloth, N.W. (1975) Indwelling catheter nursing care. *Association of Operating Room Nurses Journal*, **21**, 695–6.

Shostrom, E.L. (1973) Comment on a test review: the Personal Orientation Inventory. *Clinical Psychology*, **20**, 479–81.

Smith, M.J. (1975) Changes in judgment of duration with different patterns of auditory information for individuals confined to bed. *Nursing Research*, **24**, 93–8.

Smith, M.J. (1979) Duration experience for bed-confined subjects: a replication and refinement. *Nursing Research*, **28**, 139–44.

Smith, M.J. (1984) Temporal experience and bed rest: replication and refinement. *Nursing Research*, **33**(5), 298–302.

Smith, M.J. (1986) Human–environmental process: a test of Rogers' principle of integrality. *Advances in Nursing Science*, **9**(1), 21–8.

Sollberger, A. (1965) *Biological Rhythm Research*, Elsevier, Amsterdam.

Strumpf, N.E. (1987) Probing the temporal world of the elderly. *International Journal of Nursing Studies*, **24**(3), 210–14.

Tettero, I., Jackson, S. and Wilson, S. (1993) Theory to practice: developing a Rogerian-based assessment tool. *Journal of Advanced Nursing*, **18**, 776–82.

Warren, J.W., Platt, R., Thomas, R.J. *et al.* (1978) Antibiotic irrigation and catheter-associated urinary tract infections. *New England Journal of Medicine*, **299**, 570–3.

Whelton, B.J. (1979) An operationalisation of Martha Rogers' theory throughout the nursing process. *International Journal of Nursing Studies*, **16**, 7–20.

Witkin, H.A., Dyk, R.B., Paterson, H.F. *et al.* (1974) *Articulation of Body Concept (ABC) Scale for Evaluation of Figure Drawings*, Educational Testing Service, Princeton, NJ (mimeograph).

Yura, H. and Walsh, M.B. (1973) *The Nursing Process: Assessment, Planning, Implementing, Evaluating*, 2nd edn, Appleton-Century-Crofts, New York.

FURTHER READING

Aggleton, P. and Chalmers, H. (1986) *Nursing Models and the Nursing Process*, Macmillan, London.

Chin, P.L. and Jacobs, M.K. (1987) *Theory and Nursing*, C.V. Mosby, St Louis.

Fawcett, J. (1984) *Analysis and Evaluation of Conceptual Models of Nursing*, F.A. Davis, Philadelphia.

Fitzpatrick, J.J. and Whall, A.L. (1983) *Conceptual Models of Nursing Analysis and Application*, Prentice Hall, Englewood Cliffs, NJ.

George, J.B. (ed.) (1985) *Nursing Theories: A Base for Professional Nursing Practice*,

2nd edn, Prentice Hall, Englewood Cliffs, NJ.

Griffith-Kennedy, J.W. and Christensen, P.J. (1986) *Nursing Process Application of Theories, Frameworks and Models*, C.V. Mosby, St Louis.

Kershaw, B. and Salvage, J. (1986) *Models for Nursing*, John Wiley, Chichester.

Marriner, A. (1986) *Nursing Theorists and their Work*, C.V. Mosby, St Louis.

Parse, R.R. (1987) *Nursing Science*, W.B. Saunders, New York.

Riehl, J.P. and Roy, C. (1980) *Conceptual Models for Nursing Practice*, 2nd edn, Appleton-Century-Crofts, Norwalk, OH.

Neuman's health care systems model

7

Table of chapter contents

This chapter is an addition to the book since 1990 as it was felt that Neuman's model is important and should be included. The published work that I have found shows this to be the case.

THE AUTHOR

Betty Neuman was born in 1924 in Ohio and completed her nurse train-ing there in 1947. She then moved to Los Angeles where she held a number of posts in clinical practice in hospital as well as in school and industrial nursing. She studied for her degree in Nursing at the Univer-sity of California which she completed in 1957. In 1966 she received a Master's degree from the University of California in Mental Health, Public Health Consultation. She received a doctorate in Clinical Psychology in 1985 from Pacific Western University.

Her work in nurse education has been predominantly in mental health. At UCLA she developed a post-master's community mental health course. In 1970, she developed her systems model in response to student requests on her graduate programme: 'It included such behavioural science concepts as problem-finding and prevention' (Harris *et al.*, 1989, p. 362).

Neuman has been actively involved as a therapist in marriage and family therapy since 1970 as well as being a lecturer and consultant.

THE MODEL

Betty Neuman's model has been known since 1972 when it first appeared in the nursing press. The development of her model has been described in a number of publications: as a chapter in Riehl and Roy in both their 1977 and their 1980 editions (Neuman, 1977, 1980); in a book based on the model published in 1989 (Neuman, 1989), and in a book which develops the model particularly in relation to its application in education and in practice published in 1982 (Neuman, 1982).

The most frequently cited publications, in the papers that I found, were the 1980, 1982 and 1989 versions.

A brief outline of the model occurs here, with an indication of the changes with each publication.

SUMMARY OF THE NEUMAN HEALTH CARE SYSTEMS MODEL

This model was originally subtitled 'A total person approach to patient problems' which implied that its use is with people who are sick or who have problems. This might be off-putting to health workers who deal with prevention or with those who are well. As discussed below, this title was abandoned in 1989.

The 1980 edition of Neuman's model claims to be appropriate for use by health care workers other than nurses. It can be used 'to assist individuals, families, and groups to attain and maintain a maximum level of total wellness by purposeful interventions' (p. 119).

The aims of the model are to reduce stress and other factors associated with stress which affect the optimal functioning of individuals, groups and communities. The figure that is produced with the model is complex (Fig. 7.1), but explains its main components in diagrammatic form.

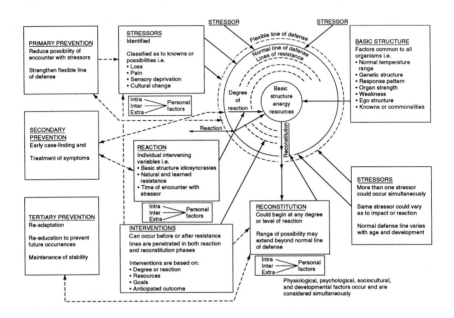

Figure 7.1 The Betty Neuman model: a total person approach to viewing patient problems. (From Neuman and Young, 1972. Reproduced with permission of the American Journal of Nursing Company.

The model sees any individual, group or community as subject to the impact of stressors. Stressors can be within oneself (intrapersonal), between one or two people (interpersonal) or outside the individual (extrapersonal). Everyone has their own characteristics and a normal range of responses which they have evolved; these are their **normal lines of defence** against stressors; so the individual is constantly adjusting him or herself to the environment, or adjusting the environment to him or herself. In this process of interaction with the environment, varying degrees of harmony are achieved. One might be able to predict a positive adjustment through knowing how the individual, group or community has adjusted in similar situations in the past.

However, amongst the possible known stressors, each has a potential to disturb the individual to a different extent. Also taking into account the nature of the individual as being a combination of physiological, psychological, sociocultural and developmental aspects, she or he will be able to use a combination of these defences against reactions to stress; these are the **flexible lines of defence**.

When the flexible line(s) of defence is unable to withstand the stressor(s), the individual's internal **lines of resistance** attempt to stabilize the individual. If this is successful the individual will be returned to a state of health. However, if the lines of resistance are unsuccessful then the individual will become incapacitated, as the basic core structure fails to support the individual.

The nurse can intervene to help the individual to stabilize and combat the stressors by primary, secondary or tertiary prevention. Neuman therefore claims that the model is dynamic. Primary prevention is important as it helps to strengthen the flexible line of defence to prevent a reaction to stress occurring. To do this the nurse must know the meaning that an individual puts on experience and also how she or he coped with it in the past.

Secondary prevention is designed to relieve the existing symptoms of stress. Thorough assessment of the meaning of the stressor for the individual is needed. Neuman describes assessment as comprising seven stages, followed by a summary of the goals and the rationale for them, then an intervention stage. Intervention uses the person's optimum resources to either stabilize or to strengthen the internal lines of resistance. At this stage a ranking of the priority of needs for the individual can occur. What is interesting in this model is its seeming lack of an evaluation phase. It appears that the assessment phase follows intervention.

Tertiary prevention is intervention after the acute stage of secondary prevention, where some stability has occurred. This stage aims at maintaining the level of adaptation already achieved and using the individual's existing energy resources.

However, following the publication in 1974, Craddock and Stanhope (1980), although finding the model very useful, were critical of it in a number of different areas:

The model can be strengthened by a clearer schematic and parsimonious discussion of the interaction of the parts of the model. The nurse's role in the system needs to be clarified and the methods of intervention at the three levels of prevention need to be identified. Notions of the role relationships of health-care providers also needs to be clarified.

(p. 166)

Despite the criticisms of Craddock and Stanhope, the 1980 version of Neuman's model received high praise from Moore and Munro (1990). They found it to have great potential in helping to assess and meet the needs of the elderly with mental health problems. They also praised the model for its focus on intervention, which has the potential for continuing to develop the body of nursing knowledge in caring for the elderly.

The 1982 version of Neuman's model saw its further development, rather than any radical changes. The additions were in the development of the person, who was now seen to comprise five interacting variables: physiological, psychological, sociocultural, spiritual and developmental. To meet their needs, the person interacts with the environment and is affected by the environment. Also in this edition is the inclusion of many case studies, which help to show the reader the potential use of the model.

However, following publication of the 1982 version, there were further criticisms of the model, among them Buchanan (1987). She criticizes the model as being 'based on signs and symptoms only, and ... antithetical to the concept of primary prevention' (p. 52). It is found not to be developed for families and groups, but only for the individual. Buchanan did however largely believe that Neuman's model was of value, but despite this she found it necessary to make some alterations to it so that the family and the community were given sufficient weight. She also agrees with the criticisms of Craddock and Stanhope outlined above.

The 1989 edition of *The Neuman Systems Model* sees further revision of the model from the 1982 version. The most striking difference is the title; gone is the subsidiary title of 'A total person approach to patient problems', which indicated a very illness-oriented approach. There is much more scope, within this edition, to develop health promotion and family care.

Previous criticisms of the model are taken into account in this edition, for example there is more emphasis on the model being used with not only the individual but also with groups, the community at large and 'even ... a social issue' (p. 16). However, although this use of the model is claimed by Neuman to be wider than the individual, the majority of the chapter explaining the 1989 edition deals with the individual.

In this edition the development of the client variables are made more explicit and the additional variable 'spiritual' is developed. The use of the model with the nursing process is also made more explicit. We see the stages of nursing diagnosis, nursing goals and nursing outcomes being clearly linked to the use of the model. Lastly, there is now considerable emphasis on health promotion which is seen as part of primary prevention 'that optimizes the client wellness potential or condition' (p. 39). Neuman also gives a nursing assessment format and intervention tool to be used with her model as an appendix to Chapter 1, combined with a helpful explanation about its use.

Since Neuman's 1989 edition there have been further reservations about her model from public health nursing in the UK. While accepting that the model 'offers a broad, flexible, inter-disciplinary framework for public health nurses, giving them clear strategies for working in partnership with the community' (p. 1921), Haggart (1993) recognizes that some aspects could be stronger and refocused. In a critical evaluation of the model in relation to public health nursing in the UK, Haggart says that the ability to assess community culture and diversity is not available, except through the client's perception of it. The model also assumes common values between the nurse and the client to promote equilibrium and defences against stressors. However, as Haggart says:

> in community work there are communities who have lines of resistance to normal lines of defence which may include behaviours or strategies considered by the nurse to be damaging to health.
>
> (p. 1919)

Furthermore, Neuman sees the client as adapting to and accepting stress in the environment, rather than helping people to change their environment, sometimes by political action, in order to improve provision and alleviate need. With these three factors in mind, Haggart says that Neuman's model, although giving a clear structure to help public health nurses' work with colleagues and clients, may not be totally congruent with current public health expectations.

The following discussion in this chapter will be devoted to the research papers that have used Neuman's model to research clinical nursing issues.

ASSESSMENT USING NEUMAN'S HEALTH CARE SYSTEMS MODEL

Many of the publications by Neuman on her model do not make a division between assessment and intervention. Indeed in the 1980 version Neuman calls her tool 'An assessment/intervention tool based upon the Neuman Health-care Systems Model: A Total Approach to Patient Problems' (pp. 132–4). Therefore although there are several categories within the tool, seven of them are devoted to collecting data from the patient and the nurse for assessment purposes.

In locating published papers in the literature I have been able to find only one that deals solely with assessment, so this will form the first section of the chapter.

PREDICTING PATIENTS' REPORTED QUALITY OF LIFE

This paper (Hinds, 1990) investigated patients who had been diagnosed as suffering from lung cancer. The research was carried out to investigate these patients' quality of life and the factors associated with this. From the paper, it appears that it was only after the research was completed that Neuman's model was assessed for the degree of fit with the data. Despite this there seems to be a good level of fit.

Hinds (1990) examined the coping abilities that some patients had achieved when they knew that they had a life-threatening illness, such as being diagnosed as having lung cancer. She felt that seven factors contributed to the reported quality of life of these patients. She tested three hypotheses:

1. patients with lung cancer who preferred information about their illness and its management would report a higher quality of life;
2. patients who reported a high level of satisfaction with family functioning would report a higher quality of life; and
3. patients who exhibited higher levels of learned resourcefulness would report a higher quality of life.

(p. 457)

She investigated 87 patients, 63 male and 24 female. All had been diagnosed as having cancer of the lung, 56% for a period of 6 months or less, 16% for 7–12 months, 11% for 13 months to 2 years and 17% for over 2 years.

The method used was to combine four instruments into a self-administered questionnaire. This collected information on the patients' demographic details and their preferences for information, their reported level of family functioning, their learned level of resourcefulness, and their reported quality of life. However, we are not told anything about validity and reliability testing of the combined questionnaires before they were administered. Some testing was undoubtedly carried out and showed that the subscales were highly correlated to the whole quality of life scale.

Two methods of data analysis were used: Pearson's correlation to test the hypotheses; and a step-wise multiple regression to assess the effect of the variables on the dependent variable (quality of life).

The patients' reported level of health suggested that if they felt in good physical health or were capable of an acceptable level of functioning then they were more likely to see their quality of life as positive ($r = 0.91$). The patients' socio-economic and psychosocial status also correlated highly with their total quality of life ($r = 0.80$). However, items dealing with the family correlated lower than the previous items ($r = 0.51$). The significance of these results will be discussed below.

The variables which were tested by Hinds to assess their effect on the patients' quality of life were:

- prognosis
- surgery
- current radiotherapy

- performance status
- learned resourcefulness (self-control)
- information preference
- age group.

These variables were entered into the regression.

However, a combination of all these variables only accounted for 30% of the variance. None of the variables contributed much more than 4% to the total variance. It was therefore clear that a number of other factors were involved in the patients' quality of life that had not been taken into account in the variables. As Hinds says:

> quality of life is a complex concept, and ... is viewed differently among various individuals. Factor or factors which may be important in determining quality of life for some individuals may not be as important as for others.
>
> (p. 458)

Hinds says that this type of serious illness disrupts people's aims for their life, which may cause them to change their goals, for example to take early retirement which they would otherwise not have done. She says that age also has a bearing on their use of resources, as with increasing age their finances, as well as the numbers of family members and friends able to give help, may be less. Also with some younger people if they have been unemployed for some time their financial position may be poor. All these individual differences lead to differences in quality of life. However, Hinds relates the individual differences that she found to differences in 'learned resourcefulness' (p. 458). She says that this is due to individuals' differences in their coping with stress and change. Furthermore, individuals' ways of responding to information related to their illness had a bearing on their reported quality of life.

Further aspects of the patients' lives which affected their quality of life were their progressive deterioration and surgery. Surgery in particular led to pain and discomfort as well as to feelings of psychological trauma – being incomplete and mutilated. These latter feelings often led to anxiety and depression. Hinds therefore found a great difference in people's responses to serious illness, however the link between this and their quality of life could not be explained in this study.

Treatment with radiotherapy was found to have many distressing side effects. These included fatigue and weakness which interfered with the normal abilities of the individuals to care for themselves as well as to carry out their normal role and to interact with others. 'They [the side effects] influence people's quality of life and self-concept and increase their social dependency' (p. 459). Also people had to cope with an environment which was new to them, in which the treatment took place.

From this Hinds continues to adhere to Neuman's model by stating that the nurses' role is one of intervention through primary, secondary and tertiary levels. In Neuman's model, Hinds sees that lung cancer and the patient's reactions to it have penetrated their flexible lines of defence, the normal line of defence and the lines of resistance. This results in disease, symptoms and other related stress factors that potentially make the core of the individual come under attack which threatens the survival of the person.

According to Hinds, treatment by radiotherapy is part of the external environment because, in order to undergo radiotherapy, the individual must have active involvement with other people. However, radiotherapy was also seen as part of the internal environment due to the effects that it had on the person; whereas the other six factors shown formed the internal environment of the individual. Hinds saw these people's coping mechanisms involving the response to their illness, the coping with the threat to their self-esteem and their struggle for survival. The patients' health was inferred by Hinds from their reported quality of life.

Hinds says that with these patients nursing intervention was at the secondary and tertiary levels, 'to assist in the recapture and maintenance of systems stability or the progress towards a peaceful death' (p. 461). She felt the stress factors to be the confirmation of the diagnosis, the radiotherapy treatment and its side effects and the circumstances that developed related to the illness. Hinds therefore felt that nursing was needed at the secondary level to reduce the stress, tension and anxiety in order to strengthen the patients' lines of resistance. For the patients who were experiencing some form of stability, intervention at the tertiary level should be directed towards preventing regression or additional stress. Nursing actions would be to support the internal and external resources and capacities of the patients and referring them, where appropriate, to other services.

Hind's paper demonstrates well the use of Neuman's model in patients with the diagnosis of lung cancer. She relates the stages of assessing stress and the patients' coping abilities using Neuman's model. She also develops Neuman's model in relation to these patients' coping abilities through using outcome measures of quality of life. Neuman's model is seen as being very useful for these types of patients and also for showing how nurses may intervene to prevent, strengthen or protect the patient. The research method is well carried out and we are given adequate information about those who took part and the tools used in the questionnaire. Therefore this study could possibly be replicated.

The research design in Hind's study was very much a cause and effect design, with the cause being the diagnosis of lung cancer and the associated stress of this and the treatment, the effect being on the quality of life of the patient. As this is a cause and effect design it is entirely appropriate that it should be testing hypothetical relationships between variables, which are well specified in the paper. It would also seem that Hinds does problematize the variables that she uses, as she queries the factors that led to the patients' quality of life, particularly when the ones she chose only accounted for 30% of the variance.

The data obtained through questionnaire were statistically analysed, with no evidence that qualitative data were sought or qualitative analysis was necessary. The fact that a questionnaire was used would lead one to question whether it was tested for validity and reliability before it was administered, as the paper gives no indication of this. However, that no qualitative analysis was necessary leads one to suppose that all the data were in predefined responses, i.e. ticking boxes was all the respondents needed to do. This may have been very sensible if they were severely ill or depressed, but it leads to some concern that responses did not allow the patients to say everything that they felt or wanted to say. Furthermore, there is always the issue with questionnaires that people may say one thing and do something else, as, particularly views, can change with time.

The paper is written to indicate that the model was not specifically being tested by the study, rather that the study was important for nursing care and to generate knowledge. However, the model was very central to the study and formed the basis of hypothesis testing. The findings do not either support or overturn the model; also, as Hinds says, the link between stress, lung cancer and quality of life is far from clear from this study.

That the study was carried out in Canada gives some indication of the acceptability of Neuman's model in North America.

ASSESSMENT THROUGH TO EVALUATION

A further study from Canada is a complete case study, from assessment to evaluation, of a young woman recently diagnosed as having multiple sclerosis (MS).

Knight (1990) says at the outset of her article that she wants to show the goodness of fit of Neuman's (1982) model to the care of patients with MS. She aims to describe some of the features of patients with MS to show the model's relevance. However, by using a single case study, she has not demonstrated the relevance of the model to every patient with MS, only to the patient she has chosen. Her method therefore seems at odds with her initial claims, although she does say that the paper 'specifically illus-trates the application of this model to a case study of a client with MS' (p. 447). The paper begins, however, by summing up the general features of people with MS, which are supported by literature, before going on to discuss the suitability of Neuman's model and to describe the 1982 ver-sion of the model in some detail. The remainder (a little over half of the paper) is then used for the case study of a 22-year-old woman who has very recently been diagnosed as having MS.

Knight uses Neuman's assessment tool as the first stage in the nursing process, although adapting it in two respects, as well as Neuman's intervention stage. However, unlike Neuman (1982), she sees the second stage of nursing care as planning nursing care and the fourth stage as evaluation. Knight therefore adopts a more traditional four-stage approach to the nursing process than Neuman has done.

The case study, of a female patient of 22 years who has been in hospital for 8 days and has recently been told of her diagnosis of MS, is begun by giving details of her symptoms. Her assessment revealed decreased right-sided motor co-ordination, some lack of equilibrium, mild weakness in both legs and nystagmus, as well as double vision, some numbness in her right leg, urinary urgency and frequency, and she also showed mild anxiety. However, although these details are given we are not told how the information was collected; we suspect some of it was from a medical examination, therefore the method of data collection for this part of the paper would not allow for replication. Neuman's adapted assessment tool is then undertaken with this patient and the findings from the assessment are given. The patient and nurse are found to have different perceptions of the substantial stressors to the patient. From this the five variables of the person, physiological, psychological, socio-economic, developmental and religious, are detailed for the patient.

From the assessment, short-term goals for the patient are set which involve primary and secondary intervention. Nursing outcomes are explained as a result of these goals.

The conclusions reached by Knight are about the health status of the patient and the stressors and threats to her. The use of the tool and the findings from it are summed up, but no mention is made of the usefulness of the model, although the author has evidently found the model gives her good information about this patient, on which she is able to plan and devise care.

The paper is evidently a good nursing care study of the use of Neuman's model with a patient with MS. The problems of a single patient are generalized to all patients with MS. However, no details are given of data collection or analysis, therefore no real conclusions can be made about how the patient's diagnosis and her treatment were arrived at. Also no conclusions can be made from this paper about any research methods suitable for use with the model, but this was not the intention of the study. The use of the model is also not problematized, so we are left with a study where the model seems ideal for this patient, with nothing left unaccounted for, except getting her to accept nursing intervention. Even getting the patient to accept nursing intervention as specified by the model gives the impression that given time the patient will see the need for this, and is starting to do so already.

The use of Neuman's model as given in this study leaves the impression that the nurse has the answers to the patient's problems, and given sufficient perseverance, the patient will come to realize that the nurse knows best.

One further paper from the USA shows the way in which Neuman's model was chosen and implemented in a general hospital.

CHOOSING NEUMAN'S MODEL FOR USE IN A GENERAL HOSPITAL

The first paper shows the very extensive programme of development, both of the systems in the hospital and of the staff, before Neuman's model was introduced into all ward areas.

Capers *et al.* (1985) undertook to implement a model of nursing throughout the hospital in order to promote quality nursing that would be goal-directed, to increase professionalism that would improve job satisfaction, which in turn would decrease trained staff turnover, and to give direction to the nursing department. A group set up for the purpose compared the models of Roy, Johnson and Neuman. Interestingly, they chose Neuman's model because 'the complexity and number of unfamiliar terms in the Johnson and Roy models precluded their feasibility as a framework for nursing practice' (p. 30). Neuman's model was 'easily understood with a manageable number of terms that would tend to decrease resistance inherent in change' (p. 30).

They document the extensive work that went into both preparation of staff and the hospital itself before implementation could begin; this includes the development of forms for assessment, diagnosis and evaluation of patient care, which are given in the article. Implementation began with a pilot project on one general surgical ward. The implementation phase for the hospital as a whole was set to take between two and a half and three years. This paper was evidently written at the time of the pilot project.

The commitment and work involved in the project is very evident, however this is a very uncritical paper and expects a considerable amount from the implementation of the model, some of which is not included in Neuman's model, such as decreasing staff turnover.

There is also evidence from two other papers that Neuman's model is becoming more popular in the UK. One is by Fulbrook (1991), and shows the process that an intensive care unit (ICU) went through in order to choose and implement a model of nursing. Neuman's model was seen as ideal by the staff for their patients. The use of an assessment tool is described in detail. This is a rather uncritical study but does represent the use of the model well in an ICU setting in the UK. The second paper is by

Parr (1993) who writes about his use of the model in pre-operative theatre visiting. He compares Neuman's model with Roper, Logan and Tierney's model, finding the former far more effective in allowing a good dialogue with the patient. He finds Neuman's model to be patient-led. However, one of his criticisms is the amount of gathered information which has to be organized. His use of Neuman's model is represented as an experiment, rather than being the model that he would normally have used.

INTERVENTION USING NEUMAN'S HEALTH CARE SYSTEMS MODEL

Neuman has three means of intervention: primary, secondary and tertiary. Primary intervention is aimed at preventing the individual's encounter with the stressor; this can be by helping the individual to strengthen their line of defence and therefore to have a decreased response to the stress.

Secondary intervention, according to Neuman, is where reactions to stress are evident. This type of intervention is concerned with making the most use of the individual's external and internal resources in order to strengthen resistance and to stabilize the situation.

Tertiary intervention occurs when the initial threat to the individual has been overcome. The individual is helped, in this stage, to maintain their level of adaptation by maximizing the use of their energy resources – re-education may be important here to prevent recurrence of the effect of the stressor(s).

We now look at the papers that use Neuman's model to provide intervention for patients and clients.

INTERVENTION WHEN GIVING WOMEN ORAL CONTRACEPTIVE ADVICE

This paper specifically sets out to show the use of Neuman's model for midwives giving information to women about contraception in Sweden, which is a legal requirement there.

Lindell and Olsson (1991) clearly state at the beginning of their paper that they wish to look at the practical application of Neuman's model 'in combined oral contraceptive counselling provided by Swedish midwives' (p. 475). Therefore this paper is an application of the model, rather than a research-based study. However, despite this I feel it warrants inclusion in this book as the model is problematized and the level of analysis of the likely problems of these women is considered in some detail. It therefore adds knowledge to the use of the model in this situation.

The authors develop the model according to Neuman's 1982 version. They give evidence of the need for contraceptive counselling among the different age groups in Sweden, showing that for the years 1975 to 1983 legal abortions for teenagers were between 23.8 and 25.2 per 100 pregnancies (National Swedish Board of Health and Welfare, 1988). They also give preliminary data for abortions for all fertile women for the years 1987 to 1988 (National Swedish Board of Health and Welfare, 1989), showing that among the 20–24 age group 26.9% of all pregnancies ended in abortion in 1987 and 27.3% in 1988.

The authors state that Sweden's capacity to offer contraceptive counselling to women is now good. It is a legal requirement for counselling on contraception to be given as part of preventive health care. Midwives act as counsellors in this respect by giving information on different contraceptive methods, by pelvic examination and by insertion of intrauterine devices for women with a normal uterus. They also undertake telephone counselling and public information. Linden and Olsson (1991) say that not only is the contraceptive pill the most reliable, but it is also the most widely used means of contraception in Sweden. However, the figures that they give do not support this statement, as their table shows that barrier methods are the most frequently used (an average percentage of 33.4% in all ages using barrier methods; 31.6% in all ages taking the pill). Women from the age of 30 show a marked preference for barrier methods.

The authors support their use of Neuman's model in primary intervention for midwives offering contraceptive counselling: 'The midwife uses Neuman's model for primary prevention at the individual level when providing counselling concerning the combination of oral contraceptives at the women's first visit to the clinic' (p. 478). They see the goal of this intervention as being to prevent the risk of unwanted pregnancy, the stress of which could threaten the core of the individual by threatening her ego, while helping to strengthen the women's flexible line of defence through giving information about oral contraception and its use.

The authors then give a summary of the main stressors which are likely to affect women; these are in receiving counselling, knowledge about their body and its normal functioning, knowledge about the use of oral contraception and its effects on their bodies including weight gain, smoking and the risks of such conditions as thrombosis, as well as the consequences of unwanted pregnancies. They divide these stressors into:

- sociological
- psychological
- physiological
- philosophical
- developmental
- interpersonal
- extrapersonal.

However, it is not clear how they arrive at this summary of the main stressors. The reader is left to suppose that it is through the experience of the authors, although they do not claim to have carried out a literature search to confirm this. However, they claim that the model can be useful:

> By helping the women to prevent different stress factors concerning birth-control pills, the model can be of positive significance both for life in general and for the relationship between women and men.
>
> (p. 479)

They advocate research to determine the effect of the model, by the decreased number of abortions. They suggest that to assess its effectiveness traditional counselling methods should be compared with counselling using Neuman's model.

This is a disappointing and somewhat frustrating paper as, although it describes the need for counselling in this situation and uses statistics to qualify this need, the authors' use of the model to provide primary intervention appears to be purely speculative, but does call for research to back this up. Therefore, while the model is adhered to, the way in which the midwife provides intervention has no basis in research. So in the absence of this evidence, one is left with a hypothetical application of the model to a real life problem. However, this paper has shown that Neuman's model is acceptable and being used in Scandinavia, as the authors are both working in Sweden.

INTERVENTION TO EVALUATION

An interesting study from the point of view of its results and also its implications for Neuman's model was conducted by Ziemer (1983).

The effects of giving different types of information on post-surgical coping

Ziemer (1983) set out to look at the effects of giving different types of information to patients, namely information on the procedure that the patients would go through; combined or not combined with information on what it would feel like; both of these combined or not combined with how the patients can cope post-operatively. She set out to test the effects of giving these different forms of information to patients, against their reported coping behaviours, and the effects of surgery in such areas as the amount of analgesia, sedatives and hypnotics they needed and their length of hospitalization.

Ziemer (1983) reviewed the literature to give an indication of the expected direction of the findings. However, she found that there was no conclusive evidence that giving information about a procedure would lead to reduction in anger or anxiety. The findings from the literature were inconsistent on this.

The study was based on Neuman's 1980 model. However, an evaluation phase was built into the study, which is not part of this version of Neuman's model, but was clearly essential to the research design. I do not interpret this as being detrimental to the model. The study considered the effects of primary prevention by building the patients' lines of defence against the stressors of abdominal surgery. So the stressor was the impending surgery; primary prevention was by providing different types of information for the patients; the effect of the stressors on the line of defence was the patients' reported coping behaviours; and the impact of the stressors was indicated by the presence of symptoms.

In this study, information was considered to be hierarchical. Information on the procedure alone was considered to be the minimal type. The second level of information was seen as the associated sensations that the procedure would give the patient, for example if the patient was told they would have an intravenous infusion (procedural information) they would also be told what the insertion of the cannula would feel like (sensory information). The third level of information was what the patients should do to cope with the procedure and the associated sensations, for example breathing, coughing and leg exercises, and why these are important for them, i.e. for their circulation and to reduce the possibility of complications.

The outcomes for the patients in Ziemer's study were:

- physical coping, as measured by the Physical Coping Behaviour Scale developed for this study – this measured deep breathing, coughing, turning, leg and foot exercises, abdominal splinting and requests for analgesia;
- psychophysiological coping, as measured by the Psychophysiological Coping Behaviour Scale which was also developed for this study – the scale was developed by asking 61 senior student nurses about their coping methods when confronted with stressful situations.

Both these scales were tested for content validity, which Ziemer found to be adequate. She also tested the Physical Coping Scale by test–retest for reliability and found this to be 0.86, i.e. a high correlation. Test–retest reliability for the Psychophysiological Coping Scale was also good at 0.87.

In addition to these scales Ziemer considered physical symptoms, by asking the patients and also through patient documentation. She considered nausea and vomiting, difficulty in passing urine, abdominal distension and problems of thrombosis and embolus. She also considered pain intensity using a five-point Pain Intensity Scale, which had previously been used but which had only face validity; however, a test–retest for reliability was conducted and reliability was found to be 0.74 – a very respectable level. The last measure of symptoms Ziemer considered was distress. She measured this using a four-point Distress Scale, previously used but which had only face validity. However, test–retest gave a mediocre level of reliability at 0.48, on which Ziemer does not comment, but she evidently found this acceptable.

The six hypotheses tested by Ziemer are listed below.

1. Information about the procedure combined with information about the associated sensations will be more effective than information about the procedure alone in the patients' physiological coping.
2. Information about the procedure combined with information about the associated sensations will be more effective than information about the procedure alone in the patients' psychophysiological coping.
3. Information about the procedure combined with information about the associated sensations and the coping strategies will be more effective than information about the procedure and associated sensations alone in the patients' physiological coping.
4. Information about the procedure combined with information about the associated sensations and the coping strategies will be more effective than information about the procedure and associated sensations alone in the patients' psychophysiological coping.
5. Patients' reporting of physiological coping behaviours will be inversely related to their development of symptoms.
6. Patients' reporting of psychophysiological coping will be inversely related to their development of symptoms.

One hundred and eleven patients' names were collected from the theatre lists the day before surgery. The patients were those admitted to a large general hospital in a metropolitan area in the USA. The patients comprised seven males and 104 females with a mean age of 35.8 years, ranging from 18 to 65 years. There were 71 Caucasians, 31 Blacks and one Asian. Using a chi-square analysis on the patients' race, employment status, education and type of surgery, the groups of patients did not differ significantly from each other.

Each patient was asked by a registered nurse if they would participate in the study which was 'designed to explore patients' responses to surgery' (p. 283). The patients were randomly assigned to one of the three information conditions (information about the procedure only; information about the procedure combined with details of the associated sensations; or information on both the procedure and the associated sensations plus information on how to cope with the effects of surgery). Each patient was then given an audiotape message corresponding to the group to which they were assigned – tapes lasted 5½, 9½ and 22 minutes, respectively. The assignment of patients to groups was such that the researcher did not know which patients belonged to which groups (a double-blind trial). The patients were told that the information on the tape recording could answer some of their questions about before and after their surgery.

Data were collected from these patients over a 5-month period. Each patient's response to surgery was tested between 2 and 4 days post-operatively by asking them to fill in the questionnaire. After discharge each patient's notes were viewed for evidence of thrombosis or embolism.

When the data were analysed using a t-test, none of the hypotheses was supported at the 0.05 level of significance and in the specified direction, although four of the hypotheses were supported at the 0.05 level but in the opposite direction. The hypotheses which were supported but in the opposite direction showed that:

- the higher the response on the Physiological Coping Scale, the higher was the score on the Pain Intensity Scale;
- the higher the score on the Physiological Coping Scale, the higher was the score on the Distress Scale;
- the higher the score on the Psychophysiological Coping Scale, the higher was the score on the Pain Intensity Scale;
- the higher the score on the Psychophysiological Coping Scale, the higher was the score on the Distress Scale.

Therefore, according to the data gathered, the patients who exhibited the most coping methods also experienced the most pain and distress.

Ziemer gives a very full discussion of her findings where she ponders over the methods of giving information to the patients, the data collection methods and their validity. She also questions the validity of Neuman's model in this situation which suggests a link between primary prevention to help the patient prepare for the impact of stressors by giving information, and the effects of these stressors on their ability to withstand stress. It is to her credit that she has published these findings, as many papers are only published when positive findings are achieved.

The study shows a strong use of hypothesis testing using a recognized nursing framework; therefore, according to Silverman (1993), the method is theoretically driven. The method shows the use of a cause and effect model of research design. The questionnaire was the primary instrument used and underwent validity and reliability testing. The data were also able to be analysed using statistical methods, therefore simple response categories were probably available for the patients' answers.

To this extent the study is very competently designed and carried out and follows a rigorous method. That the patients were examined in the environment of the hospital, rather than waiting for them to go home then asking them for their memories, is a strength of this study.

However, as Ziemer says, the results from this study not only throw doubt on the validity of the measures that she used, they also throw into question the validity of Neuman's model in providing effective intervention for these patients. However, from this study it is impossible to tease out which is causing the problem, the instruments or the model. It is also interesting to note that this is a further study in which the effects of teaching on alleviating patient problems has failed to show the expected results; further evidence is provided in the studies that use Orem's model.

CONCLUSIONS ON THE USE OF NEUMAN'S MODEL IN PRACTICE

Betty Neuman's model was first developed in 1972 and has undergone a number of revisions since that date. Her model has been widely praised, used and evaluated by nurses in the USA, Canada and the UK in many nursing situations.

To date there has been only one research study in a practice setting that has helped to support and develop the model and its concepts; this was by Hinds (1990) who assessed seven variables in patients with lung cancer to determine their effect on quality of life; however, these variables accounted for only 30% of the total variance. A further research study, by Ziemer (1983), was unable to find any link in the expected direction between giving patients information pre-operatively and their post-operative coping.

However, that the model is being evaluated and, in some areas, is being preferred to other models, is a sign of its acceptability.

REFERENCES

Beckenham and Hinds (1990)

Buchanan, B.F. (1987) Human–environment interaction: a modification of the Neuman Systems Model for aggregates, families, and the community. *Public Health Nursing*, 4(1), 52–64.

Capers, C.F., O'Brien, C., Quinn, R. *et al.* (1985) The Neuman Systems Model in practice. *Journal of Nursing Administration*, May, 29–38.

Craddock, R.B. and Stanhope, M.K. (1980) The Neuman Health Care Systems model: recommended adaptation, in *Conceptual Models for Nursing Practice* (eds J.P. Riehl and C. Roy), Appleton-Century-Crofts, Norwalk, OH.

Fulbrook, P.R. (1991) The application of the Neuman systems model to intensive care. *Intensive Care Nursing*, 7, 28–39.

Haggart, M. (1993) A critical analysis of Neuman's systems model in relation to public health nursing. *Journal of Advanced Nursing*, 18, 1917–22.

Harris, S.M., Hermiz, M.E., Meininger, M. and Steinkeler, S. (1989) Betty Neuman: systems model. In Marriner-Tomey, A. *Nursing Theorists and their Work*, CV Mosby, St Louis, pp. 361–88.

Hinds, C. (1990) Personal and contextual factors predicting patients' reported quality of life: exploring congruency with Betty Neuman's assumptions. *Journal of Advanced Nursing*, 12, 456–62.

Knight, J.B. (1990) The Betty Neuman Systems Model applied to practice: a client with multiple sclerosis. *Journal of Advanced Nursing*, 15, 447–55.

Lindell, M. and Olsson, H. (1991) Can combined oral contraceptives be made more effective by means of a nursing care model? *Journal of Advanced Nursing*, **16**, 475–9.

Moore, S.L. and Munro, M.F. (1990) The Neuman Systems Model applied to mental health nursing of older adults. *Journal of Advanced Nursing*, **15**, 293–9.

National Swedish Board of Health and Welfare (1988) The number of abortion increases. What can be done to change the development? Preliminary report about the situation of abortion and preventive work 1975–1988.

National Swedish Board of Health and Welfare (1989) Press communication of the National Swedish Board of Health and Welfare 1989 02 22.

Neuman, B. (1977) In *Conceptual Models for Nursing Practice* (eds J.P. Riehl and C. Roy), Appleton-Century-Crofts, Norwalk, OH.

Neuman, B. (1980) The Betty Neuman health-care system model: a total person approach to patient problems, in *Conceptual Models for Nursing Practice* (eds J.P. Riehl and C. Roy), Appleton-Century-Crofts, Norwalk, OH, pp. 119–34.

Neuman, B. (ed.) (1982) *Neuman Systems Model. Application to Nursing Education and Practice*, Appleton-Century-Crofts, Norwalk, OH.

Neuman, B. (ed.) (1989) *The Neuman Systems Model*, Appleton & Lange, Norwalk, OH.

Neuman, B. and Young, R.J. (1972) A model for teaching total person approach to patient problems. *Nursing Research*, **21**(3), 264.

Parr, M.S. (1993) The Neuman Health Care Systems Model – an evaluation. *British Journal of Theatre Nursing*, **3**(8), 20–7.

Silverman, D. (1993) *Interpreting Qualitative Data: Methods for Analysing Talk, Text and Interaction*, Sage, London.

Ziemer, M.M. (1983) Effects of information on postsurgical coping. *Nursing Research*, **32**(5), 282–7.

Conclusions 8

I am very pleased to have had the opportunity to follow up the developments that have accrued since 1990 through research in clinical practice using models of nursing. There has evidently been considerable development in most of the models found in this book during the 5 year period from 1990 to 1995. These developments have helped to show, with increasing clarity, the use and limitations of each model as well as each one's potential relevance to particular areas of nursing practice.

The striking developments since 1990, according to the published literature, are the following.

- Some models have failed to sustain interest, such as Roper, Logan and Tierney's model, while others have become better known and have been used in an increasing number of cultures, such as Orem's and Roger's models.
- Some models have become sufficiently interesting to researchers for them to become the basis of their research programmes, such as Roy's model. This has considerable benefits for the understanding and validation of the model and for its development in a more systematic manner through the design of a series of studies: one study can explore an area and raise questions as a result of the findings, which can then be taken on in further studies. Also, it is possible to develop a more systematic meta-analysis, where the findings of studies in a similar area are combined together to give a composite picture. However, meta-analysis needs to take into account whether the findings are sufficiently similar if different methods are used.
- There are some areas of patient care that seem to be resistant to change, despite the way in which they are perceived by the nurse and regardless of which model of nursing is used; here I am thinking particularly of the effects of patient teaching on the ability to change patients' lifestyles. There is evidence from Orem's as well as from Neuman's

model that patient teaching can make little difference to their feelings or behaviours.

- There is now considerable evidence and further understanding of the potential of the different models, as well as giving guidance to practising nurses in the results that they could expect from the use of a model in different situations. However, despite this, assessment seems to be the area where all the models find most validity; trying to link nursing actions with outcomes as specified by the model seems to be the least successful.

That some models have become known and analysed for their potential in very different cultures, for example Orem's model in Chinese culture, is evidently very good for the model. However, what will the response of the very different culture be to a model which was produced in a Western culture, and which is evidently based on Western ideals? How will it affect their culture if they take in these ideals and will it contribute to them losing their particular identity?

As to the way in which nursing models are used, there is considerable evidence from the literature that researchers have found some of the models of nursing useful as a basis for their studies or programmes. There is also evidence that some of the models have been used as the basis of education programmes, for example Roy and Roper, Logan and Tierney. Furthermore, there is some evidence that nurses working with patients are basing their care on a nursing model, particularly the assessment phase, for example articles written about the use of Neuman's model in practice. However, it would seem that the area where the use of models is less evident is in practice, which is ironic as this is what they claim to be – conceptual models for nursing practice! But it is very difficult to obtain any information on this, indeed, McKenna (1994) found only three studies (e.g. Jukes, 1988). However, from his own study (McKenna, 1994) he was able to show with a small sample, from one undergraduate programme and one RGN programme in Northern Ireland, that nursing models were generally well accepted by student nurses. They also felt that there was little problem in their use in practice, one of the main disadvantages being the amount of time the documentation took. But, as McKenna warns, this was a very small study from one particular part of Northern Ireland, the results of which should not be generalized to all students or all practice settings in the UK. A further note of caution is that students were asked for their views by a self-completion postal questionnaire which, in itself, can lead to respondents expressing certain views while doing something different in practice.

Despite my comments in the previous paragraph, it would seem that, particularly with newly trained nurses who have used conceptual models during their education and who are now, in the UK, educated to at least diploma level, their positive attitudes towards the use of models of nursing in patient care are increased; however, according to McKenna (1994), they are wanting evidence that these models are validated by research. However, the sceptics will still wonder whether nursing models are a good thing.

REFERENCES

Jukes, M. (1988) Nursing models or psychological assessment? *Senior Nurse*, **8**(11), 8–10.
McKenna, H.P. (1994) The attitudes of traditional and undergraduate nursing students towards nursing models: a comparative study. *Journal of Advanced Nursing*, **19**, 527–36.

Appendix 1: Studies of interest to particular groups of nurses

Groups of nurses	Study	Model used	Page numbers
All nurses	Assessment of sleep problems	Roper, Logan and Tierney	21
	Assessment of problems for patients with multiple sclerosis	Roper, Logan and Tierney	22
	Assessment of action to support	Orem	128–129
	The nurse as a potential self-care practitioner	Orem	135–136
	Helping in nursing	Johnson	172–174
	Assessment of the passage of time	Rogers	202–210
	Assessment of the near death experience	Rogers	222–223
	Operationalizing Rogers' model	Rogers	224–227
	The effects of therapeutic touch on headache	Rogers	231–234
	Social support as a method of stress relief	Rogers	236–238
	Self-care for people coping with cancer treatment	Orem	145–148
	The perception of time	Rogers	246
	Developing a Rogerian assessment tool	Rogers	247–248
	The experience of receiving therapeutic touch	Rogers	234–235

Groups of nurses	Study	Model used	Page numbers
All nurses	The effectiveness of giving oral contraceptive advice	Neuman	268–270
	Seriously ill patients' reported quality of life	Neuman	261–265
	A patient in early stages of multiple sclerosis	Neuman	265–267
Children's nurses	Assessment of systems imbalance in chronically ill children	Johnson	160–168
District nurses	Assessment of patients at home with chest disease	Roper, Logan and Tierney	23–24
	Assessment of adaptation in the elderly	Roy	47–49
	Assessment of patients with a right hemispheric lesion	Roy	53–56
	Planning for patients with diabetes, hypertension or rheumatoid arthritis	Roy	63–67
	Evaluation of adaptation in diabetic patients	Roy	74
	Assessment of self-care in diabetics	Orem	99–103
	Assessment of the elderly living at home	Orem	105–107
	Teaching patients about chemotherapy	Orem	114–117
	Teaching hypertensive patients	Orem	120–122
	Teaching elderly women	Orem	122–124
	Assessment of quality of care in the community	Orem	133–134
	Care of patients with urinary catheters	Rogers	238–241
	Mitral valve prolapse and its effects	Orem	140–143
Health visitors	Assessment of self-care in young children	Orem	104–105
	Analysis in relation to public health nursing	Neuman	260

Groups of nurses	Study	Model used	Page numbers
	Assessment of systems imbalance in chronically ill children	Johnson	160–168
	Assessment of the relationship between the human field and self-actualization in healthy women	Rogers	196–200
	Assessment of support experienced by new mothers	Rogers	212–214
	Assessment and evaluation of physical activity on infants' growth and development	Rogers	227–231
Community nurses	Human–environment interaction model	Neuman	260–261
Hospital nursing of adults	Assessment of a patient following a stroke	Roper, Logan and Tierney	24–26
	Assessment of pre-operative needs of patients with arterial occlusion	Roy	50–53
	The effects of information on post-surgical coping	Neuman	270–274
	Assessment of patients with a right hemispheric lesion	Roy	53–56
	Assessment of patients with a raised temperature	Roy	56–60
	Teaching patients following a myocardial infarction	Orem	111–114
	Teaching care post-operatively following pulmonary surgery	Orem	117–120
	Assessment of quality of care in the elderly	Orem	130–133
	Assessment of behavioural systems imbalance in cancer patients	Johnson	168–172
	Assessment of standards of care	Johnson	174–175

Groups of nurses	Study	Model used	Page numbers
	Assessment of wound healing	Rogers	189–193
	Assessment of ambulatory clients	Rogers	200–202
	Care of patients with urinary catheters	Rogers	238–241
	Care of the elderly using movement therapy	Rogers	241–244
Psychiatric nurses	Assessment of patients' self-care in Alzheimer's disease	Orem	107–109
	Teaching self-care for the mentally ill	Orem	124–128
	Assessment of changes in circadian rhythms affecting sleep in hospitalized psychiatric patients	Rogers	218–222
School nurses	Teaching children to self-care	Orem	110–111
Cross-cultural nursing	Applicability of Orem's model	Orem	143–145
	Testing of 'Appraisal of Self-care Agency' scale	Orem	138–140
	Validity testing of Dutch translation of 'Appraisal of Self-care Agency' scale	Orem	139–140
Midwives	Assessment of the needs of Caesarean birth parents	Roy	60–62
	Caring for mothers and babies using the birth chair	Roy	68–73
	Assessment of change in body image during and after pregnancy	Rogers	193–196
	Assessment of changes in role identity and concept from pregnancy to the postpartum	Rogers	214–218

Groups of nurses	Study	Model used	Page numbers
	Testing of Inventory for Functional Status – Fathers	Roy	83–85
	Mothers' feelings about breastfeeding in a neonatal intensive care unit	Roy	80–83

Appendix 2: Glossary of terms

Alpha-coefficient One of the most efficient methods of measuring the consistency of the items in a test. It allows for estimations of the inter-correlations between the items, and also with any test brought in to supplement a test that measures the same variable. The higher the alpha-coefficient, the more correlated are the items on the test.

Analysis of variance (ANOVA) With data that assume a normal distribution a set of statistical calculations can be made setting each variable against each other to ascertain statistical significance.

Bias Where there is more than an even chance that a certain result will be obtained, usually a result of poor experimental design.

Chi-square test A popular statistical test used to test two sets of data to ascertain if the data are independent of each other, or related. The data collected must be at the **categorical** level of measurement – in other words, what is being measured must be capable of being put into categories such as apples, oranges and bananas; or men and women.

Content analysis Involves the analysis of written or verbal communication. Categories for analysis must be decided and defined, and analysis of the communication follows the chosen categories.

Control group When an experiment is set up where subjects are split into at least two groups, the control group does not receive any of the subject matter pertaining to the experiment. Where experimental and control groups are set up the experimenter gives the former an experience that the latter does not receive, to test the resulting differences between the groups.

Correlation Where a cause and effect cannot be measured, but two results are seen to have an association; this can be shown statistically.

Dose–response curve When different strengths of a drug are measured for their different levels of reaction the dose can be calculated according to its effect.

Empirical testing Where testing of a scale or questionnaire is given to people for whom it is intended. The term refers to an experiment involving live people, rather than a study carried out in a library using results from other people's research to draw conclusions.

Ethnographic analysis In this type of data the situation is viewed by the researcher as the natural setting, with no attempt to control variables. The researcher collects data through observation or unstructured questions, and analyses it by categories centred around meanings that those being asked or observed feel are important to them.

Experimental group When an experiment is set up where subjects are split into at least two groups, the experimental group receives the subject matter of the experiment.

Extrapolation To go beyond the data and make conclusions.

Factor analysis A statistical method that allows for the isolation of factors from a large amount of data.

Forced-choice items Items on a questionnaire where the respondent has to make a choice out of two alternatives, for example 'satisfactory' or 'unsatisfactory'.

Hypothesis Assumptions made by the researcher in any experiment before data are collected that a certain outcome or number of outcomes is likely. Data will then be collected to try to refute that the opposite to those suppositions is the case. If the hypothesis is supported then the experiment has succeeded in its assumptions.

Internal consistency For a test to be valid it must be internally consistent – that is, if some of the items measure a variable, then, the other items must also be measuring the same variable. Therefore if all items in a test are highly consistent they are also highly correlated; this can be measured by the alpha-coefficient.

Inter-rater reliability When tests are carried out that involve a number of different people administering the tests, it is crucial that each person rates the responses obtained in the same manner. Statistical tests are available to show the amount of agreement between raters.

Mean The scores from a number of cases added together and divided by the number of cases, also known as an average.

Normal distribution A normal bell-shaped curve that shows the distribution of scores expected from any population on a number of tests, such as IQ.

Operationalize Where the concepts from a model are taken and made into a workable hypothesis for testing.

Pearson's correlation A statistical test that assumes data are collected from subjects forming a normal distribution. It is a popular test which allows for one set of scores to be correlated against another set.

Pilot study A small-scale study on a sample of subjects similar to those who will be involved in the main study. It allows for a questionnaire or other test instrument to be tested out to ensure validity and reliability. Instruments are frequently amended as a result of piloting.

Quasi-experimental design When experiments are taken from controlled laboratory conditions to the area where subjects are situated there are likely to be features of the situation which cannot be controlled; unexpected phenomena may impinge on the subjects in the study, causing threats to both the validity of the experiment and the results. The experimenter must be aware of these unexpected phenomena and try to minimize them as much as possible.

Randomized Each member of the population must have an equal chance of being a member of the sample.

Reactivity The design of the experiment is jeopardized as information is picked up by the subjects from the researcher or from the tools being used, suggesting a certain type of response as preferable to one the subject may have made without the information.

Regression A statistical test that has one variable as constant while the other(s) vary, so the value(s) of the variables can be tested against the constant measure.

Reliability testing Measures are reliable when they achieve the same results when administered by different people to different subjects; in other words the test is reliable and reproducible. There are statistical tests for measuring reliability, one of which is the **coefficient of correlation**, which in a well-constructed psychological test should be 0.9 or above.

Representative sample This ensures that every type of opinion to a particular topic is represented in the sample of subjects chosen. This is no easy matter, and a number of different methods have been developed to try to attain this ideal situation.

Semantic differential Assessing meanings of words by asking subjects to give a number of bipolar pairs to them, for example 'strong–weak'. The bipolar pairs are then given a 7-point scale and the subject asked to rate a word according to how 'strong' or 'weak' it is.

Significance levels The level at which an experimental result is said to be due to the experimental condition or chance. Usually the level at which significance is estimated is 5 in 100 or 0.05. Therefore a result of the probability of 0.05 ($p = 0.05$) will be taken as a case where one group is different from another by a margin that is not likely to be due to chance, but more to the experiment having produced the difference.

Split-half reliability Items in a test are split into two matched halves; scores from the two halves are then correlated.

SPSS A statistical package for use on a computer that deals with the analysis of large quantities of data. It is published by McGraw-Hill.

Standard error Any test will be efficient if the scores it achieves are sufficiently similar to each other to have a small standard deviation when the test has been administered on a large number of occasions. This is known as the standard error; the larger it is the less efficient is the test.

Standard deviation The amount that each score deviates from the mean of all the cases in the data.

t-**Test** This is one of the most commonly used statistical tests, and data used must be assumed to be normally distributed. The test allows for subjects from one group to be tested against subjects from another group, and a statistical estimation of their difference or similarity can then be made.

Test–retest A test is administered on two occasions separated by a measured amount of time so that subjects are unlikely to remember their previous responses; used to test the reliability of a measure.

Validity testing This can be tested in different ways. **Face validity** is a superficial glance to ascertain that all the items in a questionnaire contain attitudes to the subject in question. **Content validity** is more rigorous than face validity and entails ensuring that all the items in a scale or questionnaire contain features to do with the subject in question; together they should cover the full range of attitudes in a balanced way, but this will be a matter of judgment.

Variable Something that can have different values, for example, age, height, weight. In an experiment with both control and experimental groups, it is important to hold the variables of the control group constant while assessing the effect of the experiment on the variables of the experimental group. (See, for example, Porter's study, Chapter 6.)

Wilcoxon test A statistical test that assumes the population in the sample to be normally distributed. The data must be categorical, therefore measurement must only allow for the data to be put into categories, such as apples, oranges or bananas; or men and women (see also **chi-square test**). The test will show whether statistical significance has been reached between each subject's score, or between two samples of subjects' scores.

Index

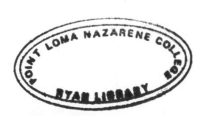

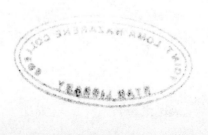